# HILLCREST MEDICAL CENTER
# BEGINNING MEDICAL
# TRANSCRIPTION

## 7TH EDITION

# HILLCREST MEDICAL CENTER
# BEGINNING MEDICAL TRANSCRIPTION

## 7TH EDITION

**PATRICIA A. IRELAND, CMT, AHDI-F**
Multispecialty Medical Transcriptionist,
Instructor, Medical/Technical Author and Editor
San Antonio, Texas

**CAROLYN K. STEIN, CMT**
Medical Transcriptionist, Author,
Instructor, Freelance Technical Editor
San Antonio, Texas

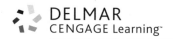
DELMAR
CENGAGE Learning™

Australia • Canada • Mexico • Singapore • Spain • United Kingdom • United States

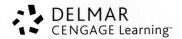
DELMAR
CENGAGE Learning™

**Hillcrest Medical Center: Beginning Medical Transcription, 7ᵗʰ Edition**

**Patricia A. Ireland, CMT, AHDI-F**
**Carolyn K. Stein, CMT**

Vice President, Career and Professional
  Editorial: Dave Garza

Director of Learning Solutions: Matthew Kane

Senior Acquisitions Editor: Sherry Dickinson

Managing Editor: Marah Bellegarde

Product Manager: Laura J. Wood

Editorial Assistant: Anthony R. Souza

Vice President, Career and Professional
  Marketing: Jennifer Baker

Marketing Director: Wendy E. Mapstone

Senior Marketing Manager: Nancy Bradshaw

Marketing Coordinator: Erica Ropitzky

Production Director: Carolyn Miller

Senior Content Project Manager:
  Stacey Lamodi

Senior Art Director: David Arsenault

Senior Technology Product Manager:
  Mary Colleen Liburdi

Technology Project Manager:
  Benjamin Knapp, Patricia Allen

For product information and technology assistance, contact us at
**Cengage Learning Customer & Sales Support, 1-800-354-9706**
For permission to use material from this text or product,
submit all requests online at **www.cengage.com/permissions.**
Further permissions questions can be e-mailed to
**permissionrequest@cengage.com**

Library of Congress Control Number: 2009938611
ISBN-13: 978-1-4354-4115-6
ISBN-10: 1-4354-4115-X

**Delmar**
5 Maxwell Drive
Clifton Park, NY 12065-2919
USA

Cengage Learning is a leading provider of customized learning solutions with office locations around the globe, including Singapore, the United Kingdom, Australia, Mexico, Brazil, and Japan. Locate your local office at: **international.cengage.com/region**

Cengage Learning products are represented in Canada by Nelson Education, Ltd.

To learn more about Delmar, visit **www.cengage.com/delmar**
Purchase any of our products at your local college store or at our preferred online store **www.CengageBrain.com**

**Notice to the Reader**

Publisher does not warrant or guarantee any of the products described herein or perform any independent analysis in connection with any of the product information contained herein. Publisher does not assume, and expressly disclaims, any obligation to obtain and include information other than that provided to it by the manufacturer. The reader is expressly warned to consider and adopt all safety precautions that might be indicated by the activities described herein and to avoid all potential hazards. By following the instructions contained herein, the reader willingly assumes all risks in connection with such instructions. The publisher makes no representations or warranties of any kind, including but not limited to, the warranties of fitness for particular purpose or merchantability, nor are any such representations implied with respect to the material set forth herein, and the publisher takes no responsibility with respect to such material. The publisher shall not be liable for any special, consequential, or exemplary damages resulting, in whole or part, from the readers' use of, or reliance upon, this material.

Printed in the United States of America
2 3 4 5 6 7 12 11

"Nothing has really happened until it has been recorded."

*Virginia Woolf, English author and critic (1882–1941)*

# CONTENTS

# SECTION 1: Introduction 1

# SECTION 2: Model Report Forms 17

# SECTION 3: References 35

# SECTION 4: Case Studies   63

# SECTION 5: Quali-Care Clinic   113

# SECTION 6: Expand Your Knowledge ....... 175

# APPENDIX ....... 233

# PREFACE

*Hillcrest Medical Center: Beginning Medical Transcription* is a text-workbook created to introduce students to the interesting and challenging world of medical transcription. The contents of the text-workbook are designed to familiarize students with: basic medical reports concerning Hillcrest Medical Center inpatients and Quali-Care Clinic outpatients; related medical terminology; appropriate formats for transcribing the reports; and specialized rules of grammar and punctuation peculiar to dictated medical reports. Users will apply these principles as they transcribe the medical reports that comprise the 10 case studies relating to inpatients, the 25 reports relating to outpatients, and their related skill-building reports.

Students of the *Hillcrest Medical Center* text-workbook and audio transcription exercises learn through a well-rounded course of beginning medical dictation and transcription. We have introduced medical editing to this edition, as transcriptionists are sometimes hired in that capacity. After the completion of this text-workbook, students may progress to *The Dictated Word*, created to provide medical transcription students and their instructors with authentic physician-recorded dictation of medical, surgical, and radiology reports—more than 15 hours of dictation. This helps the newly graduated student prepare for a job or for the Registered Medical Transcriptionist (RMT) exam. This dictation keeps transcription skills sharp in multiple medical specialties.

## NEW TO THIS EDITION— FEATURED ITEMS

**Featured Item:** The Registered Medical Transcriptionist (RMT) exam is included in our certification information in the Introduction. This designation was created by our professional association (AHDI) for level 1 transcriptionists—those newly graduated from a medical transcription program or those who have worked in only one medical specialty area. There are also some exciting new ways to earn continuing education credits for Certified Medical Transcriptionists (CMTs).

**Featured Item:** "Common Dictation Errors" was developed as a learning tool to teach students exactly what a dictated error is, how each error can be classified, how to edit these—and when not to! This information is important as medical transcriptionists are being employed as medical editors. See Expand Your Knowledge, which also contains crossword puzzles and proofreading exercises—both of which have been expanded for this edition.

We added content on the Future of Medical Transcription, including information on electronic health records (EHRs) and voice recognition technology (VRT), both of which require medical editing.

The CMTips™ section has been boosted with the addition of the ABO Blood Group, Psychology Terms, and more on Laboratory Dictation. (See References section.)

**Featured Item:** A Skill-Building Report Log keeps the 10 Transcription Skill-Building Reports and the 10 Quali-Care Skill-Building Reports organized. This log lists each patient's name and the report type with a place for the grade earned. (See References section.)

**Featured Item:** The name and specialty of each health care professional who works at Hillcrest Medical Center or Quali-Care Clinic is provided in a list intended for student and instructor quick reference. (See Section 3.)

**Featured Item:** The Hillcrest/Quali-Care Audio Dictation Information is combined into a grid—everything in one place for the instructor's convenience. Each of the 105 reports is listed separately with its accent, speed, background noise or lack thereof, difficulty level, and file length—a very organized approach for instructors' ease in assignments and testing. (See Instructor's Manual.)

**Featured Item:** In the Appendix, the Challenging Medical Words, Phrases, and Prefixes is greatly improved with the addition of more sound-alike terms.

**Featured Item:** Lastly, we have included the Official "Do Not Use" List from The Joint Commission, which shows dangerous abbreviations and what to use in their place. This is in addition to the updated Dr. Neil Davis's "HealthCare Controlled Vocabulary," which goes into dangerous abbreviations in great detail. The "Do Not Use" list is recognized worldwide by hospitals and medical professionals. (See Appendix.)

Patricia A. Ireland can be reached at:
PAItrans@sbcglobal.net

Carolyn (Carrie) K. Stein can be reached at:
cstein2@satx.rr.com

Delmar/Cengage Learning can be reached at:
800.998.7498

## PREREQUISITES

Students should be proficient in keyboarding and have a general knowledge of transcription equipment before beginning this course. English grammar and punctuation is another important part of transcription because the spoken word is turned into the written word. Even though a section of the text-workbook relates to understanding medical terminology, it is strongly suggested that students complete a course in medical terminology before beginning *Hillcrest Medical Center*.

## COURSE DESCRIPTION

This is a beginning medical transcription course designed to provide students with a working knowledge of the transcription of medical reports. Medical reports will be transcribed from 10 individual case studies, each of which concerns an inpatient with a specific medical problem. There are between 4 and 10 reports within each case study, each of which has been taken from hospital medical records. Students will be involved in the care of the patient from the date of admission to Hillcrest Medical Center through the date of discharge. The medical reports include emergency room reports, history and physical examinations, diagnostic imaging or radiology reports, operative reports, pathology reports, consultations, death summaries, and discharge summaries. Following are the case numbers and related specialty areas:

| | |
|---|---|
| Case Study 1: | Reproductive System |
| Case Study 2: | Gastrointestinal System |
| Case Study 3: | Cardiopulmonary System |
| Case Study 4: | Integumentary System |
| Case Study 5: | Psychology/Neurology System |
| Case Study 6: | Nervous System |
| Case Study 7: | Orthopedics/Endocrinology System |
| Case Study 8: | Vascular/Renal System |
| Case Study 9: | Musculoskeletal System |
| Case Study 10: | Respiratory System |

In addition, 25 outpatient medical reports and correspondence will be transcribed, each of which concerns a patient with a specific medical problem who was treated by a physician at Quali-Care Clinic. The outpatient reports and correspondence have been taken from actual patient medical records. Following are the report numbers and related specialty areas.

Report 1a&b:  Cardiology Consult and Echocardiogram
Report 2:  Genitourinary Operative Report
Report 3:  Orthopedics Operative Report
Report 4:  Surgical Pathology Report
Report 5:  Emergency Department Treatment Record
Report 6:  Interventional Radiology Report
Report 7:  Spine Clinic HPIP Note
Report 8:  Radiology Report
Report 9:  Vascular Surgery Clinic SOAP Note
Report 10:  Orthopedics Operative Report
Report 11:  Plastic Surgery Operative Report
Report 12:  Colonoscopy Procedure Note
Report 13:  Internal Medicine Clinic HPIP Note
Report 14:  Neurosurgery Operative Report
Report 15:  Urology Operative Report
Report 16:  Radiology Report
Report 17:  Pediatric Neurology Clinic Note
Report 18:  Obstetrics Operative Report
Report 19:  Orthopedics Operative Report
Report 20:  Vascular Surgery Clinic Note
Report 21:  Pediatric Dental Operative Report
Report 22:  Orthopedics Operative Report
Report 23:  Orthopedics Consult
Report 24:  Psychological/Intellectual Evaluation
Report 25a&b:  Correspondence and Consult, Cardiology

## TEACHING ENVIRONMENT

### Traditional Classroom Setting

These materials are designed to be effective in a traditional classroom setting. Laboratory time could be scheduled either individually or in groups. Each instructor would decide whether to be physically present in the lab. Estimated time to complete the case studies is 32 class hours (2 hours per week for 16 weeks) plus additional laboratory time to transcribe the medical reports (approximately 3 to 6 hours per case study). Transcription times will vary according to the length of the case study, the student's keyboarding skills, and the student's command of the English language, grammar, and punctuation. Additional lab hours should be assigned to transcribe the 25 outpatient reports and correspondence.

## Hospital In-Service Education

These materials would also be effective in a hospital in-service education department. New employees or those being cross-trained or retrained could complete the case studies plus the outpatient reports and skill-building reports. Those interested in a particular medical specialty could transcribe the reports related to that specialty or subspecialty area. Transcription lab time should be provided, allowing each employee to work at a comfortable pace, along with adequate feedback.

## Online Teaching

These materials are excellent when used in online courses. The same basic principles would apply with certain, obvious differences. Responsibility is placed on the online student for reading, understanding, and following instructions; however, an experienced mentor or facilitator assigned to each student would offer the proper guidance and feedback and provide grading. Good communication is the key to successful teaching, whether online or otherwise. Allowing about 160 hours to complete the course, at 10 hours per week, adds up to 16 weeks.

## OBJECTIVES

Upon successful completion of this course, students should be able to do the following:

1. Describe the importance of the confidential nature of medical reports. Be aware of HIPAA guidelines for the MT.
2. Describe the content and purpose of the types of inpatient medical reports used at Hillcrest Medical Center.
3. Describe the content and purpose of the 25 outpatient medical reports and correspondence used at Quali-Care Clinic.
4. Transcribe medical reports using correct report format.
5. Transcribe medical reports using correct capitalization, number, punctuation, abbreviation, symbol, and metric measurement rules.
6. Spell correctly both the English and medical terms and abbreviations presented, either by memory or by using a dictionary or medical reference book.
7. Define the medical terms and abbreviations presented, either by memory or by using a dictionary or medical reference book.
8. Define the prefixes, combining forms, and suffixes presented.
9. Identify and define the knowledge, skills, abilities, and responsibilities required of a medical transcriptionist, including medical editing.

10. Recognize the advantages of having current reference material and be able to use it effectively.

These objectives can be achieved by reading the material presented in the text-workbook, by transcribing the medical reports, and by completing the skill-building exercises, the word games, and proofreading/editing exercises provided in Expand Your Knowledge.

# STUDENT TEXT-WORKBOOK

## Section 1: Introduction

The introduction consists of both a welcome letter addressed to students and the confidentiality policy for Hillcrest Medical Center. The purpose of the letter is to inform students about their position as a medical transcriptionist at Hillcrest and to emphasize the importance of the medical transcriptionist's role in health care. The letter also describes Hillcrest as a specific medical facility. The "Confidentiality Policy" explains how important it is for employees at Hillcrest to understand and maintain confidentiality of patient records.

Information on the Association for Healthcare Documentation Integrity (AHDI), a national association representing the medical transcription profession, is also presented in this section. The AHDI Medical Transcriptionist Job Description includes a position summary for 3 distinct professional levels for medical transcriptionists (levels 1, 2, and 3). In addition, the nature of the work and the knowledge, skills, and abilities for each professional level are included in this section of the text-workbook. The AHDI Code of Ethics is presented with information about the AHDI national certification examinations, both the CMT and the RMT exams.

Also presented is information regarding the Health Insurance Portability and Accountability Act (HIPAA). This act includes standards set by the United States government for the security and privacy of patient medical records.

## Model Report Forms

The 10 model report forms included here are designed to answer frequently asked questions about set-up and formatting. By studying these model report forms, students can get a good idea of what a professional report looks like in addition to the proper name for each element found in medical reports and correspondence.

## Understanding Medical Records

The content and purpose of the model inpatient and outpatient medical report forms used at Hillcrest Medical Center are discussed in detail in this section.

## Transcription Rules for Hillcrest and Quali-Care Clinic

Rules pertaining to style variations, capitalization, numbers, punctuation, abbreviations, and symbols used to create medical reports at both Hillcrest Medical Center and Quali-Care Clinic are discussed. CMTips is included plus report formatting guidelines, a discussion of the future of medical transcription, a Skill-Building Report Log, and a list of the doctors' and other professional names used in this text-workbook for the convenience of students and instructors.

## Case Studies

Students will be required to complete 10 case studies. Each case study consists of the following:

1. A scenario including the inpatient's name and address, a summary of the inpatient's medical problem, the various specialists involved in the inpatient's care, and a list of specific reports involved.
2. A glossary of medical terms used in each case study that includes definitions and phonetic pronunciations. *NB*: The glossary words are pronounced for students on the audio files.
3. Pertinent illustrations.

## Outpatient Reports

Students will also be required to complete 25 outpatient reports and correspondence. Information about each outpatient includes the following:

1. The patient's name with a brief description of the patient's illness.
2. A glossary of medical terms used in each outpatient report and/or letter that includes definitions and pronunciations. *NB*: The glossary words are pronounced for students on the audio files.
3. Pertinent illustrations.

## Expand Your Knowledge

Additional exercises are offered in the Appendix to strengthen students' skills in medical terminology, medical transcription, and medical editing. These include crossword puzzles, proofreading exercises, and a list of common dictation errors. The Common Dictation Errors List includes what medical transcriptionists often hear dictated on the job. We classify the error, and we show when and how the transcriptionist is allowed to edit and correct each dictated error in the transcribed report. There are some dictated errors that the medical transcriptionist cannot edit or correct, and we explain what to do under those circumstances.

## Appendix

The following helpful information is included in the Appendix:
- Proofreader's Marks
- Challenging Medical Words, Phrases, Prefixes
- Sample Patient History Form
- The Lund-Browder Burn Chart
- Laboratory Test Information
- Sample Forms for Ordering Laboratory Tests, Scheduling Radiology Tests, and Consults for Physical Therapy, Sleep Studies, etc.
- Building a Reference Library
- A Healthcare Controlled Vocabulary
- Official "Do Not Use" List from The Joint Commission

## Index

The words, phrases, and abbreviations listed in each glossary are presented in alphabetic order in the index, along with the prefixes, combining forms, and suffixes. The page numbers identify their first location in the text-workbook.

**NOTE:** The terms presented *within* the Hillcrest Medical Center glossaries and *within* the Quali-Care Clinic glossaries are not duplicated. However, Hillcrest Medical Center and Quali-Care Clinic are separate entities; therefore, duplicate terms will exist between the Hillcrest Medical Center and Quali-Care Clinic glossaries.

## AUDIO TRANSCRIPTION EXERCISES

Transcription exercises are available in audio mp3 format on CD-ROM. The school has the option to purchase an institutional version of the CD-ROM that provides duplication rights to share with students, or the instructor can require each student to purchase the audio CD-ROM. Instructors can begin their students with either the 10 Case Studies or with the 25 Quali-Care outpatient reports. The text-workbook is designed for students to begin at either place.

Different regional and foreign accents and various background settings are presented in the recorded dictation—some reports will have no background noise at all. The speed of the reports within each case is mixed, varying between 80 wpm, 90 wpm, and 120 wpm, which is a conversational or officestyle speed. The variety offered represents what a student would encounter in a real-life work setting in preparation for her career.

Audio pronunciations of all Case Study and Quali-Care glossary terms included in the text-workbook are provided on the CD-ROM. Skill-Building reports are provided to enhance a student's medical transcription experience. These have the mixed speeds and similar background settings of the inpatient and outpatient reports presented in the text-workbook but have no glossary words.

## SUPPLEMENTS

### Instructor's Manual

A comprehensive Instructor's Manual is available that discusses the design of the course, suggestions for teaching the course, evaluation procedures, and production standards. Transcripts for the 10 inpatient case studies and the 25 outpatient medical reports and correspondence are provided in the manual, as well as a test bank that includes the following:

1. Ten written quizzes plus the answer keys, which correlate with the 10 inpatient case studies.
2. The answer keys to 10 transcription skill-building reports relating to inpatient case studies, which are recorded on the audio transcription exercises.
3. The answer keys to 10 Quali-Care skill-building reports relating to outpatients, which are recorded on the audio transcription exercises.
4. Answer keys to the proofreading exercises and crossword puzzles.

### Instructor Resources CD-ROM

An Instructor Resources CD-ROM containing Microsoft Word® transcripts of every dictation is included in the back of the Instructor's Manual. The CD-ROM allows instructors to make electronic comparisons of a student's transcription to the original, correct reports. This allows instructors to easily recognize student errors. For help using the comparison feature, please refer to the instructions on the CD-ROM and the help menus in Microsoft Word®.

Also included are slides created in Microsoft PowerPoint® that correspond with components of the book, including Sections 1 and 3. Use for in-class lectures, or pass out or post online as class notes. All written quizzes are presented in electronic format. Edit and print to customize for your unique student needs.

### Course Cartridge

An online course cartridge is available in the Blackboard and WebCT platforms and can easily be converted to suit the needs of your online or hybrid classroom. The course cartridge contains quizzes, discussion questions, glossary flashcards with audio pronunciations, and more!

## ACKNOWLEDGMENTS

This text-workbook is the result of the cooperation and input of many individuals. The authors would like to express their appreciation for authentic medical reports submitted for adaptation and inclusion in this text-workbook. Additionally, the authors want to thank the reviewers for their contributions and suggestions. Their feedback enabled us to develop a text-workbook to better serve your needs.

We would also like to thank Josh Herzog at Cat Trax Recording in Schenectady, NY, for his time and dedication to this project.

## ABOUT THE AUTHORS

**Patricia A. Ireland, CMT, AHDI-F,** has been in medical transcription since 1968 as both a practitioner and instructor. She lives in San Antonio, Texas, working as a multispecialty medical transcriptionist, a freelance multispecialty medical/technical editor, and as online medical transcription course facilitator since 2000.

**Carrie Stein, CMT,** has over 32 years' experience as an acute-care multispecialty medical transcriptionist at the University of Texas Medical Branch in Galveston, Texas, and for the Methodist Healthcare System in San Antonio, Texas. She has been an online medical transcription course instructor for the last 8 years.

### Content Reviewers and Contributors

**Carol Adams-Turner**
Program Director-Medical Office
    Technology
Lamar State College-Orange
Orange, TX

**Katrina Boyette Myricks**
Instructor
Holmes Community College
Ridgeland, MS

**Deborah K. Cresap, MA, MSSL**
Medical Assisting Program
    Director
West Virginia Northern
    Community College
Wheeling, WV

**Robin Douglas, BS, MS**
National Board Certified,
Medical Office Instructor
Holmes Community College
Grenada, MS

**Anita Ferguson,**
Instructor
Paris Junior College
Paris, TX

**Linda Galbraith**
Medical Transcriptionist
Branson, MO

**Deborah L. Huber, BAAS, AS**
Pulaski Technical College
Instructor of Medical
    Transcription
North Little Rock, AR

**Julie Naimi**
Medical Transcriptionist
Ft. Lauderdale, FL

**Sherwin J. Voss**
Pathology Transcriptionist
San Antonio, TX

### Technical Reviewers

**Jesse C. DeLee, MD**
Nix Orthopedic Center
San Antonio, TX

**Suzanne Gazda, MD**
Neurology Institute of San Antonio
San Antonio, TX

**Brenda J. Hurley, CMT, AHDI-F**
Medical Transcriptionist
Port Orange, FL

**Cesar James Keathley (CJ), DMD**
The Dentist Place
Clearwater, FL

**Sharon Little-Stoetzel, RN, MS**
Assistant Professor of Nursing
Graceland University
Lee's Summit, MO

**Andrew Whaley, MD**
Orthopedic Surgeon
San Antonio, TX

**Susan King, MD**
Ear Medical Group
San Antonio, TX

# How to Use StudyWARE™ to Accompany

# HILLCREST MEDICAL CENTER: BEGINNING MEDICAL TRANSCRIPTION

## 7TH EDITION

The StudyWARE™ software helps you learn terms and concepts in *Hillcrest Medical Center*. As you work on each case study and Quali-Care report in the text-workbook, be sure to explore the activities in the software designed to help increase your knowledge of medical terminology and basic medical transcription principles. Use StudyWARE™ as your own private tutor to help you learn the material in your *Hillcrest Medical Center* text-workbook.

Getting started is easy. Install the software by inserting the CD-ROM into your computer's CD-ROM drive and following the on-screen instructions. When you open the software, enter your first and last name so the software can store your quiz results. Then choose an option from the menu to take a quiz or explore one of the activities.

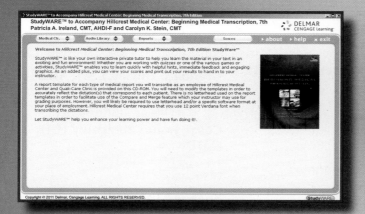

## Menus

You can access the menus from wherever you are in the program. The menus include Quizzes and other Activities.

## Quizzes

Quizzes include multiple choice and true/false questions. You can take the quizzes in both practice mode and quiz mode. Use practice mode to improve your mastery of the material. You have multiple tries to get the answers correct. Instant feedback tells you whether you're right or wrong and helps you learn quickly by explaining why an answer was correct or incorrect. Use quiz mode when you are ready to test yourself and keep a record of your scores. In quiz mode, you have one try to get the answers right, but you can take each quiz as many times as you want.

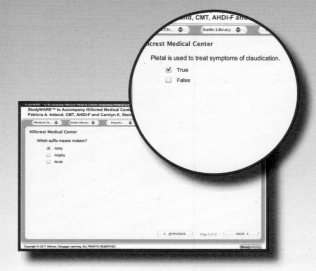

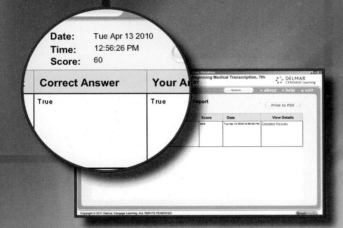

## Scores

You can view your last scores for each quiz and print your results to hand in to your instructor.

## Activities

Activities include image labeling, spelling bee, hangman, crossword puzzles, and word building. Have fun while increasing your knowledge!

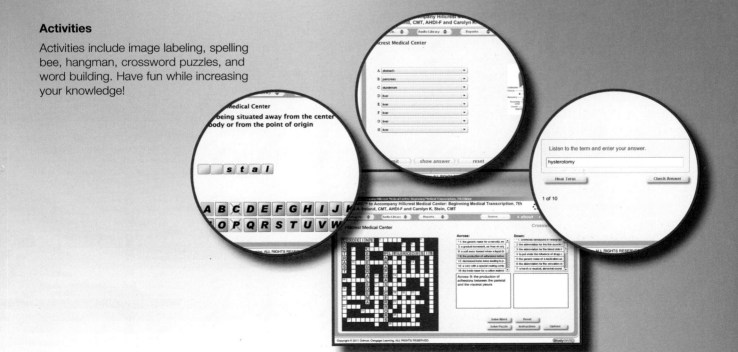

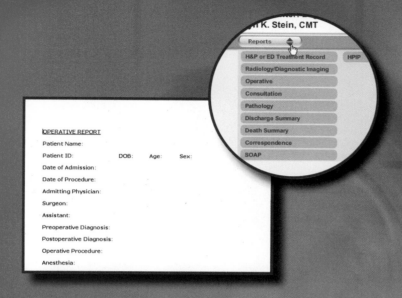

## Report Templates

Templates are provided in Microsoft Word® format for all report types you are learning in the text-workbook. You can use these templates as you work with the audio transcription exercises. NOTE: There is no letterhead used on the report templates in order to facilitate use of the Compare and Merge feature which your instructor may use for grading purposes. You will likely be required to use letterhead and/or a specific software format at your place of employment.

## Audio Library

The StudyWARE™ Audio Library is a reference that includes audio pronunciations and definitions for over 1,000 medical terms! Use the audio library to practice pronunciation and review definitions for medical terms. You can browse terms by body system or search by key word. Listen to pronunciations of the terms you select or listen to an entire list of terms. A great resource to keep as you begin your career!

| SUPPLEMENT: | WHAT IT IS: | WHAT'S IN IT: |
| --- | --- | --- |
| StudyWARE | Software program (CD-ROM in the back of the text-workbook; ISBN: 1-111-31364-4; also available for purchase separately) | • Practice Quizzes<br>• Medical Terminology Activities<br>• Audio Library of medical terminology<br>• Model Report Form templates |
| Instructor's Manual | Print (ISBN: 1-4354-4117-6) | • Transcripts for all audio recordings<br>• Answers to Skill-Building Exercises<br>• Written Quizzes<br>• Certificate of Completion |
| Instructor Resources CD-ROM | CD-ROM (located in the back of the Instructor's Manual; ISBN: 1-4354-4117-6) | • Transcripts of all audio recordings in Microsoft Word® format<br>• Instructions on Using Compare and Merge Feature<br>• All Written Quizzes in Microsoft Word® format.<br>• Course support slides created in PowerPoint® |
| Student Edition Audio Exercises on CD-ROM | CD-ROM (available for student purchase with work-textbook; no duplication rights; ISBN: 1-4354-4121-4) | • Audio recordings of all dictations and corresponding report glossaries in mp3 format |
| Audio Transcription Exercises on CD-ROM | CD-ROM (available for institutional purchase only; provides duplication rights; ISBN: 1-4354-4118-4) | • Audio recordings of all dictations and corresponding report glossaries in mp3 format |
| WebTutor | Course Management System available on Blackboard (ISBN: 1-4354-4120-6) and WebCT (ISBN: 1-4354-4119-2) platforms | • Audio glossary with flash cards<br>• Quizzes, discussion questions, Tips from the Field, web links<br>• Course support slides created in PowerPoint® |

# SECTION 1

## INTRODUCTION

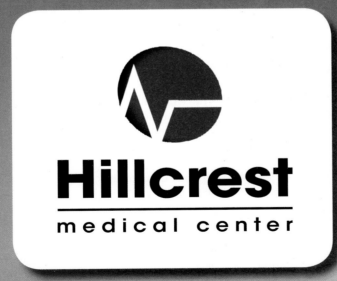

# WELCOME TO HILLCREST MEDICAL CENTER

You are now employed as a medical transcriptionist (MT) in the health information management department at Hillcrest Medical Center, transcribing reports for patients admitted to Hillcrest Medical Center and transcribing outpatient reports for patients treated at Quali-Care Clinic. MTs (medical language specialists) are a vital part of the health care team because physicians and allied health professionals rely on medical records (legal documents subject to subpoena) to maintain and document proper patient care. These documents are also involved in the revenue cycle, as diagnosis codes are the basis on which insurance claims are paid. They are important to risk management as well, as medical errors might be documented in a patient's medical records. Because of the confidential nature of these medical records, you will be asked to read the "Confidentiality Policy" and sign the "Confidentiality Statement" before beginning your duties at Hillcrest.

During your employment at Hillcrest, you will be transcribing medical reports from 10 individual case studies, each relating to an inpatient with a specific medical problem. The case studies have been taken from actual hospital medical records, and you will be involved in the care of each patient from the date of admission to Hillcrest through the date of discharge. The types of medical reports you will be transcribing include history and physical examinations, emergency department records, radiology reports, operative reports, pathology reports, consultations, discharge summaries, and death summaries.

Presented on the first page of each case study is a brief scenario including the patient's name and address, a summary of the patient's medical problem, the various specialists involved in the patient's care, and a list of the specific reports involved. In addition, a glossary of medical terms is provided for each case study. The written glossary includes phonetic pronunciations with definitions for the medical terms, phrases, and abbreviations used. The glossary words are pronounced on the audio files prior to each case to aid in student learning. Following the glossary words you will find illustrations for each case study.

The MTs who are employed by Hillcrest will also transcribe dictation for the health care providers who maintain offices at Quali-Care Clinic. This service is provided as a courtesy to the staff of Quali-Care Clinic, a freestanding medical office facility on the grounds of Hillcrest Medical Center. With the changes in insurance, the advent of health management organizations, preferred provider organizations, and managed care, the Hillcrest Medical Center Board of Directors voted to have Quali-Care Clinic built to treat a burgeoning number of outpatients—those who have no need for inpatient care.

The performance evaluations in this text-workbook will consist of skill-building reports and written quizzes. Therefore, it is important to learn the information presented in each case study and medical report, including appropriate report format and transcription rules observed by the Hillcrest health information management department. Before transcribing the medical reports, become familiar with the spellings, pronunciations, and definitions of the terms and abbreviations presented in the glossaries—both written and dictated. Words are tools of the trade for MTs.

Hillcrest Medical Center is a 300-bed general community hospital located in Miami, Florida. All patient services, the emergency room, the surgery suite, and the Hillcrest Sleep Disorders Clinic are found on the first and second floors. On the third floor are beds for 60 inpatients—20 in the pediatric unit, 20 in the coronary care unit (CCU), and 20 in the intensive care unit (ICU). Pediatric patients are usually those 14 years of age or younger. CCU is for patients—medical or surgical—who are seriously ill with heart disease. An ICU patient is either gravely ill or has had surgery on a weekend or a holiday. Otherwise, the postoperative patients are sent to the fourth floor where there are 50 surgical beds. The fifth floor has 50 beds used for medical patients, and the sixth floor has 100 beds used for geriatric patients or for those who need long-term care.

We look forward to a pleasant working relationship, and we hope your employment as an MT at Hillcrest Medical Center proves to be a rewarding experience.

Sincerely,

*Jeannette Rachel Soler*

Jeannette Rachel Soler, CMT, RHIA
Director, Health Information Management Department

**Hillcrest**
medical center

# CONFIDENTIALITY POLICY

The primary purpose of the medical record is to document the course of a patient's illness and treatment during all periods of the patient's care. The medical record is extremely important as a permanent account of the patient care provided. It serves as a means of communication between physicians and other health care professionals. As such, it is also a tool for planning and evaluating patient care. It is also important in risk management, insurance, and the revenue cycle. After all, if it was not recorded, it was not done.

For the medical record to be a useful instrument in patient care, it must contain accurate, detailed, personal information relating to each patient's medical, surgical, pharmaceutical, psychiatric, social, and family history.

Patients have the *right* to expect their medical records to be treated as *confidential*, and Hillcrest Medical Center personnel have an *obligation* to safeguard patients' medical records against unauthorized disclosure.

As an employee of Hillcrest Medical Center, you have a responsibility to ensure that each patient's right to privacy is safeguarded. You will have direct access to information contained in medical records. Information learned during the course of your work *must* be held in strictest confidence.

To ensure the confidentiality of patient information, employees of Hillcrest Medical Center must sign a statement acknowledging this confidentiality policy and must attend an orientation session regarding the Health Insurance Portability and Accountability Act of 1996 (HIPAA). Violations of this policy will result in immediate disciplinary action.

## Confidentiality Statement

I, _____, an employee of Hillcrest Medical Center, have read and reviewed the Confidentiality Policy with my supervisor. I understand the importance of each employee complying with this policy. I further understand that if I intentionally violate this policy by any unauthorized release of a patient's medical information, this violation could constitute grounds for my immediate dismissal.

| | |
|---|---|
| _____ | _____ |
| Date | Signature of Employee |
| _____ | _____ |
| Date | Witness |

# LEGAL ISSUES

In creating these medical reports, which are legal documents, what do you do if dictation is unintelligible or a section is blank? Both students and experienced MTs encounter dictation that cannot be understood, and a directive should be in place in each MT's office or workplace in this event. Some suggestions follow.

1. If you encounter a word or phrase that is unfamiliar, look it up using your medical reference materials. These would include dictionaries, word books, drug books, and other lists of medical words/phrases. (See "Building a Reference Library," Section 3: References and Appendix.)
2. If you are unsuccessful in locating the word or phrase in the reference material, have your supervisor or a coworker listen to the difficult section of dictation. One of them may be able to interpret the word or phrase.
3. If these two options are unsuccessful, the report should be flagged for the originator's attention. An underlined blank (_____) should *always* be left when dictation is omitted from a report. This lets anyone who comes in contact with the report know that there is a question about the dictation—word(s) to be filled in—and the originator of the report is the one to fill in the word(s).

A telephone call to the doctor's office could possibly yield results; however, this is not always feasible. As you work in the field of medical transcription, you will learn different tricks of the trade that can be used. As beginners, however, you must follow your supervisor's lead. The ideal report, of course, has no blanks; however, this situation is often out of the MT's control. Even so, you should *not* make up words to avoid leaving a blank. Even experienced MTs leave blanks from time to time.

The physician who originates the report and whose signature is on it is the party legally responsible for the contents thereof. This means that each report should be carefully read by the originator, corrected in the computer, reprinted, and then signed as corrected. Unfortunately, this is another situation that is not within the MT's control. The originator may make handwritten corrections on the report that never get back to the transcriptionist and, therefore, never get entered into the computer. Also, many reports are signed without being read at all. This includes electronic signatures, examples of which are in this text. Some institutions employ an electronic signature that includes the statement, "Signed but not read," which is automatically displayed on electronic records. So, even though the originator is legally responsible, some MTs buy liability (sometimes called errors and omissions) insurance to cover themselves in case of a lawsuit. (The cost of this insurance would be a valid business tax deduction.)

## OBJECTIVES

At Hillcrest Medical Center, you will learn how to transcribe medical reports. During the transcription process, you will increase your medical vocabulary, use an appropriate format for transcribing the reports, and apply specialized rules of grammar and punctuation particular to dictated medical reports. Upon successful completion of this course, you should be able to do the following:

1. Describe the importance of the confidential nature of medical records.
2. Describe the content and purpose of the medical inpatient reports used at Hillcrest Medical Center.
3. Describe the content and purpose of the outpatient medical reports and correspondence used at Quali-Care Clinic.
4. Transcribe medical reports using correct report format.
5. Transcribe medical reports using correct capitalization, numbering, punctuation, abbreviation, symbol, and metric measurement rules.
6. Spell correctly both the English and medical terms and abbreviations presented, either by memory or by using a dictionary/medical reference book.
7. Define the medical terms and abbreviations presented, either by memory or by using a dictionary/medical reference book.
8. Define the prefixes, combining forms, and suffixes presented, either by memory or by using a dictionary/medical reference book.
9. Identify and define the knowledge, skills, abilities, and responsibilities required of an MT (medical language specialist).
10. Recognize the advantages of having current reference material and be able to use it effectively.
11. Edit medical reports without changing the meaning of content dictated or the originator's style.
12. Recognize opportunities offered to MTs by the professional association, AHDI, as they pertain to beginning medical transcriptionists, including the RMT exam.

These objectives can be achieved by reading the material presented in the text-workbook, by transcribing the medical reports, and by completing the exercises in the Expand Your Knowledge section.

## LENGTH OF COURSE

You will be required to complete the 10 inpatient case studies listed below. The time estimated to complete the case studies is 32 class hours (2 days per week for 16 weeks), plus additional laboratory time to transcribe the medical reports (approximately 3 to 6 hours per case study). Transcription time will vary depending on the length of the case study, the student's keyboarding and computer skills, and the student's command of English language usage, punctuation, and transcription guidelines.

Case 1:  Reproductive System
Case 2:  Gastrointestinal System
Case 3:  Cardiopulmonary System
Case 4:  Integumentary System
Case 5:  Psychology/Neurology System
Case 6:  Nervous System
Case 7:  Orthopedics/Endocrinology System
Case 8:  Vascular/Renal System
Case 9:  Musculoskeletal System
Case 10: Respiratory System

You will be allotted additional laboratory time to transcribe the 25 outpatient medical reports and correspondence, each of which concerns a patient with a specific medical problem treated by a physician at Quali-Care Clinic. These reports have been taken from actual patient medical records. Following are the report numbers and related specialty areas:

Report 1a&b:   Cardiology Consult and Echocardiogram
Report 2:      Genitourinary Operative Report
Report 3:      Orthopedics Operative Report
Report 4:      Surgical Pathology Report
Report 5:      Pediatric Oncology Emergency Department Record
Report 6:      Interventional Radiology Report, Vascular
Report 7:      Spine Clinic HPIP Note
Report 8:      Radiology Report
Report 9:      Vascular Clinic SOAP Note
Report 10:     Orthopedics Operative Report
Report 11:     Plastic Surgery Operative Report

# TRANSCRIBING MEDICAL REPORTS

A medical record objectively records the patient's clinical course from evaluation through treatment. A clear, accurate medical record confirms both what was done and not done.

Review the following information prior to transcribing the medical reports presented in this text-workbook:

1. Become familiar with the content and format of the Hillcrest Medical Center inpatient model report forms. Also become familiar with the content and format of the Quali-Care Clinic outpatient model report forms. The structure of outpatient and inpatient medical reports will vary among health care facilities.

2. Become familiar with the prefixes, combining forms, and suffixes discussed in Section 3, "Understanding Medical Terminology."

3. Learn the spelling and definition of the medical terms, phrases, and abbreviations presented in the glossary preceding each inpatient case study and each outpatient medical report or letter. The glossaries in the case studies and medical reports are cumulative. Medical terms and abbreviations can have more than one meaning and more than one pronunciation; the definitions presented here pertain to the Hillcrest case studies and the Quali-Care medical reports and correspondence.

4. The medical terms, phrases, and abbreviations appearing in the glossaries are dictated on the audio transcription exercises that accompany the text-workbook. Listen to the pronunciation of these terms prior to transcribing each case study. Take time to become familiar with the sound of each word.

5. The pronunciation of most medical terms is indicated by a phonetic respelling that appears in parentheses immediately following each term in the printed glossary.

6. Prior to transcribing, review the rules of capitalization, numbers, punctuation, abbreviations, and symbols in Section 3, "Transcription Rules for Hillcrest Medical Center and Quali-Care Clinic." These rules are not all inclusive, and it is recommended that you use one of the standard grammar reference books. *The Book of Style for Medical Transcription* 3rd ed., published by AHDI, was created especially for our career field.

7. Review Report Formatting Guidelines. These guidelines will be important in all your transcribed reports.

8. In the case of pathology reports, the gross description is usually done on the day of scheduled surgery. The microscopic description and diagnosis are done after the tissue removed at surgery has been properly processed (at least 24 hours later). Therefore, the reference initials and dates dictated and transcribed are recorded after the gross description and again after the microscopic description and diagnosis, unless it is a "gross only" report. The physician for the two descriptions may be the same or they may be different. (The MTs could be different as well.) Whether the same or different physicians dictate the gross description and the microscopic description and diagnosis, two sets of reference initials and dates are required with one signature line at the end of the report. (See Model Report Form 4: Pathology Report.)

# EVALUATIONS

Upon completion of each inpatient case study, you may be required to take a written quiz that consists of the terms and their definitions as presented in each glossary. Each quiz is worth 20 points.

Ten transcription skill-building reports that relate to inpatients at Hillcrest and 10 transcription skill-building reports that relate to outpatients at Quali-Care are included on the audio transcription exercises. Your instructor will decide when to assign the transcription skill-building reports; however, it is advisable to have transcribed and received feedback on at least the first two inpatient case studies and/or the first five outpatient reports before going forward with the skill-building reports.

# EXPAND YOUR KNOWLEDGE: WORD GAMES AND EXERCISES

These quizzes, proofreading exercises, and common dictation errors have been provided to improve your proficiency in medical terminology, medical transcription, and medical editing.

## Crossword Puzzles

In keeping with the idea of being "word people," or those who find pleasure in working with and playing with words, Hillcrest offers crossword puzzles to reinforce knowledge of terms presented in "Understanding Medical Terminology" in Section 3 as well as the terms presented in the glossaries.

The crossword puzzles are offered as an alternate activity. They are not intended to be used as testing material or as homework assignments but as activities to be completed for your learning pleasure.

## Proofreading Exercises

"Detail-oriented" is a phrase that describes an MT. "Focal" and "word person" are others. In creating and editing medical records, students should strive to become detail-oriented, focal workers. Being able to concentrate for extended periods of time is a plus.

The MT makes several key decisions while at work, choosing: (a) the correct medical word by meaning and context, (b) the correct spelling for both medical terms and English words, (c) the correct format according to institution or client, (d) punctuation, grammar, spacing, styling of numbers and symbols, *plus* (e) editing, i.e., making additions and deletions without changing either the medical meaning or the originator's style.

To help beginning MT students in making all of the above decisions, Hillcrest offers a set of proofreading exercises. Errors incorporated into these exercises include examples of all the key decisions to be made by an MT. The standard proofreader's marks are printed in the Appendix. Using them will help MT students learn the fundamentals of proofreading and marking changes on an edited medical report. (*Note*: Not all the errors included would be caught by spellcheck. No student or practitioner should depend solely on spellcheck. Nothing takes the place of carefully proofreading your work.)

## Common Dictation Errors

This section is designed to help MT students learn dictation errors and which ones they are allowed to *fix* or edit when transcribing medical records. Originators often provide less than perfect dictation, especially when English is not their first language. Medical transcriptionists are to use their editing skills and their critical thinking skills to help create a complete and accurate medical record. The errors shown are in well-documented categories—remember, we may not change the originator's style or medical meaning. You will learn where editing is appropriate, where it is not appropriate, and where help from the originator is necessary. In today's era of voice recognition technology (VRT), speech recognition technology (SRT), and electronic health records (EHRs), these editing skills are important for every MT to learn.

# APPENDIX

The following information is included in the Appendix:

1. Proofreader's marks
2. Challenging medical words, phrases, prefixes
3. Sample patient history form
4. Lund-Browder burn chart
5. Laboratory test information
6. Sample forms for ordering lab tests, radiology tests, physical therapy consults, and sleep studies
7. Building a reference library
8. "A Healthcare Controlled Vocabulary" by Dr. Neil Davis
9. The official "Do Not Use" list from The Joint Commission

## Challenging Medical Words, Phrases, and Prefixes

This comprehensive list, developed over years of transcribing and teaching medical transcription students, represents difficult medical and English words that trouble many health care workers and/or MTs. It may be helpful to remove the list to keep at your workstation for quick referral, adding to the list as necessary.

## Lund-Browder Burn Chart

The Lund-Browder burn chart is used in hospitals and burn centers often for pediatric burn patients. This standard chart shows the anterior and posterior aspects of the human body divided into segments. It is used to estimate the percentage of burned body tissue area. One of these charts is used on admission and at each debridement, which is a surgical procedure wherein both foreign material and contaminated tissue are removed, exposing healthy tissue. The Lund-Browder burn chart is also utilized to show areas used as donor sites plus those areas covered with skin grafts and other types of grafts or dressings. This provides an ongoing picture of the progress in covering burn wounds. Published many years ago, this chart is widely used to help provide proper care for burn patients.

## A "Healthcare Controlled Vocabulary"

The safety principles regarding language used by health care professionals, as described in the article, "A Healthcare Controlled Vocabulary," by Dr. Neil Davis, are important for all MTs to understand. Dr. Davis is a pioneer in promoting these principles.

## "Do Not Use" List

The Joint Commission is a private, not-for-profit agency that since 1951 has offered voluntary evaluation and accreditation to hospitals. The agency publishes a list of dangerous abbreviations, the "Do Not Use" List, most recently updated in March 2009. It is widely regarded as a standard in medicine.

# CERTIFICATION/ CREDENTIALING

The word *certification* is used in different ways. A certificate of completion is offered after almost any course that you may take. This certifies that you have completed the required course work, and it may be beneficial to have for your résumé or personnel file. It does not mean, however, that you are either a certified medical transcriptionist (CMT) or a registered medical transcriptionist (RMT).

Credentialing by your professional association, which for MTs is the Association for Healthcare Documentation Integrity in Modesto, California, is much different. You earn status as an RMT or as a CMT by passing the examinations offered by AHDI and given at testing centers across the country. The Registered Medical Transcriptionist (RMT) exam was developed as a bridge to take students from their newly graduated status to where, as experienced medical transcriptionists, they could qualify to sit for the CMT exam. It does function quite well for single-specialty MTs, whereas the CMT exam is designed for multispecialty MTs.

Credentialing is not required for AHDI membership or to work in the field of medical transcription. It is, however, a mark of quality and professionalism that indicates a dedication to continuing education.

In addition to credentialing, a medical transcriptionist can become recognized as a fellow of AHDI. To earn fellow status, the applicant must earn at least 50 fellowship points in the five years immediately preceding the application. Points may be earned in eight different categories, demonstrating a balance between practice duties, professional experience, leadership, and community involvement.

# ASSOCIATION FOR HEALTHCARE DOCUMENTATION INTEGRITY (AHDI)

*All content in this section reprinted with permission from the Association for Healthcare Documentation Integrity.*

The Association for Healthcare Documentation Integrity (AHDI) was established in 1978 as part of an effort to achieve recognition for the medical transcription profession. In the beginning, the association focused on educating medical professionals about what medical transcriptionists do and how their work affects the quality of health care. When the U.S. Department of Labor granted medical transcriptionists their own job classification in 1999, it was an important milestone to getting the work recognized as much more than clerical.

The public as well as legislative and regulatory agencies need to understand the role MTs play in patient safety and risk management. When a knowledgeable MT works in partnership with health care providers to provide careful documentation, it is easier to identify medical inconsistencies and correct them.

AHDI works tirelessly to give thousands of medical transcriptionists a voice before legislative and regulatory agencies and to ensure MTs are recognized for their contributions to patient safety and risk management.

## MEDICAL TRANSCRIPTIONIST JOB DESCRIPTIONS: RESULTS OF A BENCHMARKING ANALYSIS OF MT PROFESSIONAL LEVELS

### Professional Levels

In an independent benchmarking study of the medical transcription profession by the Hay Management Consultants (Hay Group), three distinct professional levels for medical transcriptionists were identified and described as presented below. The Hay Group is a worldwide human resources consulting firm with extensive expertise in work analysis and job measurement.

### Compensation

Subsequent to this benchmark study of the job content levels of MTs, the Hay Group conducted a compensation survey, analyzing pay as it relates to these levels. (Hay's survey

## MEDICAL TRANSCRIPTIONIST JOB DESCRIPTION

| | Professional Level 1 | Professional Level 2 | Professional Level 3 |
|---|---|---|---|
| **Position Summary** | Medical language specialist who transcribes dictation by physicians and other health care providers in order to document patient care. The incumbent will likely need assistance to interpret dictation that is unclear or inconsistent, or make use of professional reference materials. | Medical language specialist who transcribes and interprets dictation by physicians and other health care providers in order to document patient care. The position is also routinely involved in research of questions and in the education of others involved with patient care documentation. | Medical language specialist whose expert depth and breadth of professional experience enables him or her to serve as a medical language resource to originators, co-workers, other health care providers, and/or students on a regular basis. |

*(continued)*

# MEDICAL TRANSCRIPTIONIST JOB DESCRIPTION (CONTINUED)

|  | **Professional Level 1** | **Professional Level 2** | **Professional Level 3** |
|---|---|---|---|
| **Nature of Work** | An incumbent in this position is given assignments that are matched to his or her developing skill level, with the intention of increasing the depth and/or breadth of exposure.<br>OR<br>The nature of the work performed (type of report or correspondence, medical specialty, originator) is repetitive or patterned, not requiring extensive depth and/or breadth of experience. | An incumbent in this position is given assignments that require a seasoned depth of knowledge in a medical specialty (or specialties).<br>OR<br>The incumbent is regularly given assignments that vary in report or correspondence type, originator, and specialty. Incumbents at this level are able to resolve non-routine problems independently, or to assist in resolving complex or highly unusual problems. | An incumbent in this position routinely researches and resolves complex questions related to health information or related documentation.<br>AND/OR<br>Is involved in the formal teaching of those entering the profession or continuing their education in the profession.<br>AND/OR<br>Regularly uses extensive experience to interpret dictation that others are unable to clarify. Actual transcription of dictation is performed only occasionally, as efforts are usually focused in other categories of work. |
| **Knowledge, Skills, and Abilities** | 1. Basic knowledge of medical terminology, anatomy and physiology, disease processes, signs and symptoms, medications, and laboratory values. Knowledge of specialty (or specialties) as appropriate.<br>2. Knowledge of medical transcription guidelines and practices.<br>3. Proven skills in English usage, grammar, punctuation, style, and editing.<br>4. Ability to use designated professional reference materials.<br>5. Ability to operate word processing equipment, dictation and transcription equipment, and other equipment as specified.<br>6. Ability to work under pressure with time constraints.<br>7. Ability to concentrate.<br>8. Excellent listening skills.<br>9. Excellent eye, hand, and auditory coordination. | 1. Seasoned knowledge of medical terminology, anatomy and physiology, disease processes, signs and symptoms, medications, and laboratory values. In-depth or broad knowledge of a specialty (or specialties) as appropriate.<br>2. Knowledge of medical transcription guidelines and practices.<br>3. Excellent skills in English usage, grammar, punctuation, and style.<br>4. Ability to use an extensive array of professional reference materials.<br>5. Ability to operate word processing equipment, dictation and transcription equipment, and other equipment as specified, and to troubleshoot as necessary.<br>6. Ability to work independently with minimal or no supervision.<br>7. Ability to work under pressure with time constraints. | 1. Recognized as possessing expert knowledge of medical terminology, anatomy and physiology, disease processes, signs and symptoms, medications, and laboratory values related to a specialty or specialties.<br>2. In-depth knowledge of medical transcription guidelines and practices.<br>3. Excellent skills in English usage, grammar, punctuation, and style.<br>4. Ability to use a vast array of professional reference materials, often in innovative ways.<br>5. Ability to educate others (one-on-one or group).<br>6. Excellent written and oral communication skills.<br>7. Ability to operate word processing equipment, dictation and transcription equipment, and other equipment as specified, and to troubleshoot as necessary. |

*(continued)*

## MEDICAL TRANSCRIPTIONIST JOB DESCRIPTION (CONTINUED)

| | Professional Level 1 | Professional Level 2 | Professional Level 3 |
|---|---|---|---|
| **Knowledge, Skills, and Abilities** | 10. Ability to understand and apply relevant legal concepts (e.g., confidentiality) | 8. Ability to concentrate.<br>9. Excellent listening skills.<br>10. Excellent eye, hand, and auditory coordination.<br>11. Proven business skills (scheduling work, purchasing, client relations, billing).<br>12. Ability to understand and apply relevant legal concepts (e.g., confidentiality).<br>13. Certified medical transcriptionist (CMT) status preferred. | 8. Proven business skills (scheduling work, purchasing, client relations, billing).<br>9. Ability to understand and apply relevant legal concepts (e.g., confidentiality).<br>10. Certified medical transcriptionist (CMT) status preferred. |

methodology complied with federal antitrust regulations regarding health care compensation surveys.) The results include information on transcription pay at the corporate level (health care organizations and MT businesses) and compensation for independent contractors. The data are further presented by geographic region, size of business, types of pay programs (pay for time worked and pay for production), and reward programs (benefits, etc.). The Hay report, "Compensation for Medical Transcriptionists," is contained in a 30-page booklet, available to members upon request.

# CODE OF ETHICS

*Adopted July 10, 1995*
*Revised August 2004*

## Association Membership and Professional Standards

### *Preamble*

This Code of Ethics of the Association for Healthcare Documentation Integrity (AHDI) sets forth standards of conduct and ethical principles for the medical transcriptionist professional that all members of AHDI and individuals holding the CMT designation are expected to follow. Medical transcriptionists are vigilant advocates for quality patient documentation and adhere to the highest privacy and security provisions. We uphold moral and legal rights of patients, safeguard patient privacy, and collaborate with care providers to ensure patient safety, public health, and quality of care to the fullest extent possible, through the practice of medical transcription.

AHDI is responsible for expressing the values and ethics of the profession and for encouraging its members to function in accordance with these values and ethics, especially all individuals who hold the certified medical transcriptionist credential. AHDI members are aware that it is by our standards of conduct and professionalism that the entire profession of medical transcription is evaluated. We conduct ourselves in the practice of our profession to bring dignity and honor to ourselves and to the profession of medical transcription as medical language specialists.

Instances may arise when members' and certificants' ethical obligations may appear to conflict with relevant laws and regulations. When such conflicts occur, members and certificants must make a responsible effort to resolve the conflict in a manner that is consistent with the values, principles, and standards expressed in this code of ethics. Violation of the standards in this code of ethics does not necessarily imply legal liability or violation of the law. A determination that the law has been violated can be made only in the context of legal, judicial, and/or administrative proceedings. Moreover, if this code of ethics establishes a higher standard of conduct than that required by law, members and certificants are expected to meet the higher ethical standard.

Members and certificants understand that membership and/or certification may be revoked by AHDI for failure to act in accordance with the provisions of the AHDI Code of Ethics.

Medical Transcriptionist professionals:

1. Maintain confidentiality of all patient information including but not limited to peer reviews, quality improvement, and risk management protocols with special effort to maintain data security in electronic communications.
2. Implement and maintain standards of professional transcription practice.
3. Respect the rights and dignity of all individuals.
4. Continue professional growth enhancing knowledge and skills, including continuing education, networking with colleagues, professional reading, and certification.
5. Strive to provide accurate and timely information.
6. Exercise integrity in professional practices including work or professional experience, credentials, affiliations, productivity reporting, billing charges, and payment practices.
7. Comply with all laws, regulations, and standards governing the practice of patient documentation.
8. Foster environments of employment that facilitate integrity, professionalism, and protection of patient information.
9. Strive to advance the goals and purposes of the Association and work for the advancement and good of the profession.

# HEALTH INSURANCE PORTABILITY AND ACCOUNTABILITY ACT (HIPAA)

*HIPAA for MTs* is derived from interpretation of the HIPAA privacy rule by various sources and authorities and consists of recommendations and suggestions for developing policies and procedures that demonstrate a commitment on the part of the business associate to comply with HIPAA and to protect the integrity of protected health information through all reasonable means. This information does not constitute legal advice. For answers to specific legal questions, medical transcriptionists are encouraged to consult with an attorney.

## MT's Checklist

- Be familiar with your state's privacy and confidentiality laws.
- If audiocassettes or other media containing PHI have to be shipped, designate an authorized recipient on the airbill who must sign upon receipt. This information should be sent by a carrier who can track the shipment.

- All MTs should sign a confidentiality statement.
- Databases and transcription platforms require passwords for access and only to people with an officially granted account.
- Each person is responsible for maintaining confidentiality by never sharing passwords or access and always locking or logging out of databases or transcription platform when leaving an area. Each person is accountable for all activity under their password and account. Such activity will be monitored.
- In the case of theft of software, hardware, or data at an MT remote site, immediate notification must be provided to the employer.
- The MT must provide employer signed assurance that the computer used to process PHI is used strictly for that purpose. If others have access to the use of that computer, the employer must have written assurance that acceptable measures have been taken to ensure patient confidentiality.
- Disclosure of confidential information is prohibited except when required to perform the normal requirements of one's contractual obligations. Disclosure of confidential information is prohibited indefinitely, even after termination of contract or any business agreement/relationship.
- All business associates/medical transcriptionists should be expected to uphold the Code of Ethics adopted by the American Association for Medical Transcription with regard to PHI between a patient and health care practitioner.
- The home-based MT should verify that their computer is in a secure location, facing away from the traffic flow into and out of an area.
- Use of installed screen saver when away from the computer and automatic log-off when the computer is not in use. The computer used to process PHI is a work tool and should not be shared by other family members.
- Save and store fax transmittal confirmation sheets and transmittal summaries for review and future verification.
- Each MT should have a shredder or access to a departmental shredder as a work tool and immediately shred any PHI as soon as the needed information has been utilized.
- Upon termination the MT will return all proprietary data.
- If equipment must be repaired, all PHI should be removed from the computer hard drive. A record should be kept of who made the repairs.
- Since going to each remote site would be impossible, it is suggested that a checklist (such

as this one) be sent to each remote MT. Their signature on this checklist indicates that they are aware of what your requirements are for HIPAA compliance. Keep these signed checklists on file in case of audit.

# AHDI CERTIFIED MEDICAL TRANSCRIPTIONIST (CMT) EXAM

AHDI offers a voluntary certification exam to individuals who wish to become Certified Medical Transcriptionists (CMTs). AHDI's purpose in promoting this credential is to protect the public interest by promoting high professional and ethical standards, improving the practice of medical transcription, and recognizing those professionals who demonstrate their competency in medical transcription through the fulfillment of stated requirements.

The CMT credential is awarded upon successfully passing the AHDI certification examination for medical transcriptionists.

## Eligibility Requirements

The CMT exam targets an experienced medical transcriptionist with Professional Level 2 skills and knowledge as defined in the "Medical Transcriptionist Job Descriptions." Although any candidate is "eligible" and granted permission to take the CMT certification examination, two years of transcription experience in the acute care (or equivalent) setting is strongly suggested for success on the exam. Acute care is defined as incorporating medical center dictation to include many dictators including multiple ESL dictators, many formats and report types, and all the major specialties, including and especially surgery dictation of all types, and some minor specialties.

# AHDI REGISTERED MEDICAL TRANSCRIPTIONIST (RMT) EXAM

AHDI offers a voluntary credentialing exam to individuals who wish to become Registered Medical Transcriptionists (RMTs). The RMT exam was developed to assure consumers and employers that successful candidates are qualified to practice medical transcription. It is based on the skills and knowledge described in the Medical Transcriptionist Job Description Professional Level 1 and the competencies outlined in the AHDI Model Curriculum. Many practitioners and AHDI members are recent graduates of MT education programs or work in doctors' offices and clinic settings. They do not qualify for the Certified Medical Transcriptionist (CMT) exam, designed to test for the skills and knowledge of a Professional Level 2 MT practitioner and requiring a minimum of two years of acute care experience. For successful RMTs who acquire two years of acute care experience, taking the CMT exam would, of course, be further assurance of their advanced skills and knowledge and a logical career path to follow.

The RMT credential is awarded upon successfully passing the AHDI registered medical transcriptionist examination. This credential is maintained upon the successful completion of a required online course, including a final exam, and payment of a renewal fee.

## Eligibility Requirements

The RMT exam targets the Professional Level 1 medical transcriptionist as defined in the "Medical Transcriptionist Job Descriptions." Although any candidate is eligible and granted permission to take the RMT certification examination, being a recent graduate of a medical transcription education program, an MT with fewer than two years' experience in acute care, or an MT practicing in single-specialty clinic, radiology, and pathology areas provides you with the skills suggested for success on the exam. The Credentialing Development Team titled the successful candidate a Registered Medical Transcriptionist to reflect the registries that exist within other allied health professions.

# RECREDENTIALING

The CMT credential is maintained through recertification upon the completion of continuing education requirements, earning 30 continuing education credits every 3 years and reporting them to AHDI on specialized forms, and payment of a recertification fee.

In 2009 AHDI partnered with OAK Horizons, Inc., to offer the RMT Recredentialing Course, which provides specific continuing education to individuals who have earned the entry-level RMT credential in order to ensure that their core knowledge remains current. The course includes 11 chapters with quizzes. To pass the course and renew the RMT credential, participants must complete all 11 chapters and quizzes and receive a minimum of 75% on the final exam. Successful participants will have their RMT credential renewed for an additional 3-year period.

CMTs may take the RMT Recredentialing Course to earn continuing education credits toward maintenance of their CMT credential as well. Successful participants will receive a total of 11 CECs in the following categories upon passing this course: 2 Clinical Medicine (CM), 3 Medical Transcription Tools (MTT), 3 Medicolegal (ML), 2 Technology and the Workplace (TW), and 1 Professional Development (PD).

# EMPLOYMENT POSSIBILITIES

Due to the variety of skills that MTs possess, they are employable in a variety of health care settings, including doctors' offices, public and private hospitals, teaching hospitals, psychiatric hospitals, radiology departments, clinics, medical transcription services, pathology laboratories, insurance companies, medical libraries, government medical facilities, publishing companies, research facilities, and in the legal profession.

Experienced MTs may become teachers working in adult education to train future MTs. They may become reviewers, authors, or editors working through the publishing process to provide new and improved medical publications, including course material and reference books.

Expert MTs who want to increase their professional responsibilities beyond medical transcription may become supervisors, managers, or owners of private transcription services—including those in countries other than the United States. They may aspire to quality assurance (QA) or medical editing positions.

For additional information about the medical transcription profession and the national credentialing examinations, contact the Association for Healthcare Documentation Integrity at 4230 Kiernan Ave Ste 130, Modesto, CA 95356 or visit the AHDI website at http://www.ahdionline.org.

# UNDERSTANDING MEDICAL RECORDS

Every time a patient enters Hillcrest Medical Center or Quali-Care Clinic—through the hospital admissions department, the hospital emergency room, for day surgery, or for outpatient treatment—a detailed record of the patient's care is created. Medical records are created by physicians and other health care providers recording the results of their findings on patients they see, test, and examine. They originate patient reports that may be dictated in patient care areas; in pathology, radiology, or other departments of the hospital; in the clinic; or even offsite. The hospital medical records are the property of Hillcrest Medical Center and are kept according to the regulations of The Joint Commission. Patients can get copies of their medical records; however, the information contained therein is confidential. No one has a right to obtain patient files without written permission (called an authorization or a release) from the patient.

Certain circumstances require legal disclosure of confidential information to state departments of health or social services, such as the following:

1. Birth and death
2. Blindness
3. Child abuse
4. Industrial poisoning
5. Vaccinations
6. Sexually transmitted and communicable diseases
7. Injuries resulting from criminal violence
8. Requests for plastic surgery without apparent reason (e.g., changing fingerprints or something that might indicate that the patient is a fugitive from justice)

Although laws vary from state to state relative to the length of time hospital medical records should be kept, both Hillcrest and Quali-Care Clinic chose to have each patient record microfilmed and retained for 25 years after the closure of the patient file. Because Hillcrest subscribes to voluntary accreditation by The Joint Commission, which means the hospital submits to inspections of each department by this private, not-for-profit agency every three years and follows its guidelines, the health information management department is bound by The Joint Commission regulations in many of their departmental and record-keeping decisions.

The following seven basic medical reports are used at Hillcrest Medical Center. (In medical records, the History and Physical Examination, Operative Report, Consultation, and Discharge Summary are often referred to as the "basic four.")

1. History and Physical Examinations
2. Diagnostic Imaging or Radiology Reports
3. Operative Reports
4. Pathology Reports
5. Consultations
6. Discharge Summaries
7. Death Summaries

Examples of these documents are presented in "Model Report Forms," Section 2. A brief explanation of each of these report forms follows. Additional tips for formatting your reports can be found in "Report Formatting Guidelines," Section 3. The model report forms illustrate some of these guidelines.

## HISTORY AND PHYSICAL EXAMINATION (H&P)

When a patient is admitted to the hospital for evaluation and treatment, the admitting/attending physician prepares a medical history detailing the specific complaint/illness that prompted admission to the hospital. Information about the patient's past medical history, surgery, allergies, and family and social histories, as well as psychiatric information, may be included in this report. A review of the systems of the body (a survey of possible symptoms or historical facts relating to the patient's organs) may also be included. The content of the patient's history will vary depending on the chief complaint of the patient, on the physician's specialty, and on the physician's personal style; however, the history consists largely of subjective findings. The report of the physical examination includes vital signs and other objective findings by the physician.

The H&P is a priority item in the patient's hospital course because it is the summary of the information known at the time of admission. It should be dictated and transcribed within 24 hours of admission and, according to The Joint Commission and Hillcrest regulations, must be *charted* (placed in the medical record) before surgery can be accomplished. Model Report Form 1 displays a model report form for an H&P.

# DIAGNOSTIC IMAGING OR RADIOLOGY REPORT

Radiology is that branch of the health sciences dealing with radioactive substances and radiant energy together with the diagnosis and treatment of disease by means of roentgen rays (x-rays) or ultrasound techniques. The radiology report is a description of the findings and the interpretation of radiographs and other studies done by a radiologist.

Roentgenography is the making of a record of the internal structures of the body by passage of x-rays through the body to act on specially sensitized film. Special studies of the internal organs may require the use of contrast media (dyes) taken orally or given by injection. Contrast media may be radiolucent (permitting the passage of roentgen rays) or radiopaque (not penetrable by roentgen rays or other forms of radiant energy). Ultrasonics deals with the frequency range beyond the upper limit of perception by the human ear. Ultrasound is used both therapeutically and as a diagnostic aid. MRIs (magnetic resonance imaging) and CAT scans (computed axial tomography) are also done in radiology.

At Hillcrest the numbering of these reports is done sequentially and includes the year performed. For example, a chest film from June 30, 2010, might be numbered 10-9062 to show that 9062 x-rays had been done by that date. Model Report Form 2 shows a model radiology report.

# OPERATIVE REPORT (OP)

Immediately after completion of a surgical procedure, a record of the procedure must be dictated by the physician, transcribed, and placed in the patient's file. This information is necessary for other physicians and allied health professionals who may be attending the patient. Preoperative and postoperative diagnoses are included. The body of the report (findings and procedures) is dictated in narrative form and contains information about the condition of the patient after surgery. See Model Report Form 3 for a model operative report.

# PATHOLOGY REPORT (PATH)

Pathology is that branch of medicine dealing with the study of disease. It is divided into anatomic pathology and clinical pathology. Anatomic pathology is the branch of pathology from which

tissue reports are issued. The tissue is described both grossly and microscopically by a pathologist (a physician who determines the nature and extent of disease). The gross description of the tissue is done with the naked eye before the tissue is prepared for microscopic study. The microscopic description is done after the tissue has been specially prepared and mounted on a glass slide. It is carefully examined under a microscope, and a final diagnosis is issued. Special stains and other procedures, including consultations, are sometimes necessary to make a final diagnosis.

At Hillcrest these reports are numbered sequentially and include the year performed and a letter to indicate surgical pathology (S) or cytology report (C). For example, a cytology report done on June 30, 2010, might be numbered 10-C-225 to show that 225 cytologies had been done by that date. Model Report Form 4 shows a model surgical pathology report.

# CONSULTATION (CONSULT)

Consults from physicians specializing in different fields of medicine are necessary to provide proper care for the patient; however, the admitting/attending physician is in charge and maintains continuity of care at all times. For instance, when a patient is admitted to Hillcrest by a medical doctor who later determines that surgery may be necessary, the medical doctor often requests a consultation from a surgeon. The chosen surgeon answers this request by examining the patient and dictating a complete report of the examination, including a plan for treatment or surgery and a prognosis. A consultation is shown in Model Report Form 5.

# DISCHARGE SUMMARY

A discharge summary (also called a clinical résumé or final progress note) is required for each patient who is discharged from the hospital. It contains some of the same information that is included in the patient's admission history and physical examination. It also includes information about the admitting diagnosis, surgical procedures performed, laboratory and radiology studies, consultations, hospital course, the condition of the patient at the time of discharge, the medications prescribed on discharge, instructions for continuing care and therapy (disposition), prognosis, a discharge diagnosis, and possibly a date for a followup office visit. See Model Report Form 6 for an example of a discharge summary.

## DEATH SUMMARY

If a patient expires instead of being discharged from Hillcrest, a death summary is dictated. A death summary is a standard medical report *exactly like a discharge summary* but with some important, obvious differences.

The time and date of death, for example, must be recorded. Also included in the death summary might be whether the patient's family agreed to an autopsy and whether the patient had a living will that called for no aggressive therapy, sometimes referred to as "do not resuscitate" or DNR status. Even if a patient does not have a living will, this decision is often made by the family or next of kin in an irreversible situation, and this information would be included in the death summary.

The cause of death may or may not be known when the death summary is dictated. At times, a pending surgical pathology report or autopsy report is needed before the cause of death can be confirmed. A model report form for a death summary is shown in Model Report Form 7.

## AUTOPSY REPORT

Autopsies are referred to Forrest General Hospital, the local teaching hospital, because Hillcrest does not have the proper facilities. However, information about autopsy reports is included in this text-workbook because these reports are sometimes transcribed by MTs. An autopsy is done only with permission from the next of kin of the deceased unless the patient has died within 24 hours of admission, has died of an unknown cause, or has died under suspicious circumstances. If a patient

case is determined to be medicolegal, that is, pertaining to medicine and the law (or to forensic medicine), the medical examiner or an appointed assistant is in charge of the disposition of the body. Nursing personnel, health information management personnel, and physicians on the staff of both Hillcrest Medical Center and Forrest General are familiar with the requirements of the medical examiner's office.

The complete autopsy (or necropsy) report includes the following:

1. Preliminary diagnosis
2. Clinical history or brief résumé of the patient's medical history including the course in the hospital
3. Gross examination of the body, both external and internal, including evidence of injury
4. Microscopic description of diseased organs along with final diagnoses. Special studies, special stains, summary information, and perhaps an addendum may be part of the complete autopsy report, depending upon the specific nature of the case.

## OUTPATIENT REPORTS

The outpatient medical records dictated in the Quali-Care Clinic include many of the same formats used in inpatient medical records, e.g., consults, operative procedures, radiology procedures, and specialty procedures. In addition are the subjective, objective, assessment, plan (SOAP) format; the history, physical, impression, plan (HPIP) format; and correspondence. The SOAP and HPIP formats, as well as a sample of correspondence, are included in the model report forms.

# SECTION 2

## MODEL REPORT FORMS

# Model Report Form 1

*1 inch*

## HISTORY AND PHYSICAL EXAMINATION
## OR EMERGENCY DEPARTMENT TREATMENT RECORD

*Name:*

**Patient Name**:  Roger Parks  ⟵ *2 spaces after colons*

*Avoid hyphenation "_" to join words*

**Patient ID**:  11009  *1-inch margins*

*Left justification*

**Room No.**:  812

*emergency*

*Pick one* **Date of Admission/Date of Arrival**:  12/01/- - - -  ⟵ *Format date as MM/DD/YYYY*

**Admitting/Attending Physician**:  Steven Benard, MD

**Admitting Diagnosis**:  Rule out appendicitis.

*capital* **Chief Complaint**:  Abdominal pain.

HISTORY OF PRESENT ILLNESS:  The patient is a 31-year-old white man with acute onset of right lower quadrant pain waking him up from sleep at approximately 3 a.m. on the morning of admission. The pain worsened throughout the day, radiating to his back and becoming associated with dry heaves. The patient states that the pain is constant and is worsened by walking or movement. The patient states his last bowel movement was on the previous evening and was normal. The patient is anorectic. He also gives a 1-year history of lower abdominal colicky pain associated with diarrhea. He was seen by his local medical doctor and given a diagnosis of irritable bowel syndrome; however, the pain is worse tonight and is unlike his previous bouts of abdominal pain. The patient also has had associated fever and chills to date.

*1 inch*

*double —*

PAST HISTORY:  Surgical, no previous operations. Illnesses, none. Hospitalized for epididymitis 10 years ago.

*. double*

MEDICATIONS:  None. He is ALLERGIC TO PENICILLIN. It makes him bloated.

SOCIAL HISTORY:  Carpenter. Lives with his wife and 2 children. He does not drink or smoke.

FAMILY HISTORY:  Insignificant for familial inflammatory bowel disease except for the fact that his mother has colonic polyps. Father living and well. No siblings.

REVIEW OF SYSTEMS:  Noncontributory.  *end here*

PHYSICAL EXAMINATION:  This is a 31-year-old white man with knees raised to his abdomen and complaining of severe pain. VITAL SIGNS:  Admission

*Do not leave single # sentence here*

*double space* —

(Continued)

*Use colons after brief introducers*
*First word after a colon begins with a capital letter*

*more than 1 inch*

**Hillcrest**
medical center

*Report title in all caps*
↓

HISTORY AND PHYSICAL EXAMINATION
OR EMERGENCY DEPARTMENT TREATMENT RECORD

*Name:*

*double → space*
Patient Name:  Roger Parks
Patient ID:  11009
Date of Admission:  12/01/- - - -
Page 2

**Leave blank line after title on second and subsequent page heads; single space rest of header**

*4 hard returns*

**Quadruple space between page header and text below (Text begins on fourth line following head)**

*x ④* temperature 99.6 F; 4 hours after admission it was 102.6 F. HEENT:
Normocephalic, atraumatic; EOMs intact; negative icterus, conjunctivae pink.
NECK:  Supple. No adenopathy or bruits noted. CHEST:  Clear to auscultation and
percussion. CARDIAC:  Regular rate and rhythm. No murmurs noted. Peripheral
pulses 2+ and symmetrical. ABDOMEN:  Bowel sounds initially positive but
diminished. He has positive cough reflex, positive heel tap, and positive rebound
tenderness. The pain is definitely worse in his RLQ. RECTAL:  Heme-negative.
Tenderness toward the RLQ. Normal prostate. Normal male genitalia.
EXTREMITIES:  No clubbing, cyanosis, or edema. NEUROLOGIC:  Nonfocal.

DIAGNOSTIC DATA:  Hemoglobin 14.6, hematocrit 43.6, and 13,000 WBCs.
Sodium 138, potassium 3.8, chloride 105, $CO_2$ 24, BUN 10, creatinine 0.9, and
glucose 102. Amylase was 30. UA completely negative. LFTs within normal limits.
Alkaline phosphatase 78, GGT 9, AST 39, GPT 12, bilirubin 0.9. Flat plate and
upright films of the abdomen revealed localized abnormal gas pattern in right lower
quadrant. No evidence of free air.

ASSESSMENT:  Rule out appendicitis. Some concern of whether this could be an
exacerbation of developing inflammatory bowel disease. Due to the patient's history,
increasing temperature, and localizing symptoms to his right lower quadrant, the
patient needs surgical intervention to rule out appendicitis.

**Quadruple space between last paragraph and signature rule *(line)***

*④ →*
_____
Steven Benard, MD

**Align signature block at left margin; signature rule is at least 25 underscores** *minimum*

SB:xx *— my intials AL*
D:12/01/- - - -
T:12/01/- - - -

**Double space from signature block to dictator/transcriptionist initials***

**Format dates as MM/DD/YYYY**

*2014*

*Signature block is not*

**No extra space between dictator/transcriptionist initials or dictation/transcription (D or T) and date**

*no spaces used*

**\*Either all caps or all lowercase for the initials is acceptable.**

*Today's date 09-/12/2014 exp.*

**Hillcrest**
medical center

# MODEL REPORT FORM 2

*Barua or Martinez*

## RADIOLOGY REPORT OR DIAGNOSTIC IMAGING REPORT

**Patient Name**: Marietta Mosley

**Patient ID**: 11446     **DOB**: 01/24/- - - -     **Age**: 75     **Sex**: F

**Report No.**: 03-2801

*Use 1-inch margins on sides and bottom of report*

**Ordering Physician**: John Youngblood, MD

**Procedure**: Left hip x-ray.

**Date of Procedure**: 08/05/- - - -   ◄— *Format date as MM/DD/YYYY*

PRIMARY DIAGNOSIS: Fractured left hip.

*Use left justification and avoid hyphenation*

CLINICAL INFORMATION: Left hip pain. No known allergies.

Orthopedic device is noted transfixing the left femoral neck. I have no old films available for comparison. The left femoral neck region appears anatomically aligned. At the level of an orthopedic screw along the lateral aspect of the femoral neck, approximately at the level of the lesser trochanter, there is a radiolucent band consistent with a fracture of indeterminate age that shows probable nonunion. There is bilateral marginal sclerosis and moderate offset and angulation at this site.

◄————————————————— *Double space between paragraphs*

Fairly exuberant callus formation is noted laterally along the femoral shaft.

IMPRESSION
1. No evidence for significant displacement at the femoral neck.
2. Probable nonunion of fracture transversely through the shaft of the femur at about the level of the lesser trochanter.          ◄——— *Align text at left margin*

◄——— *Quadruple space between last paragraph and signature rule*

_____
Neil Nofsinger, MD    ◄— *Align signature block at left margin; signature rule is at least 25 underscores*

◄— *Double space between signature block and dictator/transcriptionist initials*

NN:xx
D:08/05/- - - -
T:08/05/- - - -  *Transcriptionist's initials can be either all caps or all lowercase*

*10/06/2014*

*label*
*file final exam (pt name)*

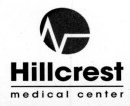

**Hillcrest**
medical center

# MODEL REPORT FORM 3

**OPERATIVE REPORT**

**Patient Name**: Kathy Sullivan

**Patient ID**: 11525      **DOB**: 08/16/- - - -      **Age**: 52      **Sex**: F

**Date of Admission**: 06/25/- - - -

**Date of Procedure**: 06/25/- - - -

**Admitting Physician**: Taylor Withers, MD

**Surgeon**: Sang Lee, MD

**Assistant**: Taylor Withers, MD

**Preoperative Diagnosis**: Urinary incontinence secondary to cystourethrocele.

**Postoperative Diagnosis**: Urinary incontinence secondary to cystourethrocele.

**Operative Procedure**: Total abdominal hysterectomy with suspension correction.

**Anesthesia**: General endotracheal.

**Specimen Removed**: None.

**IV Fluids**: 900 mL crystalloid.

**Estimated Blood Loss**: Negligible.

**Urine Output**: 100 mL by Foley catheter.

**Complications**: None.

DESCRIPTION: After an abdominal hysterectomy had been performed by Dr. Withers, the peritoneum was closed by him and the procedure was turned over to me.

(Continued)

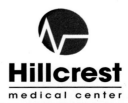

**Hillcrest**
medical center

OPERATIVE REPORT

Patient Name:  Kathy Sullivan
Patient ID:  11525
Date of Procedure:  06/25/- - - -
Page 2

← ——————————————— **Quadruple space—4 hard returns—to body of report**

At this time the supravesical space was entered. The anterior portions of the bladder and urethra were dissected free by blunt and sharp dissection. Bleeders were clamped and electrocoagulated as they were encountered. A wedge of the overlying periosteum was taken and roughened with a bone rasp. The urethra was then attached to the overlying symphysis by placing 2 No. 1 catgut sutures on each side of the urethra and 1 in the bladder neck. The urethra and bladder neck pulled up to the overlying symphysis bone very easily with no tension on the sutures. Bleeding was controlled by pulling the bladder neck up to the bone. Penrose drains were placed on each side of the vesical gutter. Blood loss was negligible. The procedure was then turned back over to Dr. Withers, who proceeded with closure.

_____

Sang Lee, MD

SL:xx
D:06/25/- - - -
T:06/26/- - - -

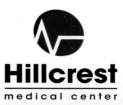

# MODEL REPORT FORM 4

**PATHOLOGY REPORT**

**Patient Name**:  Mark L. Smith   *Deanna Martinez*

**Patient ID**:  11058        **DOB**:  05/03/- - - -        **Age**:  37        **Sex**:  M  *?*

**Pathology Report No.**:  03-S-5698

**Date of Surgery**:  07/17/- - - -

**Preoperative Diagnoses**
1.  Diabetic plantar space abscess of the right foot.
2.  Grade 2 diabetic ulceration of the right foot.

**Postoperative Diagnoses**
1.  Diabetic plantar space abscess of the right foot.
2.  Grade 2 diabetic ulceration of the right foot.

**Specimen Submitted**:  Necrotic tissue, right foot.

**Date Specimen Received**:  07/17/- - - -

**Date Specimen Reported**:  07/18/- - - -

CLINICAL HISTORY:  Pain and ulceration, right foot; diabetes mellitus.

GROSS DESCRIPTION:  Received in formaldehyde labeled "necrotic material, right plantar abscess" are multiple pieces of white, tan, and yellow tissue that are irregular in size and shape. In aggregate it is about 3 cm of tissue. Selected pieces are submitted in a single cassette.

ALW:xx

D:07/17/- - - -

T:07/17/- - - -

**Double space above and below sign-off block occurring between parts of a report**

MICROSCOPIC DESCRIPTION:  There is acute and chronic inflammation and granulation tissue. These changes are consistent with an abscess cavity.

MICROSCOPIC DIAGNOSIS:  Soft tissue from plantar surface of right foot debridement: Acute and chronic inflammation and granulation tissue.

_____

Amber L. Wells, MD

*Berry J. Lozano, MD, Pathology*

ALW:xx

D:07/18/- - - -

T:07/18/- - - -

**Hillcrest**
medical center

# MODEL REPORT FORM 5

**CONSULTATION**

**Patient Name**:  Marty Gibbs

**Patient ID**:  11532        **DOB**:  03/02/- - - -        **Age**:  5        **Sex**:  M

**Room No.**:  PICU

**Consultant**:  Patrick O'Neill, MD, Plastic Surgery

**Requesting Physician**:  Diane Houston, MD, Pediatrics

**Date of Consult**:  11/25/- - - -

**Reason for Consultation**:  Please evaluate extent of burn injuries.

BURNING AGENT:  Coals in fire pit.

I have been asked to see this 5-year-old Caucasian male who appears in mild distress due to upper extremity burn after having fallen into hot coals in his backyard.

Using the Lund Browder chart,[1] the severity of burn is first and second degree. The total body surface area burned includes right lower arm 3%, right hand 1%. The joints involved include the right elbow, right wrist, right hand.

TREATMENT PLAN
1. Splinting of right hand.
2. Positioning:  Elevation with splint on.
3. Range of motion:  Good mobility.
4. Pressure therapy:  Will follow for induration, for pressure fracture.

GOALS
1. Reduce risk of contractures of involved joints by positioning, splinting, and maintaining range of motion.
2. Reduce scar tissue formation by using Jobst bandages, pressure therapy, and splinting.
3. Obtain maximum mobility and strength of upper extremities.
4. Maximize independence in activities of daily living. Activity as tolerated.
5. Provide patient and family education regarding high-calorie, high-protein diet.

←——————————————  **Double space above Continued notation**

(Continued)

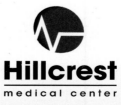

**Hillcrest**
medical center

[1] See the Lund Browder Burn Chart in the Appendix.

CONSULTATION

Patient Name:  Marty Gibbs      ◄────────── **Leave blank line after title on**
Patient ID:  11532                               **second and subsequent page heads**
Date of Consult:  11/25/- - - -                  **Single space rest of header**
Page 2


Thank you for asking me to see this delightful boy. I will follow him at the burn
clicic in 2 weeks.
                                                         ▲
                                                         │
                                          **Include at least two lines of text on the**
────────────────────────                  **top of a page with a signature block**
Patrick O'Neill, MD

PO:xx
D:11/25/- - - -
T:11/28/- - - -

C:  Diane Houston, MD      ◄────────── **Requesting physician**
                                          **receives copy of consultation**

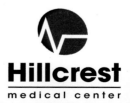

# MODEL REPORT FORM 6

**DISCHARGE SUMMARY**

**Patient Name**:  Joyce Mabry

**Patient ID**:  11709          **DOB**:  07/11/- - - -          **Age**:  21          **Sex**:  F

**Date of Admission**:  02/18/- - - -

**Date of Discharge**:  02/24/- - - -

**Admitting Physician**:  Chris Salem, DO

**Consultations**:  Tom Moore, MD, Hematology

**Procedures Performed**:  Splenectomy.

**Complications**:  None.

**Discharge Diagnosis**:  Elective splenectomy for idiopathic thrombocytopenic purpura and systemic lupus erythematosus.

HISTORY:  The patient is a 21-year-old white woman who had noted excessive bruising since last June. She was diagnosed as having thrombocytopenic purpura. At the same time, the diagnosis of systemic lupus erythematosus was made. The patient continues with the bruising. The patient had been treated with steroids, prednisone 20 mg; however, the platelet count has remained low, less than 20,000. The patient was admitted for elective splenectomy.

DIAGNOSTIC DATA ON ADMISSION:  Chest x-ray was negative. Electrocardiogram was normal. Sodium 138, potassium 5.2, chloride 104, $CO_2$ 25, glucose 111. Urinalysis negative. Hemoglobin 14.8, hematocrit 43.5, white blood cell count 15,000, platelet count 17,000. PT 11.5, INR 0.9, PTT 27.

HOSPITAL COURSE:  The patient was taken to the operating room on February 19 where a splenectomy was performed. The patient's postoperative course was uncomplicated with the wound healing well. The platelet count was stable for the first 3 postoperative days. The patient was transfused intraoperatively with 10 units of platelets and postoperatively with 10 additional units of platelets. However, on the fourth postoperative day the platelet count had risen to 77,000, which was a significant increase.

The patient was discharged for followup in my office. She will also be seen by Dr. Moore, who will follow her SLE and ITP.

(Continued)

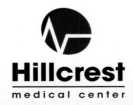

**Hillcrest**
medical center

DISCHARGE SUMMARY

Patient Name:  Joyce Mabry
Patient ID:  11709
Date of Discharge:  02/24/- - - -
Page 2

DISCHARGE DIAGNOSES
1.  Idiopathic thrombocytopenic purpura.
2.  Systemic lupus erythematosus.

DISCHARGE MEDICATIONS  ⟵————————  **No colon used unless words**
1.  Prednisone 20 mg daily.                              **follow on the same line**
2.  Percocet 1 to 2 p.o. q.4 h. p.r.n.
3.  Multivitamins, 1 in a.m. daily.

_____
Carmen Garcia, MD

CG:xx
D:02/25/- - - -
T:02/26/- - - -

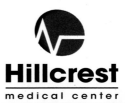

# MODEL REPORT FORM 7

**DEATH SUMMARY**

**Patient Name**:  Russell Syler

**Patient ID**:  11663          **DOB**:  12/24/- - - -          **Age**:  33          **Sex**:  M

**Date of Admission**:  05/15/- - - -

**Date Deceased**:  06/30/- - - -

**Admitting Physician**:  Anthony Zanotti, MD

**Consultations**:  Hematology/Oncology.

**Procedures Performed**:  Abdominal ultrasound and insertion of Ommaya reservoir.

**Cause of Death**:  Circulatory collapse because of overwhelming sepsis, poor immune function, pancytopenia, and diffuse lymphomatous involvement.

ADMITTING DIAGNOSES
1.  Severe headache pain of two days' duration.
2.  Non-Hodgkin lymphoma, large-cell type.

FINAL DIAGNOSES
1.  Polymicrobial sepsis.
2.  Nodular, diffuse, histiocytic lymphoma of head and neck with metastases
    to central nervous system and liver.
3.  Pancytopenia secondary to chemotherapy and sepsis.
4.  Bilateral pneumonia.
5.  Urinary tract infection due to candida organisms.
6.  Oral herpes simplex viral infection.

COURSE IN HOSPITAL:  This 33-year-old black man was originally admitted in early April with the diagnosis of nasopharyngeal mixed, nodular, histiocytic, diffuse, large-cell, noncleaved lymphoma with extensive involvement of the paranasal, parapharyngeal, and nasopharyngeal areas with erosion into the left orbit and cribriform plate and possible abdominal involvement. The patient required a tracheostomy secondary to stridor, status post radiation therapy to the neck and face in early May. He was status post chemotherapy with Cytoxan, Adriamycin, vincristine, and prednisone every 3 weeks. His last chemotherapy had been administered 1 week prior to the current admission of May 15.

(Continued)

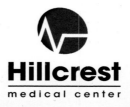

**Hillcrest**
medical center

DEATH SUMMARY

Patient Name:  Russell Syler
Patient ID:  11663
Date Deceased:  06/30/- - - -
Page 2

On admission the patient complained of intractable headache pain. He developed fever, chills, and sweats with nausea and vomiting, as well as decreased appetite for at least the past week. He also developed loose bowel movements on the day after admission. He had shortness of breath and a cough productive of yellow phlegm for the past week.

He had right upper quadrant and epigastric abdominal pain for the past week, not related to meals, with nausea and vomiting. He continued with positive frontal headache as well.

The patient's course deteriorated approximately 1 week into the hospital course, with subsequent hypotension requiring dopamine for maintenance of blood pressure.

Two days prior to his death, antituberculous medications, including INH and rifampin, were added, as well as amphotericin B for possible systemic fungal infection, after urine cultures were positive for Candida. He was treated with a 5-day course of IV acyclovir for herpes simplex viral infection of the pharynx, with resolution of lesions. The patient required multiple platelet transfusions as well as packed cells and occasional transfusions of fresh frozen plasma during his admission.

Blood cultures were positive for Pseudomonas aeruginosa. He was treated with tobramycin and penicillin G. As the sensitivity reports were returned from Microbiology, vancomycin and Fortaz were added for better pseudomonas coverage. Tobramycin was changed to amikacin when one of the patient's sputum cultures was positive for AFB, atypical, a slow grower, possible enterobacter species.

CAUSE OF DEATH was secondary to circulatory collapse because of overwhelming sepsis, poor immune function, pancytopenia, and diffuse lymphomatous involvement. The patient's wife was notified of the grim prognosis and decided to make the patient "do not resuscitate" status.

The patient was pronounced dead on June 30, - - - -, at 4:12 a.m. Permission for autopsy was requested, but the family refused.

_____

Anthony Zanotti, MD

AZ:xx
D:07/03/- - - -
T:07/05/- - - -

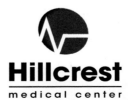

**Hillcrest**
medical center

# MODEL REPORT FORM 8

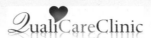

**HISTORY, PHYSICAL, IMPRESSION, PLAN (HPIP)**

**Patient Name**:  Margaret Thornton        **PCP**:  R.J. Reardon, MD

**Date of Birth**:  04/07/- - - -        **Age**:  27        **Sex**:  Female

**Date of Examination**:  09/23/- - - -

HISTORY:  Fever and some cough since 09/20/- - - - when she was started on Biaxin 500 mg 1 p.o. b.i.d. Fever has continued since that time at 101.5 Fahrenheit, taken orally as soon as her Tylenol wears off. No current pneumocystis prophylaxis; says that her T-cell count was 86 last time. She complains of headaches but denies changes in vision. She has right-sided chest pain, particularly by the end of the day and with movement. Medications include Mycostatin suspension, multivitamins, Elavil 10 mg p.r.n., Ativan 1 mg b.i.d. p.r.n., the Biaxin, and Diflucan 200 mg 1 p.o. b.i.d. Only a 2-day supply of Diflucan was given. WBC count of 5500 with differential 42% neutrophils, 34% lymphocytes, 9% monocytes, and 3% eosinophils. Hematocrit 44%, platelets 199,000. Chest x-ray:  Mild interstitial-looking fuzziness bilaterally, more on right than on left.

PHYSICAL EXAMINATION:  In general a chronically ill white female, weight down 2 pounds since her last visit, energy level is down. HEENT:  Oral cavity erythematous, no thrush. NECK:  A few small cervical lymph nodes are palpated. CHEST:  Mild decreased breath sounds on the right but no frank rales or rhonchi. No murmurs or rubs. SKIN is clear; no signs of herpes zoster reactivation. Face is somewhat flushed. ABDOMEN is scaphoid with bowel sounds present in all 4 quadrants. EXTREMITIES:  Some mild peripheral neuropathy bilaterally; reflexes and pulses intact bilaterally.

IMPRESSION:  Acquired immunodeficiency syndrome with progression of disease.

PLAN:  We had a long talk regarding her medication, her T-cell count, the possibility that she has had a progression in her disease, and that she would need to slow down. She is to be off work for this week, and we will see her back here next week.

_____

Robert Solenberger, MD
Infectious Disease

RS:xx
D:09/23/- - - -
T:09/24/- - - -

C:  R.J. Reardon, MD  ◄———————    **The primary care provider gets a copy of medical reports or letters whether or not the name is dictated (this pertains more to outpatient reports than inpatient reports)**

# MODEL REPORT FORM 9

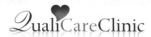

QualiCareClinic

**SUBJECTIVE, OBJECTIVE, ASSESSMENT, PLAN (SOAP)**

**Patient Name**: Mitchell Fitzpatrick          **PCP**: Norma Jacobs, MD

**Date of Birth**: 06/17/- - - -          **Age**: 53          **Sex**: Male

**Date of Examination**: 02/01/- - - -

SUBJECTIVE
Mr. Fitzpatrick presents for followup of his hemoptysis, which has improved significantly. He underwent flexible fiberoptic bronchoscopy as an outpatient at Hillcrest on 01/27/- - - -, with no endobronchial abnormalities noted. It is suspected, therefore, that his expectoration of blood is not coming from his lungs. The patient has had worsening dyspnea on exertion, according to his wife, with several episodes of nocturnal wheezing associated with mild shortness of breath.

OBJECTIVE
Spirometry shows an $FEV_1$ of 2.59, 82% of predicted. His $FEV_1$-FVC ratio is 79%. FVC is 3.26, 71% of predicted. There is mild reduction in the midflow rates. On exam, oropharynx is clear. Neck is supple without adenopathy or bruits. Lung fields are clear to auscultation. Cardiac exam:  Regular rate and rhythm with a soft systolic murmur heard best at the right upper sternal border and left apex. No significant peripheral edema or cyanosis.

ASSESSMENT
1.  Hemoptysis, no evidence of endobronchial lesions.
2.  Obesity.
3.  Probable bronchospastic lung disease.
4.  History of hypertension, remote.
5.  History of peptic ulcer disease, remote.

PLAN
1.  We will start the patient empirically on an albuterol inhaler, 2 puffs q.4 h. p.r.n. wheezing or dyspnea.
2.  He will be instructed on the proper use of his inhaler.
3.  Followup in 4 months for repeat spirometry testing.

_____

Gerald Warr Wells, MD
Pulmonology

GWW:xx
D:02/01/- - - -
T:02/02/- - - -

C:  Norma Jacobs, MD

# MODEL REPORT FORM 10: CORRESPONDENCE

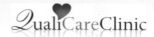

**QUALI-CARE CLINIC**
**HEMATOLOGY STE 200**
**TEN MEDICAL BLVD**
**MIAMI FL 33130**
**Phone: 305.555.2242**

June 20, - - - -

Rodney Wells, MD
Florida Center for Infectious Disease
2303 SE Military Dr
Miami FL 33173

RE:    HAL TESCH
       Date of birth:  January 24, - - - -

Dear Dr. Wells:

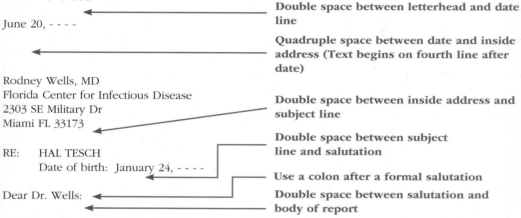

Double space between letterhead and date line

Quadruple space between date and inside address (Text begins on fourth line after date)

Double space between inside address and subject line

Double space between subject line and salutation

Use a colon after a formal salutation

Double space between salutation and body of report

Thank you for the kind referral of your patient, Hal Tesch, regarding his pancytopenia. He has a history of cirrhosis with portal hypertension. From the information you have provided me, his pancytopenia was present at the time he presented to your facility on March 6. His white blood cell count at that time was 3400 with 58 segmented forms. His WBC count dropped to 2400 on April 4 and was as low as 1900 on June 4. On June 18 the patient's WBC count was 2300; as we discussed, you gave him Neupogen. By the next day, his WBCs were up to 7400.

Physical examination has revealed evidence of hepatosplenomegaly and chronic liver disease.

As we discussed, I think the patient's pancytopenia is related to his cirrhosis and hypersplenism rather than to his antituberculous medications. He had pancytopenia at essentially the same level as he does now prior to receiving therapy for tuberculosis. I had planned to get vitamin $B_{12}$, folate, antinuclear antibody analysis, and a rheumatoid factor to look for other causes of pancytopenia; however, I suspect that these studies would be negative. I did not have them drawn in my office but decided to leave them for you to obtain in your facility, if you feel they are warranted.

(Continued)

Rodney Wells, MD
June 20, - - - -
RE: Hal Tesch
Page 2

◄——————————————— **Quadruple space between page header and text below (Text begins on fourth line following head)**

I recommend continuing the patient on Neupogen at 5 mg/kg probably about 3 times weekly. I found it impressive that he received his first dose of Neupogen on June 18 and by just the next day his white blood cell count had risen from 2300 to 7400.

Thank you for allowing me to participate in the care of this very pleasant gentleman. I will return him to your care, though I would be delighted to see him at any time I can be of further assistance.

◄——————————————— **Double space between last line of text and complimentary closing**

Sincerely,

◄——————————————— **Use 4 to 6 spaces between complimentary closing and writer's identification**

Stephen C. Gordon, MD
Hematology

SCG:xx

# SECTION 3

REFERENCES

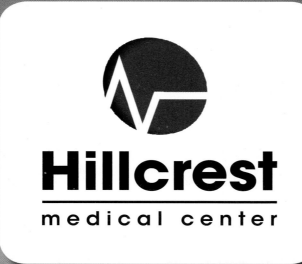

# Transcription Rules for Hillcrest Medical Center and Quali-Care Clinic

Each hospital has a process by which the abbreviations and style for its transcribed medical records are set. This process usually involves an information management committee (comprised of appointed members of the medical staff) together with representatives from both the health information management department and hospital administration. The rules adopted for medical reports at Hillcrest have been voluntarily adopted for use at Quali-Care Clinic, and they include the following.

## STYLE VARIATIONS

Flexibility in medical transcription is important. Doctors employ variations in style when dictating their records, and medical transcriptionists must be able to conform to these styles when necessary. Check for employer or client preferences and be consistent within each one's body of work. This practice is easily said but not always easily done because the originators may be inconsistent within their own work. The medical transcriptionist is charged with turning the spoken word into the written word, to create not only a legal document but also one that makes the employer or client look good. That is, transcriptionists correct dictation errors in English grammar, usage, and sentence structure when possible. Style variations that you are likely to see used both in Hillcrest and on the job are listed below.

### Headings

Headings that stand alone take *no* colon unless words follow on the same line. Headings with words that follow on the same line take a colon, and the first word that follows uses an initial capital letter. These headings, however, may be uppercase, may have an initial capital letter, may be in bold or not in bold, and may be centered, at the left margin, or tabbed. All of the above heading styles are acceptable. The AHDI *Book of Style*, 3rd ed., prefers main headings to be in all caps at the left margin with subheadings in initial caps.

The Review of Systems and Physical Examination paragraphs may be one paragraph each, or the subheadings within each paragraph may be separated out with each heading beginning a new line. Both styles are acceptable.

### Lists

Lists of medications, diagnoses, procedures, etc., may be indented, tabbed, at the left margin, or all in one paragraph. They may be numbered with the 1, 2, 3 system or with a, b, c. At times you will see (1), (2), (3) or even 1), 2), 3) used. More elaborate lists might use roman numerals with subheadings. This style is not normally utilized in the transcription of medical records; however, it is as correct as any of the above-listed numbering styles for lists. The AHDI *Book of Style*, 3rd ed., prefers lists to be numbered 1, 2, 3 at the left margin.

### Dates

Date styles are either numeric or written in words. Both are acceptable in medical transcription. Use the style as dictated by the originator. See the following examples:

01/01/2011     1 Jan 2011          1 January 2011
Jan 1, 2011     January 1, 2011

**NOTE:** Hillcrest is using a four-digit year, but *remember*, for your work at Hillcrest, use ---- instead of a year.

### Subscripts and Superscripts

Subscripts and superscripts can be used, but because it is faster to put figures on the line, some style guides recommend this style. Many transcriptionists are paid by their production of work, so time is money. (It is possible to put these in AutoText if you want the subscript or superscript without the extra time.)

> **Examples**
> $S_1$, $S_2$ *or* S1, S2
> $CO_2$ *or* CO2
> $m^2$ *or* sq m

### Continued Pages

At Hillcrest we use "(Continued)" at the end of pages that are continued. In some places of business, however, the medical transcriptionist has no control over this due to computer headers or footers that are added automatically. Some offices or facilities use the style "Page 1 of 3," "Page 2 of 3," "Page 3 of 3" on each page, which is acceptable.

Page-two headings are always used in one way or another. An on-the-job computer system may automatically add this information in a header or footer. If not, use your employer or client preference. At Hillcrest we use different page-two headings for inpatient reports, outpatient reports, and correspondence. (See the Model Report Forms in Section 2.)

## Signature Line

The signature line at Hillcrest (at least 25 underscores) is placed at the left margin; however, some facilities tab the signature line to the center of the page. Both styles are acceptable. Remember, in correspondence an actual line is not used for the signature. Just allow four to six blank lines before typing the originator's name. The signature will go in that space.

## Sign-Off Block

The sign-off block (identifying information) is always used in medical transcription but not necessarily in correspondence. The sign-off block can vary widely in style, so stay flexible. The initials can be all uppercase or all lowercase. The dates are usually numeric but can be done in a couple of styles. Hospitals and transcription companies sometimes customize their sign-off block. The sign-off block goes two spaces below the final line of text, flush left, with no spaces used.

### Examples
DI:TI        di:ti
D:1/5/----   D:01/05/----
T:1/6/----   T:01/06/----

## Copy Line

The copy line, which is typed two spaces below the sign-off block, can be C or c (copy), CC or cc (courtesy copy), PC or pc (photocopy), or BC or bc (blind copy). Any of these styles is acceptable.

## Enclosure Line

If your report or letter includes an enclosure, this information is noted by the word "Enclosure" typed two spaces below the copy line. This can be abbreviated as either Enc. or Encl.

**NOTE:** At the end of a letter or a report, to keep it from going onto another page, you can adjust the spaces between signature line, sign-off block, copy line, and/or enclosure line. You may not go to an extra page unless there are at least two lines

of text from the body of the report on the new page. (There should be no pages with just a signature line or less on them.) If you cannot arrange the information to keep it from going onto another page, then place at least two lines of text from the body of the report onto the new page.

# CAPITALIZATION

1. Use initial capital letters in eponymic terms. Eponyms are names of phrases formed from or including the name of a person. The common noun following the eponym is lowercase.

   ### Examples
   Rockey-Davis incision
   Foley catheter
   Down syndrome
   Buck fascia
   May Hegglin anomaly
   Duffy blood group
   Crohn's
   lactated Ringer's

**NOTE:** There is a trend away from using the possessive form in eponymic terms. The AHDI *Book of Style,* 3rd ed., *Dorland's Illustrated Medical Dictionary,* and *Stedman's Medical Dictionary* recognize this trend; however, the possessive form is still acceptable if your facility prefers that style. Both styles appear in this text-workbook.

2. Capitalize trade names and proprietary names of drugs and brand names of manufactured products and equipment. Do *not* capitalize generic names or descriptive terms.

   ### Examples
   Trade names of drugs include Keflex, Motrin, and Bayer. Corresponding generic terms are cephalexin, ibuprofen, and aspirin.
   Trade names of suture materials include Vicryl, Dexon, and Prolene. Generic terms include chromic catgut, silk, nylon, and cotton—either plain, braided, or twisted.
   Miscellaneous brand names include Kleenex, Vaseline, and Scotch tape. Corresponding generic terms are tissue, petroleum jelly, and cellophane tape.

3. Use an initial capital letter and italics (or underscore to indicate italics) for the name of a genus when used in the singular. Do not capitalize, italicize, or underscore when used in the plural, as an adjective, when used in

the vernacular, or when it stands alone. See "The Grammar of Microbiology." The AHDI *Book of Style*, 3rd ed., prefers no italics or underscores when transcribing medical reports.

### Examples
*Pseudomonas aeruginosa (P. aeruginosa)*
*Helicobacter pylori (H. pylori)*

**BUT**

pseudomonal appearing
helicobacter reported
strep throat
staph infection

4. Specific areas within Hillcrest Medical Center are lowercased, as common nouns.

### Examples
operating room
blood bank
postanesthesia recovery
transcription section
intensive care unit
emergency room

5. Capitalize the proper names of languages, races, religions, and sects. Do *not* capitalize the common nouns following these designations. Do *not* capitalize informal designations of race, i.e., white or black.

### Examples
Asians
Hispanic people
the English language
of Jewish ancestry
African American
Germanic languages
Seminoles
Muslim religion

6. As a courtesy, positive allergy information may be keyed in all capital letters in order to call attention to this vital information. The AHDI *Book of Style*, 3rd ed., prefers no bold type when transcribing medical records.

### Example
ALLERGIES: The patient is allergic to SULFA, which causes hives.

7. Capitalize acronyms but not the words from which the acronym is derived.

### Examples
nonsteroidal anti-inflammatory drug (NSAID)
coronary artery bypass graft (CABG)
skilled nursing facility (SNF)

# NUMBERS

1. Transcribe numbers, both ordinal (1st, 2nd, 3rd) and cardinal (1, 2, 3), in medical records and correspondence, as numeric values stand out from the text, making this vital information easier to read. When one numerical expression follows another, for clarity, spell out the one that can more easily be expressed in words. Roman numerals are used in specific instances, as in cancer stages. (See CMTips for more on roman numerals.)

### Examples
Dr. Smith removed 7 lesions from the patient's back and 2 from his 4th rib. They were diagnosed as stage II cancer.
The dietician recommended two 6-ounce cans of supplement daily.
Apgar scores were 9 and 9 at one and five minutes.
Lipoproteins included an LDL of 80 and an HDL of 50.
Vital signs showed blood pressure 120/80, pulse 72 per minute and regular, respirations 21, temperature 98 degrees F. (See "Vital Signs" for a discussion on how these may be dictated.)
Medications: Lomotil 20 mg at bedtime, diazepam 15 mg daily.

2. Always use figures with abbreviations, symbols, and technical measurements—no space comes between the number and its symbol, but use one space before and after the "x" in measurements. (See the Abbreviations and Symbols section, #2 under Symbols, for more on the lower case "x.")

### Examples
Pulses 2+, 100% oxygen, 15 mmHg, reflexes 5/5 throughout, denies x3
The uterus weighs 150 g and measures 8.0 x 4.5 x 0.9 cm.
*(handwritten: 1 space)*

**NOTE:** In the measurement above, while the whole number has a zero added for balance, the final measurement has a preceding zero added for clarity. *The preceding zero is mandatory in decimal phrases.*

3. A space should appear between an arabic number and the corresponding unit of measure abbreviation/symbol.

### Examples
9 mg%     83 mL     0.5 cm     64 g/dL
*(handwritten: space   space   space)*

4.  The smoking history is often dictated as a pack-year. The pack-year is the result of the *packs per day multiplied by the number of years of smoking*. A 50-pack-year smoking history is equivalent to smoking a pack a day for 50 years (50 × 1 = 50).

    **Example**
    > Social History: Lives with husband, they are retired. Drinks socially. Has a 25-pack-year smoking history; however, she recently quit smoking.

5.  Numbers that constitute either a series or range or span of years should not omit digits.

    **Examples**
    > The gallstones measured from 0.7 to 2.9 cm in aggregate.
    > Statistics proved the theory in 8 of 12 recipients.
    > The patient took epilepsy medication from 2010 to 2013. (*not* 2010–13)
    > The solution can be found on pages 157 through 159. (*not* 157–59)

    **NOTE:** When the phrase "from _____ to _____" is used, the "to" is spelled out. The same is true when the phrase "between _____ and _____" is used. The "and" is spelled out. No hyphen is used in these phrases to avoid unnecessary confusion.

6.  The vertebral or spinal column segments are referred to in arabic numerals (no subscripts). The 12 pairs of cranial nerves are usually referred to in roman numerals. Some places may accept arabic numerals; check with your client/employer on this.

    **Examples**
    > cervical spine = C1 through C7
    > thoracic spine = T1 through T12
    > dorsal spine = D1 through D12 (interchangeable with thoracic spine)
    > lumbar spine = L1 through L5
    > sacral spine = S1 through S5

    > Cranial nerves are usually dictated I through XII:
    > I = olfactory
    > II = optic
    > III = oculomotor
    > IV = trochlear
    > V = trigeminal
    > VI = abducens
    > VII = facial
    > VIII = vestibulocochlear
    > IX = glossopharyngeal
    > X = vagal
    > XI = accessory
    > XII = hypoglossal

7.  Titers and ratios are expressed with figures and a colon. The colon is dictated and read as "to." No spaces are used in these numeric expressions.

    **Examples**
    > Cord blood sample showed a herpes titer of 1:110.
    > Anesthesia consisted of Xylocaine and epinephrine 1:100,000.

8.  Temperature readings are expressed in either Celsius (C) or Fahrenheit (F). Use either the degree symbol or spell out the word *degrees* if the symbol is not available. Transcribe the words "zero" and "minus" regarding temperature. Each of the following examples is acceptable.

    **Examples**
    > 98.6 °F *or* 98.6 degrees Fahrenheit
    > zero degrees Fahrenheit
    > 35.4 °C *or* 35.4 degrees Celsius
    > minus 30 degrees Celsius

9.  Surgical sutures are sized by the United States Pharmacopeia (USP) system. Sizes range from 11-0 (smallest) to 7 (largest) and utilize silk, cotton, and other materials. Stainless steel sutures are sized by the Brown and Sharp (B&S) gauge system. B&S sizes are expressed in whole numbers from No. 40 (smallest) to No. 20 (largest).

    **Examples**
    > 9-0 white silk
    > 2-0 chromic
    > No. 40 stainless steel suture
    > 3-0 VEST traction sutures
    > 1-0 PDS Vicryl sutures
    > #30 wire Zytor

    **NOTE**: "No." is used at the beginning of a sentence; otherwise, the # symbol can be used in medical transcription.

10. Superscripts and subscripts are used in medical transcription; however, if the transcription equipment being used does not provide for entering characters either above or below the line, the superscript and/or subscript may be entered on the line. In either case, no spaces should be used in the superscript/subscript.

    **Examples**
    > H2O *or* $H_2O$ (water)
    > PO2 *or* $PO_2$ (partial pressure of oxygen)
    > $^{131}I$ *but* I 131 (radioactive iodine)
    > $^{198}Au$ *but* Au 198 (radioactive gold)

11. Use arabic numerals when referring to EKG leads, cancer grades, and both conventional and military time. (See CMTips™ for more on "time.")

### Examples

EKG leads V1 to V6
grade 2 tumor
1600 hours is 4 p.m.
0530 hours is 5:30 a.m.
8:45 a.m.
2 p.m.

**NOTE:** When time on a clock is dictated to describe a location, as on the breast, use the following style:

Suspicious area was tagged with a suture at 3 o'clock.

Lesions identified at 12, 3, and 6 o'clock.

# PUNCTUATION

## Apostrophe

1. The apostrophe is used to show possession.

### Examples

Patient's condition (singular possessive noun)
Doctors' opinions (plural possessive noun)

2. The apostrophe is used to form contractions, but use contractions, even if dictated, *only* when transcribing direct patient quotes.

### Examples

He's having no symptoms. (contraction of *he is*)
It's my opinion. (contraction of *it is*)
Chief Complaint: "I'm sick. I can't breathe."

### BUT

Its measurements are irregular. (possessive pronoun—no apostrophe used here)

3. Do *not* use an apostrophe to form the plural of either an all-capital abbreviation or of numerals, including years.

### Examples

DRGs          Temperature in the 20s
WBCs          Born in the 1990s
D&Cs          Three PhDs attended
DTRs
LABs
T&As

**NOTE:** When a word or letter could be misread, the apostrophe is sometimes used for clarity.

### Examples

He received all A's.
The T's were left uncrossed.
Her U's need work.
Record the patient's I's and O's.

4. The apostrophe is used with units of time and money when used as possessive adjectives.

### Examples

a week's work/a dollar's worth/in a month's time (all show singular possessive)
7 days' work/50 cents' worth/ 6 months' gestation (all show plural possessive)

## Hyphen

1. Hyphenate a compound in which a number is the first element and the compound precedes the noun it modifies.

### Examples

48-hour turnaround time
a 12-factor panel
a 15-month time period
two 6-inch lacerations

2. Hyphenate a compound adjectival phrase when it precedes the noun it modifies, but *not* when it is in the predicate.

### Examples

| | | |
|---|---|---|
| a 17-week infant | **BUT** | The infant was 17 weeks old |
| end-to-end anastomosis | **BUT** | The anastomosis was end to end. |
| a figure-of-8 suture | **BUT** | The suture was in a figure of 8. |

3. Hyphenate an adjective-noun compound when it precedes and modifies another noun.

### Examples

| | | |
|---|---|---|
| upper-range results | **BUT** | The results were in the upper range of normal. |
| third-floor burn unit | **BUT** | The burn unit was on the third floor. |

4. Hyphenate two or more adjectives used coordinately or as conflicting terms whether they precede the noun or follow as a predicate adjective.

### Examples

false-positive results (The results were false-positive.)
double-blind study (The study was done as a double-blind.)

5. Hyphenate color terms when the two elements are of equal weight.

   **Examples**
   > pink-tan tissue **BUT** pinkish tan mucosa
   > gray-brown area **BUT** grayish brown skin

6. Use a suspended (suspensive) hyphen when words or numbers are dictated without the intervening noun. One space follows each suspended hyphen, which takes the place of the missing noun.

   **Examples**
   > Patient received 1st-, 2nd-, and 3rd-degree burns to his upper torso and arms.
   > Child exhibited yellowish-, greenish-, and purplish-colored bruises across his legs.
   > Blood sugars were checked at 15-, 30-, and 60-minute intervals.

7. Use a hyphen when joining numbers or letters to form a word, phrase, or abbreviation.

   **Examples**
   | | |
   |---|---|
   | 5-FU | C-section |
   | VP-16 | X-ray |
   | SMA-12 | T-spine |
   | ICD-10 | Y-shaped incision |

8. Remember, there is a difference between a hyphen and a dash. The hyphen, as described above, joins words and phrases. A dash, typed as two hyphens with no space before, between, or after, is used to emphasize certain material within a sentence. It makes a strong break within a sentence.

   **Examples**
   > Six organs were removed at surgery 2 years ago—all apparently during the same operative procedure.
   > Decreased balance with increased lower extremity ataxia—right minimal, left moderate.

   *2 hyphens*

9. Hyphens are no longer being used between a number and its metric unit of measurement, even in a modifying situation, per the AHDI *Book of Style*, 3rd ed. This change is new from past recommendations and is per the SI Convention and metric standards. As mathematical statements, the rules of language do not apply here.

   **Examples**
   | | |
   |---|---|
   | 1800 kcal diet | 70 kg male |
   | two 3 cm pins | one 5 mL syringe |
   | a 4 g tumor | 2.0 x 12 mm stent |

# ABBREVIATIONS AND SYMBOLS

## Abbreviations

Abbreviations used in Hillcrest Medical Center case studies are listed and defined in the medical terminology glossary preceding each case. They are also listed alphabetically in the index.

The information presented in both the heading of each Hillcrest medical report and, at times, in the body of the reports will be in what is known as elliptical or "clipped" expressions, i.e., a word or words that represent a complete thought. These clipped expressions are commonly used in medical dictation and each will end with a period to show they are complete thoughts.

**NOTE:** Hillcrest medical records will have no abbreviations used in the diagnosis lines, impression lines, or preoperative or postoperative lines.

## Symbols

1. The virgule (slash or diagonal) is used to indicate the word "per" in laboratory values and other equations or the word "over" in blood pressure (BP) readings and visual acuity.

   **Examples**
   > using the virgule for "per"
   > > hemoglobin 14.1 g/dL
   > > fasting blood sugar 138 mg/dL
   > using the virgule for "over"
   > > blood pressure 110/70 mmHg in both arms
   > > 20/80 right eye and 20/40 left eye (visual acuity)

**NOTE:** When millimeters of mercury is dictated with a blood pressure reading or ocular tension, transcribe mmHg. Leave no space, and leave out the word "of." No need to transcribe this expression if it is not dictated. *mercury*

2. Lowercase $x$ is used to indicate "by" in measurements, to indicate "times" in magnification and multiplication, and to indicate "for" in other phrases. If the $x$ can be read as the word "for," then use the word *for*, not "times" and not "x."

   **Examples**
   > Sponge and instrument counts were correct x3.
   > Electron microscopy cells are magnified x100,000.
   > > (x = times above; no space is left between the $x$ and the number; do not separate at the end of a line)

*spaces*

Fetal limb length was 5.5 x 1.5 x 1.0 cm.
(x = by above; leave a space both
before and after the *x*; can be separated at the end of a line)
Dictated: Medication is to be taken *times*
six months.
Transcribed: Medication is to be taken
*for* six months.

3.  Use numerals with a symbol or an abbreviation.

    **Examples**
    Dictated: Deep tendon reflexes minus four.
    Transcribed: Deep tendon reflexes −4.

4.  Both reflexes and pulses are usually graded
    on a scale from 0 to 4+. The meanings of the
    different grades are as follows:

    *Reflexes*
    4+ = very brisk, hyperactive; may
    indicate disease; often associated
    with clonus (alternating muscular
    contraction and relaxation in rapid
    succession)
    3+ = brisker than average; possibly but
    not necessarily indicative of disease
    2+ = average or normal
    1+ = somewhat diminished; low normal
    0 = no response; may indicate
    neuropathy

    *Pulses*
    0 = completely absent
    +1 = markedly impaired
    +2 = moderately impaired
    +3 = slightly impaired
    +4 = normal

5.  Qualitative test results are usually given using
    the plus and minus symbols. Transcribe the
    word "minus" (not −) and transcribe the word
    "plus" (not +).

    | Dictated | Transcribed |
    | --- | --- |
    | − (negative) | minus |
    | + /− (very slight trace or reaction) | plus/minus |
    | + (slight trace or reaction) | plus |
    | + + (trace or noticeable reaction) | 2 plus |
    | + + + (moderate amount of reaction) | 3 plus |
    | + + + + (large amount of pronounced reaction) | 4 plus |

6.  The metric system of measurement is used in
    medicine. (See the list of metric measurements
    that follows.) Use the abbreviated forms when
    entering a number with metric measurements.
    Do not use a period following metric abbrevi-
    ations. Do not pluralize abbreviations. (*Liter*, a
    liquid measurement in this example, is abbre-
    viated with an uppercase *L*.)

    **Examples**

    | | | |
    | --- | --- | --- |
    | 1 cm | 0.9 cm | 20 cm |
    | 1 mL | 1.6 mL | 15 mL |
    | 1 g | 3.7 g | 32 g |
    | 1 L | 2.5 L | 8 L |

7.  Latin abbreviations: At Hillcrest, these are
    keyed in lowercase with periods as follows:

    a.c. (ante cibum, before meals)
    a.d. (auris dextra, right ear)
    a.m. (ante meridiem, morning)
    a.s. (auris sinistra, left ear)
    a.u. (auris utraque, each ear) (best to spell
    out)
    b.i.d. (bis in die, twice a day)
    d. (die, day)
    h. (hour)
    h.s. (hora somni, bedtime)
    n.p.o. (nil per os, nothing by mouth)
    o.d. (oculus dexter, right eye)
    o.s. (oculus sinister, left eye)
    o.u. (oculus uterque, each eye)
    p.c. (post cibum, after meals)
    p.m. (post meridiem, afternoon)
    p.o. (per os, by mouth)
    p.r.n. (pro re nata, as circumstances may
    require)
    q.d. (quaque die, every day) (dangerous
    abbreviation—transcribe either "every day"
    or "daily" per The Joint Commission's "Do
    Not Use" list, found in the Appendix.)
    q.h. (quaque hora, every hour)
    q.i.d. (quater in die, four times a day)
    q.s. (quantum satis, sufficient quantity)
    t.i.d. (ter in die, three times a day)

# LIST OF METRIC MEASUREMENTS

| Unit | Abbreviation |
|---|---|
| centimeter(s) | cm |
| cubic centimeter(s) | cc *or* cm³ (volume) (When *cc* is dictated, transcribe *mL* [for liquid volume]; see the "Do Not Use" list in the Appendix.) |
| cubic meter(s) | m³ (volume) |
| deciliter(s) | dL |
| gram(s) | g |
| kilocalorie(s) | kcal |
| kilogram(s) | kg |
| kiloliter(s) | kL |
| kilometer(s) | km |
| liter(s) | L |
| meter(s) | m |
| microgram(s) | mcg |
| milligram(s) | mg |
| milliliter(s) | mL |
| millimeter(s) | mm |
| square centimeter(s) | sq cm *or* cm² (area) |
| square kilometer(s) | sq km *or* km² (area) |
| square meter(s) | sq m *or* m² (area) |

# THE GRAMMAR OF MICROBIOLOGY

Microbiology is a fascinating field of knowledge about which transcriptionists seldom get to be experts. Here are some tips to remember. (Refer to the AHDI *Book of Style*, 3rd ed., regarding their preference in using periods, italics, and underlines in transcribing the following in medical records.)

1. Only when the full genus and species names are used is the phrase italicized.

2. In handwriting or on a keyboard an underscore indicates italics. Because of the italics feature on computers, the underline is seldom used in this manner; however, underlining a genus and species still indicates italics to a typesetter.

3. When the full genus and species names are used, the genus takes an initial cap. When the genus is referred to as a single letter, that letter is uppercase.

4. When medical jargon or slang is dictated, try to transcribe at least the short form except as noted (see following table for usage).

## JARGON OR SLANG

| Genus and Species | Short Form | Sometimes Dictated | Disease Examples |
|---|---|---|---|
| *Branhamella catarrhalis* | *B. catarrhalis* | B. cat | otitis media, URIs |
| *Clostridium difficile* | *C. difficile** | C. diff | enterocolitis |
| *Coccidioides immitis* | *C. immitis* | cox | coccidioidomycosis |
| *Escherichia coli* | *E. coli* | — | UTIs, diarrhea |
| *Haemophilus influenzae* | *H. influenzae* | H. flu | epiglottitis, pneumonia |
| *Haemophilus vaginalis* | *H. vaginalis* | H. vag | vaginal infections |
| *Helicobacter pylori* | *H. pylori* | H. py | gastric ulcers |
| *Klebsiella pneumoniae* | *K. pneumoniae* | K. pneumo | bacterial pneumonia |
| *Mycobacterium avium-intracellulare* | *M. avium-intracellulare* | MAI** | pulmonary disease |
| *Staphylococcus aureus* | *S. aureus* | MRSA** | methicillin-resistant staph aureus |
| *Staphylococcus epidermidis* | *S. epidermidis* | staph epi or MRSE** | peritonitis, endocarditis, methicillin-resistant staph epidermidis |
| *Staphylococcus pyogenes* | *S. pyogenes* | staph pyo | impetigo, scalded skin syndrome |
| *Streptococcus pneumoniae* | *S. pneumoniae* | strep pneumo | lobar pneumonia |
| *Streptococcus pyogenes* | *S. pyogenes* | strep pyo | septic sore throat, scarlet fever, rheumatic fever |

*The species "difficile" is correctly pronounced "dif fi' cil ee." We are used to hearing "dif fa ceel"; however, if you hear the first pronunciation, please know what is being dictated.*

**MAI, MRSA, and MRSE are common abbreviations, well recognized in medicine. Do not change these abbreviations, if dictated.*

# Vital Signs

In the following eight dictated vital signs, you will note different sequences *and* different criteria, even though these doctors practice in the same clinic setting. Each doctor dictates patients' vital signs in the same sequence, sometimes dictating the numbers only without using words. Transcribe what is dictated, and do not change the dictator's style. Spelling these words out is not wrong unless your client/employer prefers otherwise, but the vital signs abbreviations are accepted almost everywhere.

| Dictated Vital Signs | Originator's Initials |
|---|---|
| 1. Blood pressure, pulse, respirations, temperature BP 120/80, P 79, R 22, T 98 | SCC |
| 2. Temperature, pulse, blood pressure T 99, P 82, BP 156/90 | DHG |
| 3. Blood pressure, pulse, temperature, weight BP 90/70, P 65, T 100.1, weight 102-1/2 pounds | REB |
| 4. Temperature, pulse, blood pressure, weight T 95.5, P 82, BP 140/75, weight 190-3/4 pounds | TDF |
| 5. Weight, blood pressure, temperature, pulse Weight 264 pounds, BP 200/100, T 99.6, P 102 | JAL |
| 6. Blood pressure, temperature, pulse, respirations BP 132/78, T 97.5, P 72, R 20 | JEM |
| 7. Temperature, blood pressure, weight, height T 98.7, BP 145/69, weight 156 pounds, height 63 inches | STW |
| 8. Blood pressure alone BP 179/83 | JDMc |

Future physicians begin dictating patient records early in their training and might copy a mentor, a fellow student, or just do what comes naturally. No one teaches them exactly how to dictate their records. It is the medical transcriptionist's job to transcribe each originator's dictation correctly and in the originator's specific style.

In the previous eight examples, the transcriptionist should *not* make the styles the same and *not* add information that was not dictated. If the dictation is cut off or unclear, leave a blank and/or flag the report for the originator. If you have access to the medical record, you may look up the vitals and include the correct information. Check the date of visit *and* the date of dictation to get the correct numbers for the record.

# CMTips™

## DIFFICULT SINGULAR AND PLURAL WORDS AND PHRASES

The following words have proven to be difficult because you cannot rely on their being dictated correctly. Be aware and transcribe as follows.

| Singular | Plural |
|---|---|
| ala nasi is | alae nasi are |
| curriculum is | curricula are |
| diverticulum is | diverticula are |
| genitalis is | genitalia are |
| naris is | nares are |
| medium is | media are |
| labium | labia |
| majus is | majora are |
| minus is | minora are |
| lentigo is | lentigines are |
| focus is | foci are |
| fossa is | fossae are |
| decubitus *ulcer* is | decubitus *ulcers* are |

**NOTE:** Decubitus is *not* a noun and has no plural form.

## UNUSUAL WORDS

Spelling problems can include *yogurt*, which we eat; *solder*, as in to solder wires together; *perennial*, as in regularly repeated or renewed; and *corduroy artifact* or *pattern* (radiology). The *water hammer pulse* or *signal* is a rapid upstroke and falloff, which indicates cardiac problems. A *wrinkle test* is done in orthopedics. Do not assume a dictated word must be impossible—research it to make sure of its relevance in your report.

## TEMPERATURE VERSUS FEVER

If a dictator says, "Patient has some headache but no temperature," remember that we *always* have a temperature, it just may not be elevated. Correctly transcribed, the phrase should read either, "Patient has some headache but no elevated temperature" or "Patient has some headache but no fever."

## A TONGUE TWISTER

The following changes are found in patients with chronic muscle spasm. The difference between chronic spasm and newly acquired spasm can be palpated on physical exam and may be described as either:

tense, tender tissue texture changes

**OR**

tender tissue texture changes

## DERMATOLOGY TERMS

Hair cycles or phases include (1) anagen, (2) catagen, and (3) telogen. Examples include anagen effluvium, a loss of hair after chemotherapy, and telogen effluvium, a loss of hair due to the trauma of surgery, high fever, stress, etc.

pyknotic nuclei = a thickening of the nuclei

arrectores pilorum = muscles in the connective tissue of the upper dermis, attached to the hair follicles below the sebaceous glands

delling = the formation of a slight blister or dimpling

## PULMONARY TERMS

I-E ratio (dictated "eye to E")

The ratio of inspiratory to expiratory time.

E → A (dictated "E to A")

When the patient saying "E, E, E" comes out as sounding like "A, A, A" upon auscultation of the lung by the physician, this shows consolidation of the lung.

## RACE/AGE

When transcribing race, *Caucasian* and *African American* are properly capitalized; however, *white* and *black* are properly lowercased.

### Examples

This 45-year-old black female . . .
This 72-year-old white male . . .
A 15-month-old Caucasian girl . . .
A 25-year-old black Cuban male . . .

**OR**

This black male patient is 15 years old.
My Anglo gardener is 74 years old.
An African American girl, 9 months old . . .
His boy, a Native American, is 7 years old.

**NOTE:** "45-year-old" is a single modifier adjective and needs hyphens. "74 years old" does not use hyphens. Clue: If the term dictated is "years," then no hyphen is needed; if the term dictated is "year," then hyphens are needed.

In age references, it may be helpful to remember that:

- Neonates or newborns are people from birth to 1 month of age.
- Infants are people 1 month to 24 months of age.
- Children are people 2 years to 13 years of age, also boys or girls.
- Adolescents are people 13 to 17 years of age, also teenagers, boys, or girls.
- Adults are people 18 years of age or older, also men or women.

## ZERO SAFETY

Preceding zeros with decimals: These are important safety factors in transcription. In either typewritten or handwritten records, a decimal point on the line is hard to see, is easily missed, and incorrect dosing can result. The preceding zero is essential in transcription.

### Examples
Dictated: "Xylocaine point 1 percent"
Transcribed: Xylocaine 0.1%.
A drug dosage dictated as "point two five" should be transcribed as 0.25.

**NOTE:** This pertains only to zeros in front of decimals (preceding zeros), and not to those behind the decimal. Trailing zeros are dangerous in medications. See "A Healthcare Controlled Vocabulary" in the Appendix.

## THE DIGITS

When roman numerals are used in dictating digits, they mean the following:

| | |
|---|---|
| I (one) | digitus primus manus = digit I (thumb) |
| II (two) | digitus secundus manus = digit II (index finger) |
| III (three) | digitus tertius manus = digit III (long finger) |
| IV (four) | digitus quartus manus = digit IV (ring finger) |
| V (five) | digitus quintus manus = digit V (little finger) |

## TIME

When transcribing time followed by a.m. or p.m., use no zeros and no colon when the full hour is given.

### Example
Take the medication at 8 a.m., noon, and 4 p.m.; however, take a meal at 7:30 a.m., 11:30 a.m., and 3:30 p.m.

When 12 o'clock is specified as *time,* use noon or midnight. No numerals are necessary. See #11 under Numbers for when 12 o'clock is used as a location.

## ABDUCTION VERSUS ADDUCTION

Abduction means moving away from the midline. (To *ab*duct is to take away.) Adduction means moving toward the midline. (To *ad*duct means to draw toward.) These two words are often dictated using letters at the beginning; for example, "a-b duction" or "a-d duction," since it is hard to hear the difference between "ab" and "ad" when spoken.

## CLASS AND STAGE

Numbers used in the class and stage of disease can vary widely; however, in cancer terminology, class is generally given in arabic numerals with stage given in roman numerals. In rheumatoid arthritis terminology, however, both class and stage are given in roman numerals, for example, stage I (early disease), stage II (moderate disease), stage III (severe disease), and stage IV (terminal). Class I would indicate complete functional capacity, class II adequate functional capacity, class III the ability to perform few to no activities of daily living (ADLs), and class IV an incapacitated patient—either bedridden or confined to a wheelchair.

## CONNECTIVE TISSUES

Connective tissues can attach, bind, and/or support.

### Examples
Fascia attaches muscle to muscle.
Tendons bind muscle to bone.
Ligaments attach bone to bone.
Cartilage supports, covers, and provides firmness, but does not connect.

## SUBJECTIVE VERSUS OBJECTIVE

The chief complaint, history of present illness, and review of systems are subjective paragraphs.

That is, the patient describes his or her feelings, symptoms, etc., which the doctor records. The subjective examination, therefore, consists of data reported by the patient (opinion). The physical examination is objective; that is, the doctor dictates what he or she sees and feels and hears on direct physical exam (facts).

# Surgical Terms

## Sharp and Blunt Dissection

The phrase "sharp and blunt dissection" takes a singular verb. The idea is that the surgeon is separating tissues by a process alternately involving *sharp* use of instruments (snipping with scissors or cutting with a scalpel) and *blunt* use (inserting scissors or clamp with blades closed, then opening them to establish a plane of separation; or using a finger, sponge, or instrument to develop a separation already started). Hence, the whole process is just one dissection, but it involves two different types of activity. A singular verb is appropriate.

# Obstetric Terms

GPMAL = *g*ravida, *p*ara, *m*ultiple births, *a*bortions, *l*ive births
TPAL = *t*erm infants, *p*remature infants, *a*bortions, *l*iving children

In dictating the number of children a woman has had, various styles may be used. A woman with 3 pregnancies, 2 full-term deliveries, 1 miscarriage or abortion, and 2 living children can be dictated in any one of the following ways:

(a) gravida 3, para 2, ab 1, LC 2
(b) gravida 3, para 2, abortus 1, living children 2
(c) gravida 3, para 2, a 1
(d) G3, P2, A1
(e) gravida 3, para 2-0-1-2

(Style "e" shows 3 pregnancies, 2 full-term deliveries, 0 premature deliveries, 1 miscarriage or abortion, and 2 living children.)

Transcribe the style as dictated by the originator of the report. The words *gravida* and *para* are not capitalized except at the beginning of a sentence, and arabic numerals are used.

To "add up" the numbers and make sure they are correct, when using one of the first four styles above, add the number of deliveries and abortions/miscarriages. That number should equal the number of pregnancies.

For the fifth style (e), add the number of full-term deliveries, premature deliveries, and abortions/miscarriages. That number should equal the number of pregnancies.

If the numbers do not "add up," check the medical record if you have access to it, contact the originator of the report, or flag the report to let the originator know that there is a discrepancy in the numbers. The transcriptionist cannot assume which number is wrong, if any. Multiple births can throw the count off.

# Cardiology Terms

Heart murmurs are written in arabic numerals. An abnormal heart sound heard on auscultation is a bruit (broo-ee), plural bruits (broo-ees).

> **Example**
> A grade 3/6 systolic ejection murmur was heard at the left sternal border with multiple bruits.

Murmurs go up from grade 1 (barely audible, a low-grade murmur) to grade 6 (the loudest, a high-grade murmur). The virgule, dictated as "over," is placed between the murmur grade and the scale used. The murmur above would equal a grade 3 murmur on a scale of 6.

If a partial unit is dictated, transcribe as follows:

Dictated: "grade 2 and a half over 6 murmur"
Transcribed: grade 2.5 over 6 murmur *or* grade 2.5/6 murmur

Dictated: "grade 4 to 5 over 6 murmur"
Transcribed: grade 4/6 to 5/6 murmur *or* grade 4 to 5 over 6 murmur.

# The ABO Blood Group

- Almost 40% of the population has O+ blood.
- Patients with type O blood must receive type O blood.
- Type O blood is the universal blood type and is the only blood type that can be transfused to patients with other blood types.
- Only about 7% of all people have type O, Rh-negative blood.
- Type O, Rh-negative blood is the preferred type for accident victims and babies needing exchange transfusions.
- There is always a need for type O donors because their blood may be transfused to a person of any blood type in an emergency.

## IF YOUR BLOOD TYPE IS

| Type | You Can Give Blood To | You Can Receive Blood From |
|------|----------------------|----------------------------|
| A+   | A+ AB+               | A+ A- O+ O-                |
| O+   | O+ A+ B+ AB+         | O+ O-                      |
| B+   | B+ AB+               | B+ B- O+ O-                |
| AB+  | AB+                  | Everyone                   |
| A-   | A+ A- AB+ AB-        | A- O-                      |
| O-   | Everyone             | O-                         |
| B-   | B+ B- AB+ AB-        | B- O-                      |
| AB-  | AB+ AB-              | AB- A- B- O-               |

# PSYCHOLOGY/PSYCHIATRY TERMS

The multiaxial system consists of five axes, which are dictated using roman numerals, as follows:

Axis I — clinical syndromes

Axis II — developmental disorders and personality disorders

Axis III — physical disorders and conditions

Axis IV — severity of psychosocial stressors

Axis V — Global Assessment of Functioning or GAF—a numeric scale from 1 to 100

# LABORATORY DICTATION

## Tube Tops

Some doctors, especially hematologists, dictate the exact tube to be used in collecting blood, referring to the color of the stopper in the top of the tube. Here is a brief explanation of what some of that dictation means:

| | |
|---|---|
| red-top tube | Used for chemistry or serology testing |
| purple-top tube | Used for hematology testing; these tubes contain an anticoagulant, EDTA |
| blue-top tube | Used for coagulation testing; these tubes contain a liquid anticoagulant, sodium citrate |
| tiger-top tube | Used for chemistry or serology testing; these tubes contain a gel separator |

All types of evacuated blood collection tubes are used to collect whole blood directly from a patient's vein. Blood may be collected using a syringe, then transferred into an appropriate tube or tubes, depending upon the testing required.

## Platelet Count

This information is reported in thousands, but doctors often fail to mention the ending zeros in their dictation. We might hear "platelets 366" or "platelet count 90" when the values are actually 366,000 or 90,000. If the results are greater than 1,000,000, the *exact* results must be dictated and transcribed.

## Urinalysis

Dictation of UA with C&S (urinalysis with culture and sensitivity) is a bit redundant because a sensitivity is automatically done if and when bacteria are cultured from a urine sample. At some hospitals, the urinalysis is automatically ordered as UA with C&S.

## Specific Gravity

The urine specific gravity is often dictated as "ten-ten" or some other arrangement of two whole numbers. The "ten-ten" dictation is correctly transcribed as 1.010 because it actually is a whole number and a fraction with the decimal coming after the first number. Specific gravity normal values can range from 1.000 to 1.035. If the results are greater than 1.035, they may be reported as just that—greater than 1.035. You may hear "SG greater than ten thirty-five." Just make sure to get that decimal in the correct place.

## Oxygen Saturation

This pulmonary information may be dictated in several ways—O2 sat, SaO2, SpO2, satting, or pulse ox. Any of these would be acceptable—with its numeric value in percentage.

O2 sat = oxygen saturation

SaO2 = arterial oxygen percent saturation

SpO2 = oxygen saturation by pulse oximeter

satting = saturating

pulse ox = pulse oximetry

# JR, SR, II, AND III

The use of a comma before and a period after *Jr* and *Sr* is optional, but use both or neither. At Hillcrest we use *neither*. Roman numerals used with proper names take no comma *before* the numeral.

### Examples

| | |
|---|---|
| Ronald DeVittori Jr | Steve Dittman III |
| Kevin King Jr, PhD | Sigmund Klein II |
| Dafnis Panagides Sr | Magnus Flaws III, CPA |

CMTips are compiled by Patricia A. Ireland, CMT, AHDI-F; references include the AHDI *Book of Style*, 3rd ed., *The Gregg Reference Manual*, 10th ed., *Dorland's Illustrated Medical Dictionary*, 31st ed., *Stedman's Medical Dictionary*, 28th ed., and *Merriam Webster's Collegiate Dictionary*, 11th ed.

# REPORT FORMATTING GUIDELINES

*✳ Commonly used advise*

1. Use two spaces after all colons. Exceptions include titers, ratios, and sign-off block.
2. The use of either one space or two spaces after a period at the end of a sentence is acceptable; however, consistency is required in your spacing throughout the entire report.
3. Double space between all paragraphs.
4. Display all dates on report headings and in the sign-off block as MM/DD/YYYY (*not M/D/YYYY or M/DD/YY*). Dates appearing within the body of a report should be transcribed as dictated (e.g., May 14 or 24 August).
5. Use left justification on reports.
6. Avoid hyphenation at the end of lines in reports. If necessary, use a hard hyphen or a hard space to keep figures on the same line (e.g., 6-pound baby or 12.5 mg dose).
7. When using enumerated lists in transcribed reports, align the items in the list by using the automatic numbering feature of the word processing software or by placing a tab after each numeral in the list.
8. Use a 1-inch margin on sides, top, and bottom of report pages.
9. Double space between the last line on a page and the "(Continued)" notation.
10. All page breaks should take place between paragraphs or in the middle of a paragraph with at least *two* lines of text on the bottom of one page and *two* lines of text at the top of the next page. Avoid "widows" and "orphans." An orphan is the first line of a paragraph printed by itself at the bottom of a page. A widow is the last line of a paragraph printed by itself at the top of a page.
11. Use either a colon or a verb for brief introducers within the body of a report (e.g., "HEENT: Normocephalic" *or* "SKIN is warm and dry to the touch" as used in History and Physical Exam).
12. Use a double space above and below sign-off blocks occurring between two parts of a report.
13. Subsequent page headers should contain report title in all caps, patient name, hospital number, date, and page number. Double space between report title and patient name. Use a quadruple space to the paragraph below (4 hard returns).
14. Do not include the signature block alone on a page. Include at least *two* lines of text on the top of the page containing the signature block.
15. Quadruple space (four hard returns) between the ending paragraph of a report and the signature rule (or line). We use no signature line in correspondence.
16. The signature rule should begin at the left margin and should be long enough to extend past the length of the dictator's name and title.
17. Do not include extra lines between the physician's name and the signature rule. The physician's name should be entered on the line under the signature rule and positioned at the left margin to align with the signature rule.
18. Use a double space between the physician's name and the sign-off block at the end of a report.
19. Use a double space between the transcribed date and copy line (if applicable) at the end of a report.
20. Use a double space between the copy line and an "Enclosure" notation (if applicable) at the end of a report.
21. In correspondence, the spacing of the date can be adjusted up or down in order to balance the length of the letter on the page.

*10/06/2014*

*p. 234        Orphan – the first line*
*Widow the last line*

# The Future of Medical Transcription

The electronic health record (EHR) is mandated by the current presidential administration, as it was by the previous administration, with an impact date of 2012. This means that medical information on every patient (their medical records) is to be computerized and available to hospitals, doctors' offices and clinics, and pharmacies across the country in an electronic format with access on demand. Although in reality the terms are being used interchangeably, EHR is supposed to be the compilation of various EMRs (electronic medical records, i.e., pediatric, obstetric, orthopedic, geriatric, etc.).

The EHR includes electronic signatures—remember, these are neither dictated nor transcribed. They are entered into the medical record automatically when the dictating physician "signs" the report by entering commands on the computer.

With baby boomers retiring, the impact this will have on health care in this country and others will be profound. Having EHRs will be important, and there will be an ongoing need for qualified medical transcriptionists, who may transition into medical transcription editors (MTEs). Even now, there is a shortage of qualified MTs throughout the country.

Please see the AHDI website for more information on this: http://www.ahdionline.org

## Speech Recognition Technology

Speech (or voice) recognition technology has been a factor in medical transcription for more than two decades. It has been expected to save time, reduce transcription costs, accelerate billing and collection, and offer more flexibility and accuracy to the originator of the dictation. Many promises have been made and few have been realized; however, the Medical Transcription Industry Association (MTIA) and the Association for Healthcare Documentation Integrity (AHDI) have formed a joint task force to study this. The goal of this task force and its subsequent white paper is to help healthcare organizations separate fact from fiction when trying to choose a vendor to provide them with the most up-to-date technology—and to make objective and comparative assessments on its use and benefits.

When implemented in a medical practice, speech recognition necessitates that the medical transcriptionist become a medical transcription editor (MTE) who can correct the speech-recognized drafted reports—a big difference from transcribing a report dictated by a physician. One important difference here is critical thinking, which is best performed by a human being. Contact George Catuogno, the founding chair of the Work Group on Speech Recognition Adoption and Impact, and the white paper's primary author, at george.catuogno@sten-tel.com for the most current information. AHDI position statements on this and other issues that impact medical transcriptionists can be found at http://www.adhionline.org under "Advocacy" then "About AHDI."

# UNDERSTANDING MEDICAL TERMINOLOGY

Medical terminology appears to be complicated until one learns the principles of basic word structure. Medical terminology consists of the following components:

* prefix, word beginning
* suffix, word ending
* root word, the foundation of a word
* combining vowel, a vowel (usually *o*) connecting a root word to a suffix or a root word to another root word
* combining form, the combination of a root word and a combining vowel

The combining vowel aids in pronunciation.

## PRINCIPLES

1. Generally speaking, begin reading a medical word from the suffix to the root word or prefix.

    **Example**

    | hemi/ | gloss/ | ectomy |
    |---|---|---|
    | ⬆ | ⬆ | ⬆ |
    | half | tongue | removal |
    | (prefix) | (root) | (suffix) |

    *Definition:* removal of half (one side of) the tongue

2. Drop the combining vowel before a suffix beginning with a vowel.

    **Example**

    | gastr/ | itis | NOT | gastr/ | o/ | itis |
    |---|---|---|---|---|---|
    | ⬆ | ⬆ | | | | |
    | stomach | inflammation | | | | |
    | (root) | (suffix) | | | | |

    *Definition:* inflammation of the stomach

3. Retain the combining vowel before a suffix beginning with a consonant.

    **Example**

    | gastr/ | o/ | megaly | NOT | gastr/ | megaly |
    |---|---|---|---|---|---|
    | | | ⬆ | | | |
    | | | enlargement | | | |
    | | | (suffix) | | | |

    *Definition:* enlargement of the stomach

4. Retain the combining vowel between two root words even if the second root word begins with a vowel.

    **Example**

    | electr/ | o/ | encephal/ | o/ | graphy |
    |---|---|---|---|---|
    | ⬆ | | ⬆ | | ⬆ |
    | electricity | | brain | | process of recording |
    | (root) | | (root) | | (suffix) |

    *Definition:* process of recording the electricity of the brain

# PREFIXES, PRONUNCIATION

| Prefixes/Pronunciation | Meaning | Example |
|---|---|---|
| **A** | | |
| a- (ā, ă) | not, without | apnea—not breathing |
| ab- (ăb) | away from | aberrant—deviating from the normal |
| ad- (ăd) | to, toward | adhere—to cling together |
| ambi- (ăm′ bĭ) | on both sides | ambilateral—affecting both sides |
| an- (ăn) | not, without | anoxia—without oxygen |
| ante- (ăn′ tē) | before | antefebrile—before the onset of fever |
| anti- (ăn′ tī, an′ tĭ) | against | antiemetic—an agent that prevents nausea |
| auto- (aw′ tō) | self | autohypnotic—pertaining to self-induced hypnotism |
| **B** | | |
| bi- (bī) | two | biarticular—pertaining to two joints |
| brady- (brăd′ē, brād′ē) | slow | bradycardia—slowness of the heartbeat |
| **C** | | |
| cata- (kăt′ ah) | down | cataphoria—a permanent downward turning of the visual axes of the eyes |
| co- (kō) | with, together | cohesive—uniting together |
| con- (kŏn) | with, together | confluent (kon′ floo-ŭnt)—becoming merged |
| contra- (kŏn′ trah) | against, opposite | contraceptive—an agent that prevents conception |
| **D** | | |
| de- (dē) | lack of | dehydrate—to remove water from |
| di- (dī) | two, twice | diplopia—double vision |
| dia- (dī′ ah) | complete, through | dialysis—complete separation |
| dis- (dĭs) | reversal, separation | disacidify—to remove an acid from |
| dys- (dĭs) | bad, painful, difficult | dysmenorrhea—painful menstrual flow |
| **E** | | |
| ecto- (ĕk′ tō) | out, outside | ectopic—out of normal position |
| en- (ĕn) | in, within | encephalic—within the skull |
| endo- (ĕn′dō) | within | endocrine—pertaining to secretions within |
| epi- (ĕp′ĭ) | above, upon | epibulbar—upon the eyeball |
| eu- (ū) | good, well, easily | eupepsia—good digestion |
| ex- (ĕks) | out, outside | excision—removal |
| exo- (ĕk′ sō) | outside, outward | exocardial—situated outside the heart |
| **H** | | |
| hemi- (hĕm′ ē) | half | hemiglossitis—inflammation of one half of the tongue |
| hyper- (hī′ pĕr) | above, excessive | hyperactivity—excessive activity |
| hypo- (hī′ pō) | deficient, below | hypotension—abnormally low blood pressure |
| **I** | | |
| in (ĭn) | not | incurable—not able to be cured |
| infra- (ĭn′ frah) | below, inferior | infrasternal—below the sternum (breast bone) |
| inter- (ĭn′ tĕr) | between | intercostal—between the ribs |
| intra- (ĭn′ trah) | within | intracutaneous—within the skin |

*(continued)*

| Prefixes/Pronunciation | Meaning | Example |
|---|---|---|
| **M** | | |
| macro- (măk′ rō) | large | macrocyte—an abnormally large erythrocyte (red blood cell) |
| mal- (măl) | bad | malnutrition—any disorder of nutrition |
| meso- (měz′ ō) | middle | mesonasal—situated in the middle of the nose |
| meta- (mět′ ah) | beyond, change | metamorphoses—change of shape |
| micro- (mī′ krō) | small | microcyst—a very small cyst |
| **N** | | |
| neo- (nē′ ō) | new | neonate—a newborn infant |
| **P** | | |
| pan- (păn) | all | panhysterectomy—total hysterectomy |
| para- (păr′ ah) | near, beside | paraesophageal—near the esophagus |
| per- (pěr) | through | percutaneous—performed through the skin |
| peri- (pěrē) | around, surrounding | perihepatic—occurring around the liver |
| poly- (pŏl′ē) | many | polyneuritis—inflammation of many nerves |
| post- (pōst) | after, behind | postoperative—after a surgical procedure |
| pre- (prē) | before, in front of | preprandial—before meals |
| pro- (prō) | before | prognosis—a forecast as to the probable outcome of a disease |
| **R** | | |
| re- (rē) | back, again | reabsorb—to absorb again |
| retro- (rět′ rō) | behind, backward | retronasal—behind the nose |
| **S** | | |
| semi- (sěm′ ē) | one half, partly | semiprone—partly prone (lying face downward) |
| sub- (sŭb) | under, below | subabdominal—situated below the abdomen |
| supra- (soo′ prah) | above, over | suprarenal—situated above a kidney |
| sym- (sĭm) | together, with | sympodia—fusion of the lower extremities |
| syn- (sĭn) | together, with | syndrome—a set of symptoms that occur together |
| **T** | | |
| tachy- (tăk′ē) | fast, rapid | tachycardia—rapid heartbeat |
| trans- (trăns) | across, through | transepidermal—occurring through or across the epidermis (top layer of skin) |
| **U** | | |
| ultra- (ŭl′trah) | beyond, excess | ultrastructure—the structure beyond the resolution power of the light microscope |

# Combining Forms

| Combining Form | Meaning | Example |
|---|---|---|
| **A** | | |
| aden/o (ăd′ ĕn-ō) | gland | adenodynia—pain in a gland |
| angi/o (ăn′ jē-ō) | vessel | angiectomy—surgical excision of a vessel |
| arteri/o (ăr-tē′ rē-ō) | artery | arterioplasty—surgical repair of an artery |
| arthr/o (ăr′ thrō) | joint | arthrotomy—surgical incision of a joint |
| **B** | | |
| blephar/o (blĕf′ ăr-ō) | eyelid | blepharoplegia—paralysis of an eyelid |
| brachi/o (brā′ kē-ō) | arm | brachiocephalic—pertaining to the arm and head |
| bucc/o (bŭk′ ō) | cheek | buccolingual—pertaining to the cheek and tongue |
| burs/o (bŭr′ sō) | bursa (fluid-filled sac) | bursopathy—any disease of a bursa |
| **C** | | |
| carcin/o (kăr′ sĭn-ō) | carcinoma | carcinolysis—destruction of carcinoma cells |
| cardi/o (kăr′ dēō) | heart | cardiogenic—originating in the heart |
| cephal/o (sĕf′ ah-lō) | head | cephaledema—edema of the head |
| cerebr/o (sĕr′ ĕ-brō) | brain, cerebrum | cerebrospinal—pertaining to the brain and spinal cord |
| cervic/o (sĕr′ vĭ-kō) | neck | cervicoplasty—plastic surgery of the neck |
| coccyg/o (kŏk′ sĭ-gō) | tailbone, coccyx | coccygodynia—pain in the coccyx |
| cost/o (kŏs′ tō) | ribs | costoclavicular—pertaining to the ribs and clavicle (collar bone) |
| crani/o (krā′ nē-ō) | skull | craniopathy—any disease of the skull |
| cutane/o (kūt-tā′ nē-ō) | skin | subcutaneous—beneath the skin |
| cyst/o (sĭs′ tō) | urinary bladder | cystogram—an x-ray of the urinary bladder |
| **D** | | |
| dactyl/o (dăk′ tĭl-ō) | finger or toe | dactylospasm—spasm of a finger or toe |
| dent/i (dĕn′tē) | tooth | dentibuccal—pertaining to the teeth and cheek |
| dips/o (dĭp′sō) | thirst | dipsosis—morbid thirst |
| dors/o (dōr′sō) | back of the body | dorsolateral—pertaining to the back and side |
| **E** | | |
| electr/o (e-lĕk′ trō) | electricity | electrotome—a surgical cutting instrument powered by electricity |
| encephal/o (ĕn-sĕf′ ah-lō) | brain | encephalomyelitis—inflammation of the brain and spinal cord |
| enter/o (ĕn′ tĕr-ō) | intestine | enterorrhaphy—repair or suture of the intestine |
| esophag/o (ĕ-sŏf′ ă-gō) | esophagus | esophagomalacia—softening of the walls of the esophagus |
| **F** | | |
| fasci/o (făsh′ ē-ō) | fascia (fibrous tissue) | fasciitis—inflammation of fascia |
| femor/o (fĕm′ ō-rō) | femur (thigh bone) | femoroiliac—pertaining to the femur and ilium (hip bone) |
| fibul/o (fĭb′ ū-lō) | fibula (the smaller of the two lower leg bones) | fibulocalcaneal—pertaining to the fibula and calcaneus (heel bone) |

*(continued)*

| Combining Form | Meaning | Example |
|---|---|---|
| **G** | | |
| gastr/o (găs′ trō) | stomach | gastrostenosis—contraction or shrinkage of the stomach |
| gingiv/o (jĭn′ jĭ-vō) | gums | gingivolabial—pertaining to the gums and lips |
| gloss/o (glŏs′ ō) | tongue | glossopharyngeal—pertaining to the tongue and pharynx (throat) |
| gynec/o (gī′ nĕ-kō) | woman, female | gynecology—that branch of medicine that treats diseases of the female genital tract |
| **H** | | |
| hemat/o (hēm′ ah-tō) | blood | hematuria—blood in the urine |
| hepat/o (hĕp′ ah-tō) | liver | hepatologist—a specialist in the study of the liver |
| hist/o (hĭs′ tō) | tissue | histolysis—destruction of tissue |
| hypn/o (hĭp′ nō) | sleep | hypnogenic—inducing sleep |
| hyster/o (hĭs′ tĕr-ō) | uterus, womb | hysterosalpingectomy—excision of the uterus and uterine (fallopian) tubes |
| **I** | | |
| idi/o (ĭd′ ē-ō) | individual, self | idiopathic—self-originated condition of unknown causation |
| ile/o (ĭl′ ē-ō) | ileum (portion of the small intestine) | ileocecal—pertaining to the ileum and cecum |
| ili/o (ĭl′ ē-ō) | ilium (expansive superior portion of the hip bone) | iliocostal—pertaining to the ilium and ribs |
| **J** | | |
| jejun/o (jĕ-joo′ nō) | jejunum (portion of the small intestine) | jejunectomy—excision of the jejunum |
| **K** | | |
| kerat/o (kĕr′ ah-tō) | cornea | keratomycosis—fungal infection of the cornea |
| kinesi/o (kĭ-nē′ sē-ō) | movement | kinesiotherapy—treatment of disease by movements or exercise |
| **L** | | |
| labi/o (lā′ bē-ō) | lip | labiolingual—pertaining to the lips and tongue |
| laryng/o (lah-rĭng′ ō) | larynx (voice box) | laryngoparalysis—paralysis of the larynx |
| later/o (lăt′ ĕr-ō) | side | lateroversion—a turning to one side |
| lip/o (lĭp′ ō) | fat, lipid | lipiduria—lipids in the urine |
| lith/o (lĭth′ ō) | stone, calculus | lithogenous—producing or causing the formation of calculi |

*(continued)*

| Combining Form | Meaning | Example |
|---|---|---|
| **M** | | |
| mamm/o (măm′ ō) | breast | mammoplasty—plastic reconstruction of the breast |
| mast/o (măs′ tō) | breast | mastography—the making of an x-ray of the breast |
| my/o (mī′ ō) | muscle | myobradia—slow, sluggish reaction of muscle to electric stimulation |
| myel/o (mī′ ĕ-lō) | spinal cord, bone marrow | myelopoiesis—formation of bone marrow |
| **N** | | |
| nas/o (nā′ zō) | nose | nasopalatine—pertaining to the nose and palate (roof of the mouth) |
| nephr/o (nĕf′ rō) | kidney | nephrorrhagia—hemorrhage from a kidney |
| neur/o (nū′ rō) | nerve | neuroallergy—allergy in nervous tissue |
| noct/i (nŏk′ tē) | night | nocturia—excessive urination at night |
| **O** | | |
| onc/o (ŏng′ kō) | mass, tumor | oncogenesis—the production or causation of tumors |
| oo/o (ō′ ō-ō) | egg, ovum | oocyte—an immature egg |
| oophor/o (ō-ŏf′ ō-rō) | ovary | oophorohysterectomy—excision of the ovaries and uterus |
| ophthalm/o (ŏf-thăl′ mō) | eye | ophthalmodynia—pain in the eye |
| orchi/o (ŏr′ kē-ō) | testis, testicle | orchitis—inflammation of the testicle |
| or/o (ō′ rō) | mouth | oral—pertaining to the mouth |
| oste/o (ŏs′ tē-ō) | bone | osteodystrophy—abnormal, defective bone formation |
| ot/o (ō′ tō) | ear | otorrhea—a discharge from the ear |
| ox/o (ŏk′ sō) | oxygen | anoxia—absence of oxygen |
| **P** | | |
| path/o (păth′ ō) | disease | pathoanatomic—pertaining to the anatomy of diseased tissue |
| poster/o (pŏs′ tĕr-ō) | back (of the body) | posterolateral—behind and to one side |
| pseud/o (sū′ dō) | false | pseudocyesis—false pregnancy |
| psych/o (sī′ kō) | mind | psychogenesis—mental development |
| py/o (pī′ ō) | pus | pyosalpinx—pus in the uterine tube |
| **R** | | |
| radi/o (rā′ dē-ō) | rays, x-rays | radioimmunity—diminished sensitivity to radiation |
| ren/o (rē′ nō) | kidney | renal—pertaining to the kidney |
| retin/o (rĕt′ ĭ-nō) | retina | retinomalacia—softening of the retina |
| rhin/o (rī′ nō) | nose | rhinotomy—incision of the nose |
| roentgen/o (rĕnt′ gĕn-ō) | x-rays | roentgenotherapy—treatment with roentgen rays |

*(continued)*

| Combining Form | Meaning | Example |
|---|---|---|
| **S** | | |
| sacr/o (sā′ krō) | sacrum | sacrodynia—pain in the sacral region |
| salping/o (săl-pĭng′ gō) | uterine tubes | salpingo-oophorectomy—excision of a uterine tube and an ovary |
| secti/o (sĕk′ shē-ō) | to cut | section—a cut surface |
| sphygm/o (sfĭg′ mō) | pulse | sphygmometer—an instrument for measuring the pulse |
| stomat/o (stō′ mah-tō) | mouth | stomatomycosis—fungal disease of the mouth |
| **T** | | |
| thorac/o (thō′ rah-kō) | chest | thoracoscopy—examination of the pleural cavity with an endoscope |
| tibi/o (tĭb′ ē-ō) | tibia, shin bone (the larger of the two lower leg bones) | tibialgia—painful shin bone |
| top/o (tŏp′ ō) | place, position, location | ectopic—located away from normal position |
| tox/o (tŏk′ sō) | poison | toxicity—the quality of being poisonous |
| trache/o (trā′ kē-ō) | trachea (windpipe) | tracheolaryngotomy—incision of the larynx (voice box) and trachea |
| **U** | | |
| ur/o (ū′ rō) | urine, urinary tract | urolith—a calculus (stone) in the urine |
| uter/o (ū′ tĕr-ō) | uterus | uteroplacental—pertaining to the placenta and uterus |
| **V** | | |
| vagin/o (văj′ ĭ-nō) | vagina | vaginovesical—pertaining to the vagina and urinary bladder |
| vas/o (văs′ ō) | vessel, duct | vasomotion—change in the caliber of a (blood) vessel |
| ven/o (vē′ nō) | vein | veno-occlusive—pertaining to obstruction of the veins |
| viscer/o (vĭs′ ĕr-ō) | internal organs | viscerad—toward the viscera |
| **X** | | |
| xanth/o (zăn′ thō) | yellow | xanthemia—presence of yellow coloring matter in the blood |
| xer/o (zēr′ rō) | dry | xerosis—abnormal dryness |
| **Z** | | |
| zyg/o (zī′ gō) | yoked, joined | zygal—shaped like a yoke |

# SUFFIXES

| Suffix | Meaning | Example |
| --- | --- | --- |
| **A** | | |
| -ac (ăk) | pertaining to | cardiac—pertaining to the heart |
| -al (ăl) | pertaining to | postnatal—pertaining to after a birth |
| -algia (ăl′ jē-ah) | pain | otalgia—pain in the ear |
| -asthenia (ăs-thē′ nē-ah) | lack of strength | myasthenia—lack of muscular strength |
| **C** | | |
| -cele (sēl) | hernia | cystocele—hernial protrusion of the urinary bladder through the vaginal wall |
| -centesis (sĕn-tē′ sĭs) | surgical puncture to remove fluid | amniocentesis—surgical puncture to remove fluid from the amnion |
| -cidal (sī′ dăl) | killing | bactericidal—destructive to bacteria |
| -clysis (klī′ sĭs) | irrigation, washing | enteroclysis—irrigation of the bowel |
| -coccus (kōk′ ŭs) | bacterial cell | staphylococcus—microorganism that causes localized suppurative infections |
| -cyte (sīt) | cell | leukocyte—white blood cell |
| **D** | | |
| -desis (dē′ sĭs) | binding | arthrodesis—surgical fixation of a joint |
| **E** | | |
| -ectasis (ĕk′ tah-sĭs) | stretching, dilation | angiectasis—lengthening of a blood vessel |
| -ectomy (ĕk′ tō-mē) | removal | appendectomy—removal of the vermiform appendix |
| -emesis (ĕm′ ĕ-sĭs) | vomiting | hyperemesis—excessive vomiting |
| -emia (ē′ mē-ah) | blood condition | septicemia—blood poisoning |
| **G** | | |
| -genesis (jĕn′ ĕ-sĭs) | producing, originating | pathogenesis—the development of disease or a morbid condition |
| -gram (grăm) | record | myelogram—the record produced by an x-ray of the spinal cord |
| -graph (grăf) | instrument for recording | gastrograph—an instrument for recording the motions of the stomach |
| -graphy (grăf′ ē) | process of recording | myelography—process of recording an x-ray of the spinal cord |
| **I** | | |
| -ia (ē′ ah) | condition, process | dyspepsia—condition of bad digestion |
| -ic (ĭk) | pertaining to | thoracic—pertaining to the chest |
| -ist (ĭst) | specialist | nephrologist—a specialist in the study of the kidney |
| -itis (ī′ tĭs) | inflammation | osteitis—inflammation of a bone |
| **L** | | |
| -logy (lō′ jē) | study of | ophthalmology—study of the eye |
| -lysis (lī′ sĭs) | separation, destruction | splenolysis—destruction of splenic tissue |

*(continued)*

| Suffix | Meaning | Example |
|--------|---------|---------|
| **M** | | |
| -malacia (mah-lā′ shē-ăh) | softening | osteomalacia—softening of bone |
| -megaly (měg′ ah-lē) | enlargement | acromegaly—enlargement of extremities |
| **O** | | |
| -odynia (ō-dĭn′ ē-ah) | pain | gastrodynia—pain in the stomach |
| -ole (ōl) | little, small | arteriole—a minute arterial branch |
| -oma (ō′ mah) | tumor | carcinoma—a malignant new growth |
| -opia (ō′ pē-ah) | vision | amblyopia—dimming of vision |
| -orrhaphy (ŏr′ ah-fē) | suture | herniorrhaphy—suture of a hernia |
| -orrhea (ō′ rē-ah) | flow, discharge | menorrhea—discharge of the menses |
| -osis (ō′ sĭs) | abnormal condition | arthropyosis—abnormal condition of pus in a joint cavity |
| -osmia (ŏz′ mē-ah) | smell | anosmia—absence of the sense of smell |
| -ostomy (ŏs′ tō-mē) | new opening | colostomy—surgical creation of a new opening in the colon |
| **P** | | |
| -pepsia (pĕp′ sē-ah) | digestion | dyspepsia—bad digestion |
| -phagia (fā′ jē-ah) | eating, swallowing | polyphagia—excessive eating |
| -phobia (fō′ bē-ah) | fear | hydrophobia—fear of water |
| -plasia (plā′ zē-ah) | formation, development | chondroplasia—the formation of cartilage |
| -plasty (plăs′ tē) | surgical repair | rhinoplasty—surgical repair of the nose |
| -plegia (plē′ jē-ah) | paralysis | hemiplegia—paralysis of one side of the body |
| -pnea (nē′ ah) | breathing | dyspnea—difficult breathing |
| -ptosis (tō′ sĭs) | drooping, prolapse | blepharoptosis—drooping of the eyelid |
| -ptysis (tĭ′ sĭs) | spitting | hemoptysis—spitting blood |
| **S** | | |
| -sclerosis (sklē-rō′ sĭs) | hardening | arteriosclerosis—hardening of the arteries |
| -scope (skōp) | instrument for visual examination | cystoscope—an instrument for visual examination of the urinary bladder |
| -stasis (stā′ sĭs) | control, stop | hemostasis—stopping the flow of blood |
| -stenosis (stĕn-ō′ sĭs) | narrowing, stricture | angiostenosis—narrowing of a vessel |
| **T** | | |
| -therapy (thĕr′ ah-pē) | treatment | thermotherapy—therapeutic use of heat |
| -tocia (tō′ sē-ah) | labor, birth | dystocia—abnormal labor |
| -tome (tōm) | instrument to cut | osteotome—an instrument to cut bone |
| -tomy (tō′ mē) | incision | tracheotomy—incision of the trachea |
| -trophy (trō′ fē) | nourishment, development | hypertrophy—excessive development |
| **U** | | |
| -ule (ūl) | little, small | venule—a small vein |
| -uria (ū′ rē-ah) | urination, urine | pyuria—pus in the urine |

# DOCTORS' AND OTHER PROFESSIONAL NAMES USED IN HILLCREST AND QUALI-CARE CLINIC*

| | | | |
|---|---|---|---|
| Carl Erickson Avalon, MD<br>Anesthesiology | Male | Robert P. Johnson, DDS, MD<br>Pediatric Dentistry (British) | Male |
| Marie Aaron, DO<br>Family Practice (Korean) | Female | Trevor Jordan, MD<br>Nephrology (Eastern Indian) | Male |
| Beth Brian, MD<br>Infectious Disease | Female | Sachi Kato, MD<br>Dermatology (Chinese) | Female |
| Rosemary Bumbak, MD<br>Obstetrics/Gynecology (Swedish) | Female | Patrick Keathley, MD<br>Endocrinology (Irish) | Male |
| Tomas Burgos, MD<br>Vascular Surgery (Russian) | Male | Bernard Kester, MD<br>General Surgery (Upstate NY) | Male |
| Tommy Edward Burnett, MD<br>Radiology | Male | Berry J. Lozano, MD<br>Pathology (Puerto Rico) | Female |
| Chuck Delaney, MD<br>Anesthesiology | Male | J. K. McClain, MD<br>Cardiology (Upstate NY) | Male |
| Stella Rose Dickinson, PhD<br>Psychology (Russian) | Female | Alex McClure, MD<br>Hillcrest ER Physician (Russian) | Female |
| Carol Dodd, MD<br>Orthopedic Surgery | Female | Leon Medina, MD<br>Internal Medicine (Upstate NY) | Male |
| Diana K. Easterly, MD<br>Pediatric Neurology (British) | Female | Reed Phillips, MD<br>Pediatrics | Male |
| Martha C. Eaton, MD<br>Family Practice/Geriatrics (Boston) | Female | Paula Reddy, MD<br>Radiology (Dutch) | Female |
| Linda Garibaldi, RN, FNP<br>Family Nurse Practitioner | Female | Chris Salem, DO<br>Family Practice | Male |
| Michael Gerard, DO<br>Obstetrics/Gynecology | Male | Gary Shelton, DPM<br>Podiatry | Male |
| Sheila Goodman, MD<br>Neurosurgery (Jamaican) | Female | Jesse D. Smith, MD<br>Orthopedic Surgery (Upstate NY) | Male |
| Donna Harrison, MD<br>Radiology (Upstate NY) | Female | Lyndon F. Talcott, MD<br>Neurology (Upstate NY) | Male |
| Max L. Hirsch, MD<br>Orthopedic Surgery (Upstate NY) | Male | Georgia Tamayo, MD<br>Pathology (Hispanic) | Female |
| Anna Marie Iaccarino, RN<br>Scrub Nurse | Female | Jason Wagner, PA-C<br>Surgical Assistant | Male |
| Jimmy Dale Jett, RN<br>Circulating Nurse | Male | Simon Williams, MD<br>Pulmonary/Thoracic Surgery (British) | Male |
| Markus LeRoy Johnson, PA-C<br>Surgical Assistant | Male | | |

***A Word About Accents:** Medical transcription reflects the global reach of today's technology by bringing dictators to your ears who do not speak American English (such as someone from England or Ireland) or for whom English is not the first language. Words may be spoken with an accent on a different syllable or the vowels may be pronounced differently from American English. For example, the word "urine" may be pronounced "you ryne." Some cultures pronounce the letter "z" as the word "zed." You may not understand the words at first, but the more you listen, the more you will understand. Keep an open mind, stay flexible, and keep the context in mind.*

## SKILL-BUILDING REPORT LOG

Student Name: _____

*Attach this sheet (or a copy) to your transcribed work; give to your instructor for grading.*

| SB Report Number/Patient Name/Report Type | Grade |
|---|---|
| Trans SB Report 1  Robert Randall (Operative Report, Neurosurgery) | _____ |
| Trans SB Report 2  Sharon Garcia (Operative Report, Oral) | _____ |
| Trans SB Report 3  Ricardo Benavidez (Operative Report, Orthopedics) | _____ |
| Trans SB Report 4  Sadako Sasaki (Operative Report, GYN/GU) | _____ |
| Trans SB Report 5  Ralph Gleason (Operative Report, Gastroenterology) | _____ |
| Trans SB Report 6  Copernicus Boclair (Operative Report, Urology) | _____ |
| Trans SB Report 7  Olivia Carpenter (Operative Report, Plastic Surgery) | _____ |
| Trans SB Report 8  Clarita J. Wilson (Operative Report, Orthopedics) | _____ |
| Trans SB Report 9  J. Richard Feeley (Operative Report, Neurosurgery) | _____ |
| Trans SB Report 10  Jack Towles (Operative Report, Pedi Dental) | _____ |
| QC SB Report 1  Priscilla L. Pate (Consult, Orthopedics) | _____ |
| QC SB Report 2  Carlos Noriega (Emergency Dept Treatment Record) | _____ |
| QC SB Report 3  Natalie P. Hall (Electrophysiology Study) | _____ |
| QC SB Report 4  Elaine Kabbas (Emergency Dept Treatment Record) | _____ |
| QC SB Report 5  Mark M. Stettler (Clinic SOAP Note, Internal Medicine) | _____ |
| QC SB Report 6  Ryan Boscoe (Consult, Orthopedics) | _____ |
| QC SB Report 7  Holly Lorzano (Electroencephalogram Report) | _____ |
| QC SB Report 8  Karen A. Meyer (Clinic HPIP Note, Internal Medicine) | _____ |
| QC SB Report 9  Charles Nobles III (Consult, Cardiothoracic) | _____ |
| QC SB Report 10  James T. Ward (Preop H&P, Orthopedics) | _____ |

# SECTION 4

## CASE STUDIES

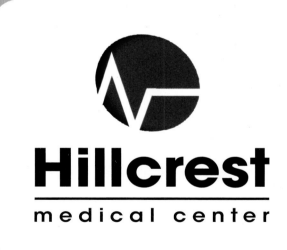

# CASE STUDY 1: REPRODUCTIVE SYSTEM

**Patient Name**

Brenda C. Seggerman

**Address**

701 Dadeland Blvd.
Miami FL 33133-5017

**Situation**

Brenda Seggerman's vaginal spotting and abdominal pain had increased during the night until she was in an emergent situation, and her husband called an ambulance. Once in the Hillcrest emergency room, the patient was assessed. A pregnancy test was found to be positive. Further testing by Radiology revealed an ectopic pregnancy. Her gynecologist was called by the emergency room physician, and the patient was prepared for immediate surgery. Tissues removed at surgery were sent to pathology for examination and final diagnosis. After 3 days, Mrs. Seggerman was discharged to office followup in improved condition.

Review Figure CS1-1A, The female reproductive system; Figure CS1-1B, The female anatomy external genitalia; Figure CS1-2, Continuous sutures; Figure CS1-3, Sites of ectopic pregnancy; Figure CS1-4, Tubal ligation.

**Student Name** _____

**Patient:  Brenda C. Seggerman**

| SEQUENCE OF REPORTS | Date Completed | Grade |
|---|---|---|
| Emergency Services Admission Report | _____ | _____ |
| Diagnostic Imaging Report | _____ | _____ |
| Operative Report | _____ | _____ |
| Pathology Report | _____ | _____ |
| Discharge Summary | _____ | _____ |

**NOTE**: Study the glossary for Case Study 1. Enter the date each report is completed in the space provided. When you have transcribed all reports, tear this sheet out and attach it to the front of the reports (in the order listed above); give the completed reports to the instructor.

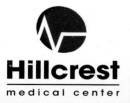

**Hillcrest**
medical center

# Glossary for Case Study 1

**adhesions** (ăd-hē'zhens)—fibrous bands or structures by which body parts abnormally adhere, as in wound healing

**adnexa** (sing. and pl.) (ăd-nĕk'sah)—appendages or adjunct parts; in gynecology, used to describe the tubes and ovaries (primarily used in the plural form)

**adnexal mass** (ăd-nĕk'sĕl)—an abnormality in the uterine adnexa

**approximate** (v.) (ah-prok'sĭ-māt")—to bring close together or into apposition

**arthralgia** (ar-thrăl'jē-ah)—pain in a joint

**beta-hCG** (bā'tuh)—*h*uman *c*horionic *g*onadotropin; the pregnancy hormone found in blood

**bimanual** (bī-man'-ye-wel)—performed using both hands

**blood type O**—blood type O has neither A nor B antigens (blood type O is in 40% of the population)

**chromic suture** (krō'mĭk)—absorbable catgut suture material

**Claforan** (klăh'for-ăn)—antibiotic against gram-negative bacteria, trade name

**crown-rump length**—the length between the top of the head to the buttocks or gluteal region

**cul-de-sac** (from the French) (kŭl'-duh-săk)—a blind pouch

**Demerol** (dĕm'er-all)—trade name for meperidine hydrochloride, a drug to sedate and relieve pain

**distal** (dĭs'tal)—situated away from the center of the body, or from the point of origin; specifically applied to the extremity or distant part of a limb or organ

**ectopic pregnancy** (ĕk-tŏp'ĭk)—a pregnancy in which the fertilized ovum becomes implanted on tissue outside of the uterine cavity

**edema** (ĕ-dē'mah)—abnormal accumulation of fluid in the intercellular tissue spaces of the body, resulting in swelling

**embedding** (ĕm-bed'ing)—fixating a tissue specimen in a firm medium to keep it intact during sectioning of the tissue

**endovaginal** (ĕnd"dō-văj'ĭ-nal)—within the vagina

**EtOH**—abbreviation for ethyl alcohol, ethanol, grain alcohol; each letter is pronounced individually

**exploratory laparotomy** (lăp"ah-rŏt'ō-mē)—surgical entry into the abdomen to examine the abdominal contents

**fallopian tube** (făl-lō'pē-ăn)—also called oviduct or uterine tube; transports the ovum from the ovary to the uterus

**fascia** (făsh'ē-ah)—supportive layer of thin connective tissue within the muscles and organs of the body

**figure-of-8 stitches**—sutures in which the thread follows the contours of the figure 8

**fundus** (fŭn'dŭs)—the bottom or base of anything; the part of an organ opposite the opening into that organ

**general endotracheal tube** (ĕn"dō-trā'kē-ăl)—referring to the tube inserted within the trachea through which to administer general anesthesia

**gravida 2, para 1, abortus 1** (grăv'ĭ-dah) (păr'ah) (ah-bor'tŭs)—from the Latin; 2 pregnancies, 1 live birth, 1 abortion or miscarriage

**gravida 3, para 1-0-2-1**—three pregnancies, 1 live birth, no premature births, 2 abortions or miscarriages, and 1 living child

**GYN**—abbreviation for gynecology; pronounced "jin" or G-Y-N

**Heaney clamp** (hā'nē)—medical tool used to grasp and manipulate tissue

**HEENT**—abbreviation for *h*ead, *e*yes, *e*ars, *n*ose, *t*hroat; each letter is pronounced individually

**hematemesis** (hēm"ăh-tĕm'ĕ-sĭs)—the vomiting of blood

**hematochezia** (hēm-ăh"tō-kē'zē-ah)—the passage of bloody stools

**hematocrit** (Hct) (hē-măt'ō-krĭt)—the volume percentage of erythrocytes in whole blood

**hematuria** (hēm"ah-tū'rē-ah)—blood in the urine

**hemoglobin** (Hgb) (hē'mō-glō"bĭn)—carries oxygen from the lungs to the tissues and carbon dioxide from the tissues to the lungs

**hemoperitoneum** (hē"mō-per"ĭ-tō-nē'um)—an effusion of blood in the abdominal cavity

**hemostasis** (hē"mō-stā'sĭs)—the arrest of bleeding by surgical means

**ICD Code 633.1**—International Classification of Diseases; a standard list of identifying codes used in statistics, billing, etc. (This code refers to an ectopic pregnancy.)

**informed consent**—a patient gives written permission for surgery, clinical treatment, and to release his or her records to a 3rd party after a thorough discussion of the issues with the physician involved

**lactated Ringer's** (solution)—a fluid and electrolyte replenisher given to a patient by intravenous infusion

**lyse** (v.) (līs)—to cut or separate, as at surgery

**lysis of adhesions** (lī'sĭs)—disintegration or destruction of adhesions (a surgical procedure)

**melena** (mĕl'ĕ-nah)—the passage of black stools

**mesosalpinx** (mēz"ō-săl'pĭnks)—layers that enclose a uterine tube, which are composed of the broad ligament of the uterus and are located above the mesovarium

**milliliter(s)** (mĭl'i-lē'tĕr)—unit of volume in the metric system, being one thousandth of a liter; abbreviated mL, sometimes dictated "mils"

**mucopurulent** (mū"kō-pū'roo-lĕnt)—containing both mucus and pus

**No. 1** (suture)—referring to the size of suture materials

**normal saline**—a 0.9% solution of sodium chloride (salt water)

**oriented x3**—neurologic terminology meaning that a patient is aware of person, place, and time

**packing laps**—cloths used to pack off the tissues and aid in hemostasis during surgery; also called laparotomy pack

**palpable** (păl'pah-b'l)—perceptible by touch

**pelvic** (pĕl'vĭk)—referring to the pelvis, the basinlike structure formed by the hips, and all it contains

**pelvic ultrasound**—an imaging study of the pelvic area in which the deep structures of the pelvis are scanned by way of ultrasonic waves for diagnostic purposes

**peritoneum** (per"ĭ-tō-nē'um)—the serous membrane lining the abdominal walls and investing the viscera

**Pfannenstiel incision** (făn'ĕn-stēēl")—abdominal incision across the abdomen curved in a "smile" at the bikini line; named for Dr. Hermann Johann Pfannenstiel, a German gynecologist

**Phenergan** (fĕn'ĕr-găn)—medicinal sedative and antinauseant; trade name

**pilonidal cyst** (pī'lō-nī'dal)—a cyst containing a tuft of hairs, usually found at the base of the spine

**positive cardiac activity**—medical term for "the heart is beating" and all that the statement implies

**proximal**—nearest the trunk or point of origin, said of part of a limb, artery, or nerve

**pseudodecidual sign** (soo"dō-dē-sĭd'ū-al)—a false response of the lining of the uterus in the absence of pregnancy

**pseudogestational sac** (soo"dō-jĕs-tā'shĕn-al)—false pregnancy; the gestational sac surrounds the embryo, but in a false pregnancy, there is a "pseudo" or false gestational sac

**retractor**—instrument used to hold wound edges or tissues apart during surgery

**Rh-negative**—describes blood with *no* Rh antigen

**Rh-positive**—describes blood *with* the Rh antigen

**RhoGAM** (rō'găm)—trade name for a preparation of $Rh_0(D)$ immune globulin, required in an Rh-negative mother

**ruptured tubal pregnancy**—a pregnancy in a fallopian tube that has burst through the walls of the tube

**salpingectomy** (săl"pĭn-jĕk'tō-mē)—surgical removal of a uterine tube

**serosal abrasion** (sē-rō'săl)—wearing away of the serous membrane due to friction or pressure

**speculum** (spĕk'ū-lŭm)—instrument used to spread open a passage or cavity for ease in its examination; most often dictated in relation to spreading the vaginal canal

**staple gun**—an instrument by which one accomplishes the process of closing a surgical opening with staples

**subcutaneous** (sŭb"kū-tā'nē-ŭs)—beneath the skin

**tetanus** ('tĕt-nŭs)—acute infectious disease (commonly called lockjaw) caused by the toxin of the bacterium Clostridium tetani; easily prevented by immunization

**transabdominal** (trăns-ăb-dŏm'ĭ-năl)—across or through the abdominal wall

**transvaginal ultrasound** (trăns-văj'ĭ-nal)—an imaging study utilizing sound waves performed through the vagina (radiologic procedure)

**tubo-ovarian** (too"bō-ō-vā'rē-ŭn)—pertaining to a uterine tube and ovary

**tubo-uterine** (too"bō-ū'ter-ĭn)—pertaining to a uterine tube and the uterus

**urinalysis** (ū"rĭ-năl'ĭ-sĭs)—physical, chemical, or microscopic analysis or examination of urine

**Vicryl** (vī'krĭl)—trade name for an absorbable suture made of multifilament braided material

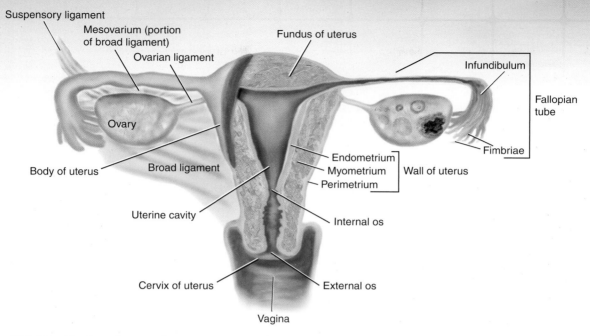

**Figure CS1-1A** The female reproductive system. (*Delmar/Cengage Learning*)

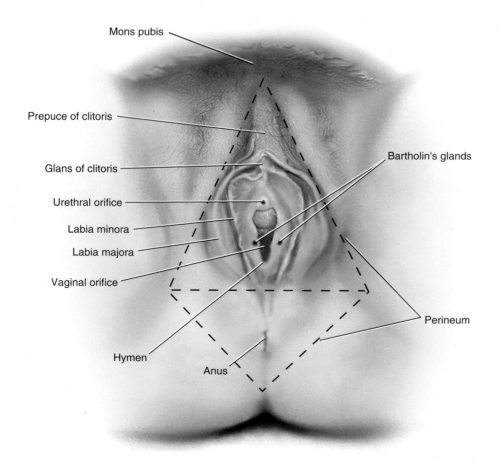

**Figure CS1-1B** The female anatomy external genitalia. (*Delmar/Cengage Learning*)

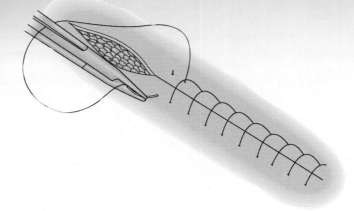

**Figure CS1-2** Continuous sutures. (*Delmar/Cengage Learning*)

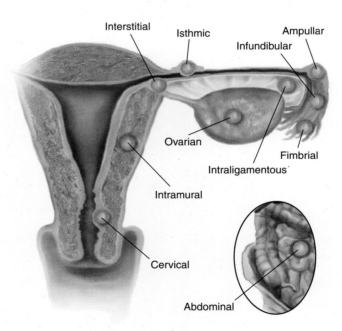

**Figure CS1-3** Sites of ectopic pregnancy. (*Delmar/Cengage Learning*)

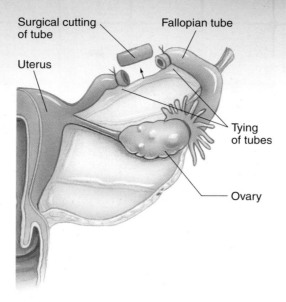

**Figure CS1-4**  Tubal ligation. (*Delmar/Cengage Learning*)

# Case Study 2: Gastrointestinal System

**Patient Name**

Benjamin Engelhart

**Address**

938 Shore Road
Ocean View FL 33140-4989

**Situation**

Benjamin Engelhart, who had had abdominal pain for 3 days, was taken to Hillcrest emergency room where CT scan results were consistent with acute appendicitis. Emergency surgery was necessary, and the patient was taken to the operating room where the surgeon was able to complete his surgery laparoscopically. The patient was discharged with a drain in place after 3 days' hospitalization. He returned to his doctor for drain removal after 1 week. Patient was advised to have no heavy lifting for 4 weeks after surgery and to complete his entire course of antibiotics.

Review Figure CS2-1, Small and large intestine; Figure CS2-2A, Computed tomography (CT) scanning; Figure CS2-2B, Patient instructed to breathe deeply and to relax during the procedure. Patient is reassured that whirring and clicking sounds are normal; Figure CS2-3, Digestive system.

**Student Name** _____

**Patient: Benjamin Engelhart**

| SEQUENCE OF REPORTS | Date Completed | Grade |
| --- | --- | --- |
| Emergency Services Admission Report | _____ | _____ |
| Diagnostic Imaging CT Scan | _____ | _____ |
| Operative Report | _____ | _____ |
| Pathology Report | _____ | _____ |
| Discharge Summary | _____ | _____ |

**NOTE**: Study the glossary for Case Study 2. Enter the date each report is completed in the space provided. When you have transcribed all reports, tear this sheet out and attach it to the front of the reports (in the order listed above); give completed reports to the instructor.

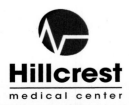

**Hillcrest**
medical center

# GLOSSARY FOR CASE STUDY 2

**0.5% Marcaine** (mar'-kān)—dictated "half percent"; brand name for local anesthetic

**19-French**—French is a scale used to denote catheter sizes and other tubular instruments; each unit is approximately 0.33 mm in diameter; 19-French indicates a diameter of approximately 6.2 mm

**89% shift**—"shift to the left" on CBC differential indicates an increase in the number of band cells or bands; 89% represents the percentage of band cells compared to the total number of white cells counted; this often indicates acute infection

**anorexia** (an"ō-rek'sē-ă)—diminished appetite; aversion to food

**appendicitis** (ă-pen"dǐ-sī'tǐs)—infection or inflammation of the vermiform appendix (see definition of vermiform appendix)

**auscultation** (aws"kul-tā'shŭn)—the act of listening for sounds within the body

**benzoin** (ben'zō-in)—a topical skin protectant

**Blake drain** (blāk)—silicone drain placed in wound to encourage drainage of fluids from wound

**cecum** (sē'kum)—any blind pouch; used to describe the closed end of the large intestine

**clot** (klot)—a soft mass formed when a liquid (blood or lymph) thickens

**clubbing** (klŭb-ing)—a condition of thickening and widening of the fingers and toes with abnormally curved nails

**colonoscopy** (kō"lon-os'kǒ-pē)—examination by means of a flexible, elongated scope that permits visual examination of the colon

**contrast** (kon'-trast)—chemical substances introduced in radiography to increase the difference between different tissue types or between abnormal and normal tissues

**coronal reconstructions** (kuh-rō'năl rē"-kǒn-strŭk'shŭn)—term used in CT scanning to mean three-dimensional view looking at the image from the front of the body

**CPT Code A 88304**—(Current Procedural Terminology)—a set of codes that describes medical, surgical, and diagnostic services; Code A 88304 is the CPT code for surgical pathology, gross and microscopic examination

**cranial nerves**—referred to by either roman or arabic numerals (2 through 12 or II through XII), the 12 pairs of nerves connected with the brain; cranial nerve 1 or I (olfactory) is not always included in the routine physical examination

**crystalloid** (kris'tăl-oyd")—a hydration solution containing only electrolytes

**CT scan**—a procedure in which x-ray images are analyzed and combined by a computer to yield views representing thin slices of the parts examined

**cyanosis** (sī"ă-nō'sĭs)—bluish discoloration of the skin or mucous membrane due to deficient oxygenation of the blood

**degenerative joint disease**—arthritis characterized by softening and fraying of the cartilage and mainly affecting weightbearing joints

**desufflated** (dē'-sŭf-lāt"ed)—air or gas removed from a cavity or chamber of the body

**dilatation** (dil"ă-tā'shŭn)—stretching or enlarging an opening of a hollow structure

**edema, extremity** (e-dē'mă)—swelling of the extremity

**electronically signed**—a statement that specifies the physician has electronically signed the report; this statement is added to the end of a report by a computerized system when the physician "signs" the report by pressing a key

**emesis** (em'ě-sis)—vomiting

**Endo GIA**—a type of surgical stapler

**Endo Catch bag**—a bag used in laparoscopic surgeries to remove the resected specimen (see laparoscopic appendectomy)

**extraocular motions**—eye movements; these are examined by having the patient look in all directions without moving the head

**fibrinous** (fĭ'brin-ŭs, fī'brin-ŭs)—pertaining to or composed of fibrin

**fistula** (fis'tyū-lă)—an abnormal passage between 2 organs in the body or between an organ and the outside of the body

**fistulogram** (fis'tyū-lă-gram")—radiograph after infusion of the fistula with contrast

**flatus** (flā'tŭs)—gas or air in the gastrointestinal tract passed through the anus

**Foley catheter**—tube that is passed into the bladder through the urethra to collect urine

**free air**—air in the abdomen, not trapped within tissues, as a result of perforation of a hollow organ

**gentamicin** (jĕn"tă-mī'sĭn)—antibiotic used to treat many types of infections; sometimes dictated "gent" as medical jargon

**guarding**—tensing of muscles in response to touch

**Hasson trocar** (Hăs'-sŏn trō'-kar)—a blunt instrument used to enter the abdominal cavity; used for insufflation and introduction of laparoscope

**hemicolectomy** (hĕm"ē-kō-lĕk'-tō-mē)—removal of the right or left side of the colon

**hemorrhagic** (hĕm'ŏ-raj'ik)—relating to or marked by hemorrhage

**hepatobiliary** (hep"-ă-tō-bĭl'-e-ar"-e)—related to the liver and bile or biliary ducts

**illicit** (ĭ-lĭs'ĭt)—unlawful

**in toto** (in tō'tō)—entirely, in the whole

**inflammatory bowel disease**—general term for disorders of the small and large intestine

**integument** (in-teg'yū-ment)—enveloping membrane of the body, including skin, hair, and nails

**JP drain**—abbreviation for *Jackson-Pratt* drain; suction drain with tubing inside the body and a bulb reservoir which, when squeezed empty, applies suction and pulls fluid out of the body; used in thoracic or abdominal surgery

**JVD**—abbreviation for *jugular venous distension* or distension of the neck veins

**Kelly clamp**—a curved instrument used for arresting hemorrhage by compression of the bleeding vessel

**laparoscopic appendectomy** (lap"a-rō-skŏp'ic ap"en-dek'-tuh-mē)—removal of vermiform appendix using several scopes placed into the abdomen as opposed to using a right lower quadrant abdominal incision (see open appendectomy)

**LFTs**—abbreviation for *liver function tests*; a lab study

**localized** (lō'kăl-īzd")—restricted or limited to a definite part

**lymphadenopathy**—enlargement of lymph nodes, which may indicate infection

> **cervical lymphadenopathy**—on the back of the neck
>
> **supraclavicular lymphadenopathy**—above the collar bones
>
> **axillary lymphadenopathy**—in the armpit
>
> **inguinal lymphadenopathy**—in the groin

**McBurney sign**—tenderness at a point on the abdomen that indicates appendicitis

**mesoappendix** (mēz"-ō-uh-pĕn-diks)—fold of tissue attaching the appendix to the small bowel

**necrotic** (nĕ-krot'ik)—dead, as in dead tissue

**necrotizing** (nĕk'ro-tīz"ing)—causing death of cells

**normocephalic** (nōr"mō-sĭ-fal'ik)—having a head of medium length

**obturator sign** (ob'tū-rā"tŏr sīn)—pain in the lower abdomen or inside of thigh when the hip is flexed and internally rotated; a sign of appendicitis

**open appendectomy**—removal of vermiform appendix through a right lower quadrant abdominal incision, going through muscle layers and underlying tissue until reaching the abdominal cavity

**OR**—abbreviation for *operating room*

**osseous** (os'ē-us)—of the nature or quality of bone; bony

**p.o.**—Latin abbreviation meaning by mouth (per os)

**PAR**—abbreviation for *postanesthesia recovery*, where patients are sent immediately after surgery (the recovery room); each letter is pronounced separately

**pedal pulses** (pē'-dul)—the 2 arterial pulses able to be felt in the foot; 1 pulse is on the arch of the foot and the other is on the back of the ankle

**periappendiceal** (per"ē-a-pen"-dĭ-cēl')—near the appendix

**pericecal** (per"ē-sē'kal)—near the cecum

**perioperative antibiotics**—antibiotics given either immediately before or immediately after surgery

**phlegmon** (flĕg'mŏn)—a spreading inflammatory reaction to infection that can form multiple pus pockets

**piroxicam** (pĭ-roks'-ĭ-kam) (fel-dēn)—generic nonsteroidal anti-inflammatory drug (brand name Feldene)

**pneumoperitoneum** (new"mo-pĕr-ĭ-tō-nē'um)—air within the peritoneal cavity

**psoas sign** (sō'as)—flexion of or pain on hyperextension of the hip caused by contact of the psoas muscle plus inflammation; often seen in appendicitis

**purulent** (pyūr'ū-lĕnt, pyūr'ŭ-lĕnt)—containing, consisting of, or forming pus

**radiate** (rā'dē-āt)—to spread out in all directions from a center, such as pain radiated from the abdomen

**rebound**—when the abdomen is pressed, then released, more pain is felt upon release than when it is applied

**representative sections**—in gross pathology, pieces of tissue that represent the overall appearance of the specimen

**RLQ**—abbreviation for *right lower quadrant* (of the abdomen)

**saturations 96%**—blood oxygen saturation is measured in percentages with 100% being the most saturated

**SCDs**—abbreviation for *s*equential *c*ompression *d*evices (devices that are wrapped around the legs and inflate and deflate to prevent blood clots in the legs)

**seminal vesicles**—structures in the male about 2 inches long, located behind the bladder. The seminal vesicles contribute fluid to the ejaculate.

**Steri-Strips**—sterile skin closure strips that are made of a porous, nonwoven backing coated with a pressure-sensitive, hypoallergenic adhesive and reinforced with polyester filaments for added strength

**supine** (sū-pīn')—lying face upward

**terminal ileum** (ĭl'ē-ŭm)—the end of the small intestine

**thrills**—large areas of sustained outward motion of the chest felt when performing a heart examination

**thyromegaly** (thī"rō-meg'ă-lē)—enlargement of the thyroid gland

**TMs**—abbreviation for *t*ympanic *m*embranes (eardrums)

**vermiform appendix** (ver'mĭ-fōrm ă-pĕn'dĭks)—a small, tube-like structure attached to the first part of the large intestine

**WNL**—abbreviation for *w*ithin *n*ormal *l*imits

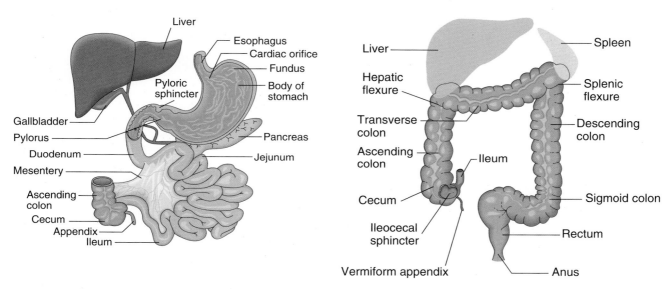

**Figure CS2-1**  The small and large intestine. (*Delmar/Cengage Learning*)

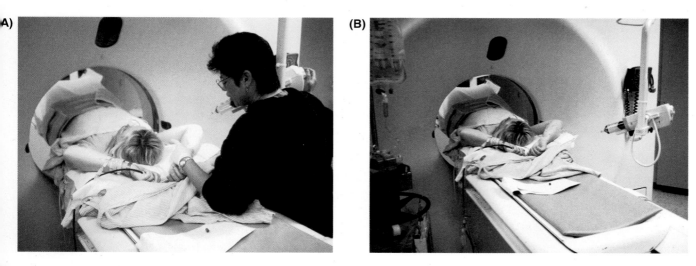

**Figure CS2-2**  Computed tomography (CT) scanning. (A) The patient is instructed to lie still and (B) patient is instructed to breathe deeply and to relax during the procedure and is reassured that whirring and clicking sounds are normal. (*Delmar/Cengage Learning*)

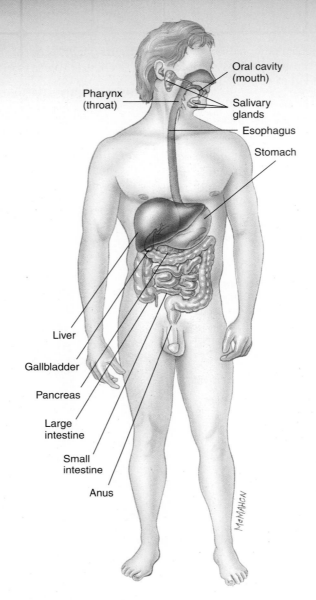

**Figure CS2-3**   Digestive system. (*Delmar/Cengage Learning*)

# Case Study 3: Cardiopulmonary System

**Patient Name**

Putul Barua

**Address**

3506 NW 56th Court
North Miami Beach FL 33160-5938

**Situation**

Putul Barua, a male patient from Bangladesh, presented to Hillcrest Medical Center with signs and symptoms of a possible myocardial infarction. He was admitted to Cardiac Care and evaluated by both Cardiology and Pulmonology. Workup showed the patient to have hemoptysis with a history of tuberculosis. Further testing included bronchoscopy, CT scan of chest, chest x-ray, CT scan of brain, and an open-lung biopsy. The patient developed renal failure, which was managed by Nephrology. Even with the efforts of these 3 specialty services, Mr. Barua did not improve; he was pronounced dead on hospital day 8. Permission for autopsy was denied.

Review Figure CS3-1, Lungs and supporting structures; Figure CS3-2, Position of diaphragm during (A) inhalation and (B) expiration; Figure CS3-3, Apex/base of heart; Figure CS3-4, Coronary arteries; and Figure CS3-5, Internal anatomy of the kidney.

**Student Name** _____

**Patient: Putul Barua**

| SEQUENCE OF REPORTS | Date Completed | Grade |
|---|---|---|
| History and Physical Examination | _____ | _____ |
| Operative Report | _____ | _____ |
| Diagnostic Imaging Report 1 | _____ | _____ |
| Diagnostic Imaging Report 2 | _____ | _____ |
| Diagnostic Imaging Report 3 | _____ | _____ |
| Death Summary | _____ | _____ |

**NOTE**: Study the glossary for Case Study 3. Enter the date each report is completed in the space provided. When you have transcribed all reports, tear this sheet out and attach it to the front of the reports (in the order listed above); give completed reports to the instructor.

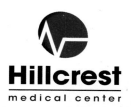

**Hillcrest**
medical center

# GLOSSARY FOR CASE STUDY 3

**acute hepatic failure** (ah-kūt' hě-păt'ĭk)—the sudden onset of liver failure

**advanced cardiac life support**—a set of interventions for urgent treatment of cardiac arrest; these interventions include medications, CPR, and defibrillation (delivery of electrical energy with defibrillator)

**alveolitis** (ăl"vē-ō-lī'tĭs)—inflammation of the alveoli (air sacs in the lung)

**amphoric** (ăm-for'ĭk)—describing a hollow sound resulting from percussion over a lung cavity

**ancillary** (ăn'-sĭ-lěr'ē)—supplementary

**asystolic** (ā"sĭs-tol'ĭk)—pertaining to asystole (absence of cardiac contraction)

**atrial fibrillation** (ā'trē-al fī"brĭ-lā'shun)—rapid, irregular contractions of the atria (upper chambers of the heart)

**atrial flutter**—rapid contractions of the atria, more regular than fibrillation

**axial sections** (ăk'sē-ăl)—referring to cross sections obtained in a horizontal plane of a structure of the body, either by slicing or by imaging techniques

**axillary** (ăk'sĭ-ler"ē)—pertaining to the armpit

**basal ganglia calcifications** (bā'săl gang'lē-ah)—deposits of calcium in basal ganglia (groups of nerve cells in the brain)

**bilateral** (bī-lăt'er-al)—occurring on both sides

**bleb** (blĕb)—an abnormal air-filled or fluid-filled sac

**bronchoscopy** (brŏng-kŏs'kō-pē)—visual examination of the bronchial passages of the lungs through a bronchoscope; a surgical procedure

**brushings** (brŭsh'ĭngs)—cell samples that are obtained with a brush; this material is sent for examination of the cells for carcinoma or other disease processes, such as tuberculosis

**carina** (kah-rī'nah)—a downward and backward projection of the lowest tracheal cartilage, forming a ridge between the openings of the right and left main bronchi

**cavitary lesions** (kăv'ĭ-tār"ē)—abnormal tissue areas containing cavities

**cerebral edema** (sě-rē'brăl ě-dē'mah)—excessive accumulation of fluid in the brain substance that causes swelling

**Code Blue**—medical jargon meaning a patient's heartbeat and/or respirations have ceased, calling for immediate resuscitation procedures (CPR)

**congestion**—swelling of blood vessels due to engorgement with blood

**cords**—referring to the vocal cords, 2 small bands of muscle within the larynx; the vocal cords vibrate to produce the voice

**cortical atrophy** (kor'tĭ-kal ăt'rō-fē)—death of cells in the cerebral cortex (part of the brain)

**Coumadin** (koo'mah-dĭn)—trade name for warfarin sodium, an anticoagulant drug

**CT**—abbreviation for computerized tomography

**dialysis catheter** (dī-al'ĭ-sĭs)—tubular instrument inserted into a major vein in order to filter the blood of impurities; dialysis is done in patients whose kidneys have less than normal function

**echocardiogram** (ĕk"ō-kăr'dē-ō-grăm)—the record obtained by using ultrasound to bounce back ultrasonic waves from the heart

**effusion** (ē-fū'zhŭn)—the escape of fluid into a body part or tissue

**ejection fraction**—the proportion of the volume of blood in the ventricles at the end of diastole that is ejected during systole

**EKG leads**—conductors connected to an electrocardiograph (EKG) machine

**embolectomy** (ĕm"bō-lĕk'tō-mē)—surgical removal of a blood clot (embolus) from a blood vessel

**endobronchial** (ĕn"dō-brŏng'kē-ăl)—within the bronchi or bronchial tubes

**epiglottis** (ĕp'ĭ-glŏt'is)—the lidlike cartilaginous structure that folds back over the larynx during swallowing and that prevents food from entering the lungs

**ET tube**—abbreviation for endotracheal tube, a tube inserted into the trachea (windpipe) to assist in ventilating the patient

**etiology** (ē'tē-ŏl'o-jē)—cause or origin of a disease or disorder

**fungemia** (fŭn-jē'mē-ah)—the presence of a fungal growth in the blood stream

**glottis** (glŏt'is)—the vocal apparatus of the larynx consisting of several structures that form the supporting structures of the vocal cords

**Hemoccult** (hē'mō-kŭlt)—trade name for test to discover occult (hidden) blood in the stool

**hemodialysis** (hē"mō-dī-ăl'ĭ-sis)—the removal of waste substances from the blood by means of a hemodialyzer (machine)

**hemoptysis** (hē-mŏp'tĭ-sis)—the expectoration or spitting up of blood or blood-stained sputum from the bronchial tubes as a result of pulmonary or bronchial hemorrhage

**hepatosplenomegaly** (hĕp-ă'-tō-splĕ'-nō-mĕg'ă-lē)—enlargement of the liver and spleen

**high-flow oxygen**—oxygen administered via the highest setting on the oxygen machine (as opposed to low-flow oxygen, which is at a lower level)

**hilar** (hī'lĕr)—pertaining to the depression, notch, or opening where the vessels and nerves enter an organ

**HPI**—abbreviation for *h*istory of *p*resent *i*llness

**hydrocephalus** (hī"drō-sĕf'ah-lŭs)—an increase in the volume of cerebrospinal fluid in the ventricles of the cerebrum (brain)

**hypokinesia** (hī"pō-kĭ-nē'zē-ah)—abnormally decreased motor function or activity

✓ **hypoxic** (hī"pŏk'sĭk)—pertaining to deficient oxygenation of the tissues

✓ **idiopathic pulmonary fibrosis** (ĭd"ē-ō-păth'ik pŭl'mō-ner-ē fī-brō'sĭs)—hardening of the pulmonary (lung) structures of either unknown or spontaneous origin

**infiltrate** (n.) (ĭn'-fĭl-trāt)—a collection of inflammatory cells, foreign organisms, and cellular debris; when present on chest x-ray it indicates pneumonia

**INR**—abbreviation for *i*nternational *n*ormalized *r*atio—one of the clotting studies performed along with PT (prothrombin time) and PTT (partial thromboplastin time)

**intravenous** (ĭn"trah-vē'-nŭs)—within or into a vein

**intravenous contrast**—material inserted into a vein that allows differences in tissues to be delineated; used in radiology and cardiology procedures

**intubated** (ĭn'tū-bāt-ĕd)—the condition of having a tube inserted into a body canal or hollow organ

**intubation**—the insertion of a tube into a body canal or hollow organ

**Klebsiella pneumoniae** (klĕb"sē-ĕl'ah nū-mō'-nē-ī)—one etiologic agent of acute bacterial pneumonia (microbiology genus and species name)

**lesion** (lē'zhŭn)—any abnormality involving an organ or tissue due to a disease process or injury

**low-flow oxygen**—oxygen administered via the lowest setting on the oxygen machine (as opposed to high-flow oxygen, which is at a higher setting)

**malaise** (mal-āz')—a vague feeling of bodily discomfort

**mechanical ventilation**—ventilation (breathing) supported or provided by a machine

**mediastinal** (mē"dē-ah-stī'năl)—pertaining to the membranous partition separating the lungs or the 2 pleural sacs

**MVA**—abbreviation for *m*otor *v*ehicle *a*ccident

**myocardial infarction** (mī"ō-kăr'dē-ăl ĭn-fărk'shŭn)—injury or necrosis of the heart muscle due to lack of blood supply to the area (heart attack)

**nasoduodenal feeding tube** (nāz'ō-dū'ō-dē'năl)—a tube that goes through the nose and down through the esophagus and stomach to sit at the first part of the intestine; the patient is fed nutritional supplementation through the tube

**nephrologist** (nĕ-frŏl'ō-jĭst)—a medical specialist in diagnosing and treating kidney disease

**open-lung biopsy**—taking a small sample of apparently diseased tissue in surgery while the lungs are exposed (as opposed to a brush biopsy or a procedure with the lungs not exposed)

**palpitations** (păl"pĭ-tā'shŭns)—rapid or irregular heartbeats; primarily used in the plural form

**parenchymal** (pah-rĕng'kĭ-mal)—pertaining to the essential elements of an organ, i.e., the functional elements of an organ

**pleural** (ploo'răl)—pertaining to the serous membrane that covers the lungs and lining of the thoracic cavity

**prothrombin time** (prō-thrŏm'bĭn)—a test for coagulation factors of the blood; also dictated and written pro time

**pseudocords** (soo"dō-kords)—false cords; part of the anatomical structure of the larynx (voice box)

**pulmonary** (pŭl'mō-ner"ē)—pertaining to the lungs

**pulmonary vascular congestion**—engorgement of pulmonary vessels occurring in cardiac disease, infections, and certain bodily injuries

**rhonchi** (sing. rhonchus)—sounds with a musical pitch (heard on auscultation) in bronchial tubes due to inflammation, spasm of muscle, or presence of mucus; used most commonly in the plural form

*flash cards*     *some words final exam*

**S₁, S₂, S₃, S₄** *or* **S1, S2, S3, S4**—first, second, third, and fourth heart sounds; may be heard while listening to the heart via stethoscope; S1 and S2 are normal sounds, S3 and S4 are not normally heard

**septicemia** (sĕp"tĭ-sē'mē-ah)—toxins in the blood, formerly called "blood poisoning"

**sputum** (spū'tŭm)—material coughed up from the lower respiratory tract

**subarachnoid hemorrhage** (sub"ah-răk'nōid)—hemorrhage at or between the arachnoid and pia mater of the brain

**supraventricular cardiac arrhythmias** (soo"prah-vĕn-trĭk'ū-lar kăr'dē-ak ah-rĭth'mē-ahs)—irregularity in the rhythm of the heart starting from a focus above the ventricles

**tachycardia** (tăk'ē-kăr'dē-ah)—fast heart rate

**thorax** (thō'răks)—chest

**thrombosis** (thrŏm-bō'sĭs)—formation or presence of a thrombus or blood clot

**tuberculosis** (too-ber"kū-lō'sĭs)—an infectious disease of the lung

**ventricles** (vĕn'trĭ-k'ls)—lower chambers of the heart

**Versed** (vĕr'-sĕd, vĕr-sĕd')—trade name for a drug given intravenously either before or during surgery to produce sedation and amnesia

**Xylocaine** (zī'lō-kān)—trade name for lidocaine, a topical anesthetic drug

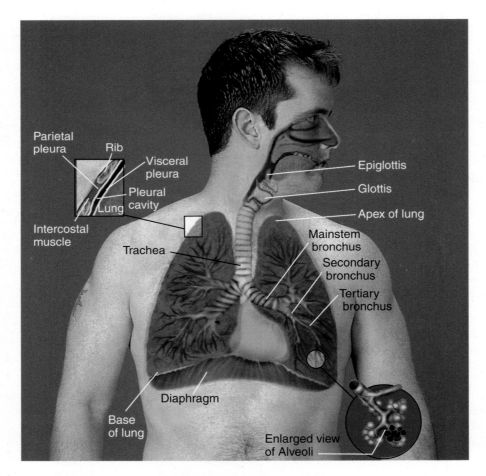

**Figure CS3-1**   Lungs and supporting structures. (*Delmar/Cengage Learning*)

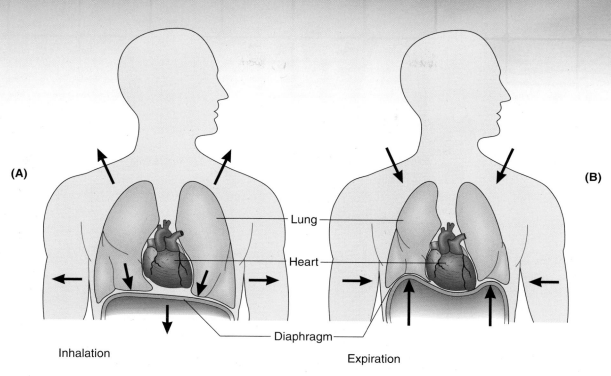

(A)

(B)

Lung

Heart

Diaphragm

Inhalation

Expiration

**Figure CS3-2** Position of diaphragm during (A) inhalation and (B) expiration. (*Delmar/Cengage Learning*)

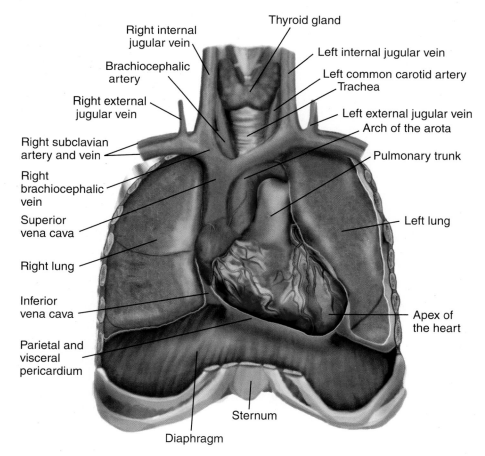

Right internal
jugular vein

Brachiocephalic
artery

Right external
jugular vein

Right subclavian
artery and vein

Right
brachiocephalic
vein

Superior
vena cava

Right lung

Inferior
vena cava

Parietal and
visceral
pericardium

Thyroid gland

Left internal jugular vein

Left common carotid artery
Trachea

Left external jugular vein
Arch of the arota

Pulmonary trunk

Left lung

Apex of
the heart

Sternum

Diaphragm

**Figure CS3-3** Apex/base of the heart. (*Delmar/Cengage Learning*)

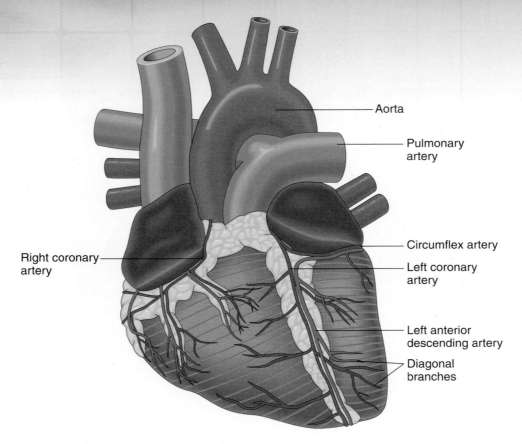

**Figure CS3-4**   Coronary arteries. (*Delmar/Cengage Learning*)

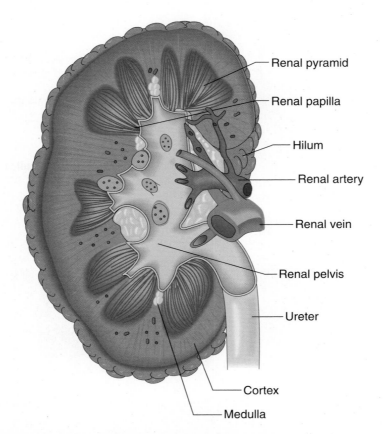

**Figure CS3-5**   Internal anatomy of the kidney. (*Delmar/Cengage Learning*)

# Case Study 4: Integumentary System

**Patient Name**

Adela Torres

**Address**

5900 SE 22ⁿᵈ Avenue
Miami Beach FL 33156-5937

**Situation**

Adela Torres, a middle-aged woman with multiple medical problems, developed painful ulcerations of her mouth and lips, making eating and drinking difficult. She sought medical treatment at her internist's office, and he admitted her to Hillcrest Medical Center. Ms. Torres had a routine chest x-ray on admission, and she was referred to Dermatology Services in consultation. She was offered the services of Psychology due to anxiety issues, but she deferred. The dermatologist and internist agreed on a treatment plan for the patient, and after a few days, marked improvement was noted in her condition. She was discharged in improved condition to be followed by the internist, to see the dermatologist as needed, and to consult with the psychologist if her anxiety continues.

Review Figure CS4-1, Glands of the skin; Figure CS4-2, Aphthous stomatitis; and Figure CS4-3, Fissure.

**Student Name** _____

**Patient: Adela Torres**

| SEQUENCE OF REPORTS | Date Completed | Grade |
| --- | --- | --- |
| History and Physical Examination | _____ | _____ |
| Radiology Report | _____ | _____ |
| Consultation | _____ | _____ |
| Discharge Summary | _____ | _____ |

**NOTE**: Study the glossary for Case Study 4. Enter the date each report is completed in the space provided. When you have transcribed all reports, tear this sheet out and attach it to the front of the reports (in the order listed above); give completed reports to the instructor.

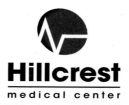

**Hillcrest**
medical center

# Glossary for Case Study 4

**albeit** (ăl-bē'ĭt)—even though

**albumin** (ăl-bū'mĭn)—a necessary protein substance produced in the liver; levels are reduced in malnutrition and in liver and kidney diseases

**Arava** (ah-rā'vah)—trade name for medicine used to treat rheumatoid arthritis

**arthritis** (ăr-thrī'tĭs)—inflammation of the joints

**azathioprine** (ā'zah-thī'ō-prĕn)—generic drug used in treating rheumatoid arthritis and other autoimmune diseases

**Azulfidine** (ā-zŭl'fĭ-dēn)—trade name for sulfasalazine, an antibacterial agent

**chlorambucil** (klō-răm'bū-sĭl)—generic name of drug used in chemotherapy

**compression fracture**—any break or rupture of bone due to compression, e.g., the bones of the spine

**conjunctival injection** (kŏn'jŭnk-tī'văl)—increased blood flow to the conjunctiva (mucous membrane covering the eyeball and inside of the lids), making it appear swollen

**corticosteroids** (kor"tĭ-kō-stĕ'roids)—a group of steroids (or lipids) used clinically in immune suppression or in hormonal replacement

**cyclophosphamide** (sī"klō-fŏs'fah-mīd)—generic drug used in chemotherapy

**debilitating**—causing weakness or a lack of strength

**dehydration** (dē"hī-drā'shŭn)—condition resulting from either excessive loss of or inadequate intake of water

**dermatology** (dĕr"mah-tŏl'ō-jē)—the study of the skin

**diffuse** (adj.) (dĭf-fūs')—widely distributed, not concentrated

**distally** (dĭs'tăl-lē)—in a remote direction; opposite of proximally or near

**dysphagia** (dĭs-fā'jē-ah)—difficulty swallowing

**ecchymosis** (pl. ecchymoses) (ĕk"ĭ-mō'sis)—a purplish patch on the skin caused by blood passing from a vessel into the tissues

**enteritis** (ĕn"tĕr-ī'tĭs)—inflammation of the intestine, particularly the small intestine

**erosion** (ē-rō'zhŭn)—destruction of the surface of the skin, as by friction or pressure

**erythema** (ĕr"ĭ-thē'mah)—redness of the skin produced by abnormal accumulation of blood

**erythema multiforme** (mŭl"tĭ-form"ay)—a symptom complex including multiple skin discolorations and raised lesions; may be caused by allergic reaction or virus

**estradiol** (ĕs"tră-dī-ăl)—estrogen produced by the ovaries; used as hormone replacement therapy and marketed under multiple trade names

**exophthalmos** (ĕk"sŏf-thăl'mus)—abnormal protrusion of the eyeball

**exudate** (ĕks'ū-dāt)—any fluid that has escaped from blood vessels and deposited in tissues, usually due to an injury or inflammation

**fissuring** (fĭsh'ūr-ing)—splitting of the skin; can include painful ulcerations

**flare** (v.)—to intensify suddenly

**folic acid** (fō'lĭk)—a B-complex vitamin necessary for normal production of red blood cells; used to treat certain types of anemia

**gingiva** (jĭn'jĭ-vah)—the pale pink tissues of the oral mucosa, otherwise known as the gums

**HCTZ**—abbreviation for *h*ydrochloro*t*hia*z*ide, a generic name for a diuretic medication used to treat edema and hypertension

**hydroxychloroquine** (hī-drŏk"sē-klō'rō-kwĭn)—generic name of drug used to treat rheumatoid arthritis

**hyperpigmentation** (hī"pĕr-pig"men-tā'shun)—abnormally increased coloration

**hyporeflexia** (hī"pō-rē-flĕk'sē-ah)—decreased reflexes

**IV hydration**—receiving fluids *intra*venously

**kyphosis** (kī-fō'sis)—abnormally increased curvature of the thoracic spine; humpback

**leucovorin** (loo"kō-vō'rĭn)—generic name of drug used to treat both anemia and malignances

**Lidex gel** (lī'dĕks)—trade name for topically applied gel, which has anti-inflammatory properties

**liver enzymes**—those protein molecules that induce necessary chemical reactions in the liver; a group of laboratory tests done on blood or serum that give the values of these proteins

**macular** (măk'ū-lăr)—pertaining to a macule, which is a nonelevated, discolored spot on the skin

**methotrexate**—generic name for chemotherapy drug; used also in treatment of immune disorders, such as rheumatoid arthritis

**Mobic** (mō'bĭk)—trade name for anti-inflammatory drug used to treat arthritis

**nephrocalcinosis** (nĕf"rō-kăl"sĭ-nō'sis)—diffusely scattered calcifications in the kidneys leading to renal insufficiency

**NSAID**—abbreviation for *non*steroidal *a*nti*i*nflammatory *d*rug; often dictated "n-sed"

**osteoporosis** (ŏs"tē-ō-pō-rō'-sis)—reduction in quantity of bone; decreased bone mass leading to pathologic fractures

**palate** (păl'ăt)—roof of the mouth

**penicillamine** (pĕn"ĭ-sĭl'ah-mēn)—generic name for drug, a product of penicillin, used to treat rheumatoid arthritis

**perimalleolar** (pĕr"ĭ-măl-ē'ō-lăr)—around the bony protuberances on each side of the ankle

**pitting edema**—indentations (pitting) when a finger is pressed on the skin; occurs when excessive fluid is in the tissues

**posterior pharynx** (făr'ĭnks)—the back of the throat

**prednisone** (prĕd'nĭ-sōn)—generic name for a type of steroid used as an anti-inflammatory agent

**quiescent** (kwī-ĕs'sent)—at rest; inactive

**regimen** (rĕj'ĭ-mĕn)—a strictly regulated plan of therapy, diet, exercise, or other activity designed to achieve a certain goal

**rheumatoid arthritis** (roo'mah-toid)—chronic systemic, painful joint disease that can result in deformities

**serum cholesterol** (sē'rŭm kō-lĕs'tĕr-ŏl)—the level of cholesterol (a complex organic compound synthesized in the liver and other tissues) found in the serum; high levels of cholesterol can clog arteries and can form gallstones

**stasis edema** (stā'sĭs ĕ-dē'mah)—stagnation of the flow of blood or fluids resulting in swelling

**Stevens-Johnson syndrome**—a severe, sometimes fatal multisystemic form of erythema multiforme

**stomatitis** (stō-mah-tī'tĭs)—inflammation of the oral mucosa, the mucous membranes of the mouth

**t.i.d.** [L.]—*t*er *i*n *d*ie (three times a day)

**topically**—applied to the skin

**total protein**—a laboratory test to determine the level of all proteins in the serum

**vertebral body** (vĕr'tĕ-brăl) (vĕr-tē'brăl)—main portion of each of the bones of the spine; bears about 80% of the load while standing and provides an attachment for the disks between the vertebrae

**volume depletion**—dehydrated state

**Westergren sedimentation rate**—standard laboratory test to determine the rate of settling of red blood cells in anticoagulated blood; procedure designed by Alf Westergren, a Swedish physician born in 1891

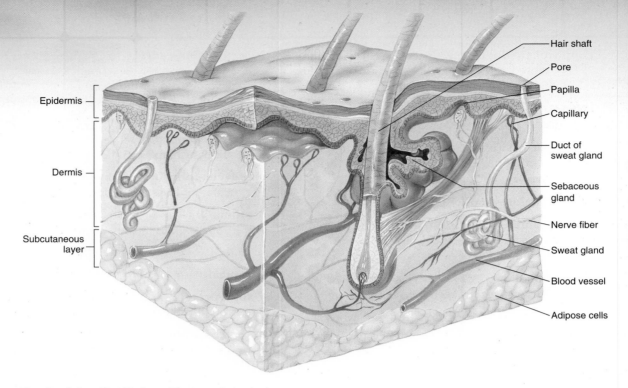

Epidermis
Dermis
Subcutaneous layer

Hair shaft
Pore
Papilla
Capillary
Duct of sweat gland
Sebaceous gland
Nerve fiber
Sweat gland
Blood vessel
Adipose cells

**Figure CS4-1**    Glands of the skin. (*Delmar/Cengage Learning*)

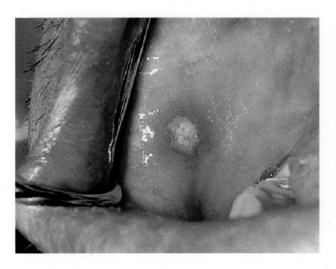

**Figure CS4-2**    Aphthous stomatitis. (*Courtesy of Dr. Joseph Konzelman, School of Dentistry, Medical College of Georgia*)

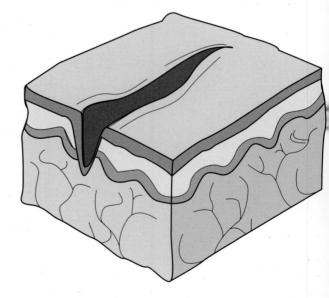

**Figure CS4-3**    Fissure. (*Delmar/Cengage Learning*)

# CASE STUDY 5: PSYCHOLOGY/NEUROLOGY SYSTEM

**Patient Name**

Fanny Copeland

**Address**

509 Red Road
Miami FL 33114-0229

**Situation**

Fanny Copeland is a middle-aged lady who was admitted to Hillcrest Medical Center through the emergency room after she presented with suicidal thoughts and memory problems. She was referred to Neurology for a consult and a full workup, which included a CT scan and laboratory work. Her workup was within normal limits, but her personal situation included stressors that resulted in depression, which can lead to memory problems.

Review Table CS5-1, Categories of mental disorders; and Figure CS5-1, Adjustment—a relative state that shifts according to life experiences.

**Student Name** _____

**Patient: Fanny Copeland**

| SEQUENCE OF REPORTS | Date Completed | Grade |
|---|---|---|
| History and Physical Examination | _____ | _____ |
| Consultation | _____ | _____ |
| Diagnostic Imaging Report | _____ | _____ |
| Discharge Summary | _____ | _____ |

**NOTE**: Study the glossary for Case Study 5. Enter the date each report is completed in the space provided. When you have transcribed all reports, tear this sheet out and attach it to the front of the reports (in the order listed above); give completed reports to the instructor.

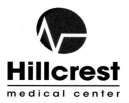

**Hillcrest**
medical center

# GLOSSARY FOR CASE STUDY 5

**bilateral salpingo-oophorectomy** (săl-pĭng'gō-ō'of-ō-ĕk'tŏ-mē)—removal of both fallopian tubes and ovaries

**buccofacial apraxia** (bŭk'ō-fā'shăl ă-prăk'sē-ă)—inability to coordinate and carry out facial and lip movements on command, such as whistling or winking

**carotid bruits** (kă-rŏt'-id brū-ēz', brū'-ēz)—harsh or musical abnormal sounds in the carotid artery produced by turbulent blood flow

**curt** (kŭrt)—rudely abrupt; blunt; brief; gruff

**dementia** (dĕ-men'shē-ă)—the progressive loss of cognitive and intellectual functions without impairment of perception or consciousness

**Detrol** (dĕ'trol)—trade name prescription medicine used to treat symptoms of overactive bladder

**drift**—a gradual movement, as from an original position; dictated in neurologic exam

**dysphoric** (dis-for'-ic)—an emotional state characterized by anxiety, depression, or unease

**dysthymic personality disorder** (dis-thī'mik)—a chronic disturbance of mood characterized by mild depression or loss of interest in usual activities

**fasciculation** (fă-sik'yū-lā'shun)—involuntary contractions, or twitching, of groups of muscle fibers

**frontal release signs**—the primitive reflexes normally present in infants that appear in adults with frontal lobe (brain) lesions; frontal release signs (primitive reflexes) are grasp, snout, root, and suck

**Geriatric Depression Scale** (jer'ē-at'rik)—a 30-item self-report assessment designed specifically to identify depression in the elderly

**homicidal ideations**—thoughts about killing another person

**hysterectomy** (his'ter-ek'tŏ-mē)—removal of the uterus

**ibuprofen** (ī'bū-prō'fen)—a generic nonsteroidal anti-inflammatory agent

**impulsivity**—inclined to act on impulse rather than thought

**limb gestural apraxia** (jĕs'tūr-al ă-prăk'sē-ă)—inability to move a limb in a specific way on command, such as a finger, even though the person understands what must be done and has moved the limb in the past

**limb manipulation apraxia**—inability to use an object such as to open a door with a key or flip a coin

**major depressive disorder**—condition characterized by one or more major depressive episodes not due to a medical condition, medication, abused substance, or psychosis

**Mattis Dementia Rating Scale**—test that identifies individuals at risk for Alzheimer disease; also used to study efficacy of drugs given for dementia in Parkinson disease

**meningismus**—condition characterized by neck stiffness, headache, and other symptoms of meningeal irritation but without meningitis

**MMPI**—abbreviation for *M*innesota *M*ultiphasic *P*ersonality *I*nventory—psychological test most commonly used by health professionals to assess and diagnose mental illness

**MMSE**—abbreviation for *M*ini-*M*ental *S*tatus *E*xamination—screening tool to assess overall brain function and often used to evaluate patients with possible Alzheimer disease or other related dementia

**Omnipaque** (ahm'nē-pāk')—x-ray contrast medium for use in computerized tomography (CT), brand name

**osteoarthritis** (os'tē-ō-ar-thrī'tis)—arthritis characterized by erosion of the articular cartilage

**paraphasic errors** (par'ă-fā'sik)—substitution of an incorrect sound (e.g., tree for free) or related word (e.g., chair for bed)

**passive-aggressive**—passive-aggressive personality disorder is a chronic condition in which the person seems to passively comply with the desires and needs of others but actually passively resists them, in the process becoming increasingly hostile and angry

**passive-dependent**—a personality characterized by helplessness, indecisiveness, and a tendency to cling to and seek support from others

**praxis** (prăk'sĭs)—conception and planning of a motor act in response to an environmental demand

**Romberg** (rŏm'bĕrg)—test performed for balance; the patient stands with feet together (touching) with eyes closed; if the patient cannot maintain the position, this may indicate lesions in the brain or nervous system

**suicidal ideations**—thoughts of killing oneself

**sullen** (sŭl'lĕn)—implies a silent ill humor and refusal to be sociable

**tandem walking**—on stepping forward, placing the heel of the foot in front against the toe of the foot in back

**tetracycline** (tĕt-ră-sī'klēn, -klĭn)—generic name for an antibiotic

**TMJ**—abbreviation for *temporomandibular joint*; the joint of the jaw

**tonsillectomy** (ton'si-lĕk'tŏ-mē)—removal of the entire tonsil (usually both faucial tonsils)

**Trail Making Test Parts A and B**—test given to identify brain function impairment. The test consists of two parts, A and B, and is a test of speed. Part A consists of encircled numbers from 1 to 25 randomly spread across a sheet of paper. The object of the test is for the subject to connect the numbers in order, beginning with 1 and ending with 25, in as little time as possible. Part B is more complex than A because it requires the subject to connect numbers and letters in an alternating pattern (1-A-2-B-3-C, etc.) in as little time as possible.

**visual fields**—the entire scope of vision of each eye

**Wechsler Logical Memory** (weks'lĕr)—test given to measure immediate and delayed narrative memory; comprised of 2 short prose stories. The first is composed of 24 units or ideas, and the second is composed of 22 units or ideas. One point is awarded for each idea that is recalled verbatim, and a half-point is awarded for each time the participant recalls the gist of an idea utilizing a different word or phrase.

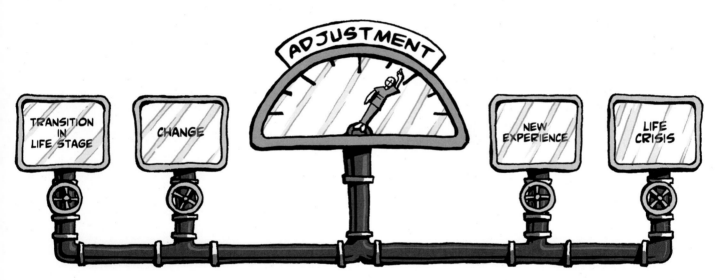

**Figure CS5-1**  Adjustment—a relative state that shifts according to life experiences. (*Source: Milliken, Mary Elizabeth and Honeycutt, Alyson. [2004]. Understanding Human Behavior: A Guide for Health Care Providers, 7th ed. Clifton Park, NY: Delmar Cengage Learning.*)

## TABLE CS5-1.   CATEGORIES OF MENTAL DISORDERS

| Cognitive Disorders (Axis I) | Substance-Related Disorders (Axis I) | Schizophrenia (Axis I) | Mood Disorders (Axis I) | Anxiety Disorders (Axis I) | Somatoform Disorders, Sleep Disorders, & Factitious Disorders (Axis I) | Dissociative Identity Disorders (Axis I) | Sexual and Gender Identity Disorders (Axis I) | Eating Disorders (Axis I) | Personality Disorders (Axis II) |
|---|---|---|---|---|---|---|---|---|---|
| Amnesia | Substance abuse | Paranoid schizophrenia | Major depressive disorder | Panic disorder | Conversion disorder | Dissociative identity disorder (formerly multiple personality disorder) | Gender identity disorder | Anorexia nervosa | Antisocial personality disorder |
| Delirium | Substance dependence | | Cyclothymic disorder | Phobic disorder | Pain disorder | Dissociative amnesia (formerly psychogenic amnesia) | Transvestic fetishism | Bulimia | Borderline personality disorder |
| Dementia | Substance intoxication | | Bipolar disorders | Obsessive-compulsive disorder | Hypochondriasis | Dissociative fugue (formerly psychogenic fugue) | Sexual sadism | Narcissistic personality disorder | |
| | | | | | Posttraumatic stress disorder | Narcolepsy | Sexual masochism | Paranoid personality disorder | |
| | | | | | | Munchausen syndrome | Exhibitionism | Schizoid personality disorder | |
| | | | | | | Malingering | Frotteurism | | |
| | | | | | | | Pedophilia | | |

Source: Jones, Betty Davis. (2008). *Comprehensive Medical Terminology*, 3rd ed. Clifton Park, NY: Delmar Cengage Learning.

# CASE STUDY 6: NERVOUS SYSTEM

**Patient Name**

Deanna Martinez

**Address**

7334 Kendall Avenue
Miami FL 33156-5948

**Situation**

After suffering with long-term pain in both her low back and right leg and receiving no benefit from chiropractic manipulation, Ms. Martinez sought advice and treatment from Neurosurgery Services. She was admitted to Hillcrest for radiology testing and lumbar puncture, which revealed her to have a herniated disk. She was taken to surgery where the herniated disk was removed and the tissue sent to Pathology for examination and diagnosis. After an uneventful, afebrile hospital course, the patient was discharged in improved condition with her pain resolved.

Review Table CS6-1, The cranial nerves; Figure CS6-1, Cranial nerves numbered by roman numerals or name, indicating distribution or function; Figure CS6-2, Nervous system—brain, spinal cord, nerves; Figure CS6-3, Prone position; Figure CS6-4, Herniated disk.

**Student Name** _____

**Patient:  Deanna Martinez**

| SEQUENCE OF REPORTS | Date Completed | Grade |
|---|---|---|
| History and Physical Examination | _____ | _____ |
| Radiology Report 1 | _____ | _____ |
| Radiology Report 2 | _____ | _____ |
| Operative Report | _____ | _____ |
| Pathology Report | _____ | _____ |
| Discharge Summary | _____ | _____ |

**NOTE**:  Study the glossary for Case Study 6. Enter the date each report is completed in the space provided. When you have transcribed all reports, tear this sheet out and attach it to the front of the reports (in the order listed above); give completed reports to the instructor.

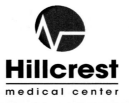

**Hillcrest**
medical center

# Glossary for Case Study 6

**aggregating**—crowding or clustering together

**ambulating** (ăm"bū-lā'ting)—walking

**blunted**—less sharp; dull

**cesarean section** (sē-sār'ē-ăn, sē-zăr-ē-ăn)—delivery of a fetus by making an incision in the abdominal wall and uterus

**chiropractor** (kī'rō-prăk'tŏr)—a practitioner of chiropractic, a conservative science of applied neurophysiology; chiropractic theory is that irritation of the nervous system is the cause of disease

**Cloward saddle** (klow'erd)—surgical equipment in which a patient is placed for back surgery, trade name

**contrast medium** (pl. contrast media)—any substance administered internally that has a different opacity from soft tissue, allowing visualization of structures on radiography or CT

**contused** (kon-tūzd')—bruised

**convex** (kon'-věks')—having a surface that is rounded and somewhat elevated

**curette** *or* **curet** (kū-rět')—spoon-shaped surgical instrument for removing tissue from a cavity wall or other bodily surface

**Darvocet** (dăr'vō-sět)—trade name for drug used to treat mild to moderate pain

**denies x3** (dictated "denies times three")—used in the Social History to refer to the fact the patient denies the use of alcohol, tobacco, or illicit drugs

**discrete** (dĭs-krēt')—made up of separate and distinct parts or defined by lesions that do not become unified

**diskectomy** (dĭs-kěk'tō-mē)—removal of an intervertebral disk

**epinephrine** (ěp"ĭ-něf'rĭn)—drug used as a vasoconstrictor, cardiac stimulant, and bronchodilator; generic name

**exacerbate** (ěg-zăs'ěr-bāt")—to worsen or make more severe

**facet arthropathy** (fă-set' ăr-throp'ah-thē, fă'-sět)—disease or abnormality of the joints (facet joints) of the vertebrae

**Flexeril** (flěks'ěr-ĭl)—trade name for drug used to treat muscle spasm

**focal degeneration**—main area or center of deterioration

**formalin** (fŏr'mah-lĭn)—a powerful disinfectant gas, used in water as a fluid to preserve tissue removed at surgery for pathologic evaluation; same as formaldehyde

**Gelfoam sponge**—trade name for absorbable gelatin sponge; sterile, they are used in surgery to stop the flow of blood

**gutter**—low area, trough, or groove (posterior gutter: area deep and low in the chest where fluid accumulates when in the erect position)

**herniated disk** (hěr'nē-āt"ěd)—rupture of the intervertebral disk cartilage, allowing contents to protrude through it, putting pressure on the spinal nerve roots; can cause pain

**ICD Code 540.9**—the diagnosis code for necrotizing acute appendicitis

**i.e.** [L.]—abbreviation for *id est* (that is)

**intermittent**—periodically stopping and starting again at separated intervals

**intervertebral** (ĭn"ter-věr'tě-brăl, ĭn"ter-věr-tē'-brăl)—located between two adjoining vertebrae

**Kantrex** (kăn'treks)—trade name for an antibiotic

**2+ knee and ankle jerks**—this phrase refers to the sudden reflex or involuntary movements made when the examiner uses a rubber hammer to tap the reflex points of the knees and ankles; part of the neurologic exam; in this case they are graded as 2+, which means average or normal

**L1-2**—*l*umbar spine; denotes disk space between the 1st and 2nd lumbar vertebrae

**L2-3**—*l*umbar spine; denotes disk space between the 2nd and 3rd lumbar vertebrae

**L3-4**—*l*umbar spine; denotes disk space between the 3rd and 4th lumbar vertebrae

**L4-5**—*l*umbar spine; denotes disk space between the 4th and 5th lumbar vertebrae

**L5-S1**—*l*umbar spine and *s*acral spine; denotes space between 5th lumbar vertebrae and 1st sacral vertebra

**lamina** (pl. laminae) (lăm'ĭ-nah)—part of the back of the bony arch of each vertebra

**laminectomy** (lăm"ĭ-něk'tō-mē)—removal of a lamina

**lateral recess syndrome**—in spinal anatomy, the lateral recess is within the spinal canal; narrowing of the lateral recess causes compression of the nerve roots, which causes pain in the back and legs and difficulty walking

**ligamentum flavum** [L.] (lĭg"ah-mĕn-tŭm flāv'ŭm)—band of yellow elastic tissue that assists in maintaining or regaining the erect position between 2 adjoining vertebrae (sometimes called yellow ligament)

**light touch**—when an examiner lightly strokes a part of the body, such as the extremities, to determine the patient's ability to feel; used in evaluation of the central nervous system

**lumbosacral** (lŭm"bō-sā'krăl)—pertaining to the lumbar region of the spine and the sacrum; low back and pelvis

**myelogram** (mī'ĕ-lō-grăm)—the record produced by an x-ray of the spinal cord obtained after injection of dye into the spinal canal

**nipple retraction**—the inward displacement of the nipple below the level of the surrounding breast tissue

**Norflex** (nŏr'flĕks)—trade name for a drug used to treat muscle spasms

**Pap smear**—a smear of cells taken from the vagina or cervix to be studied for evidence of cancer; named for Dr. George N. Papanicolaou, 1883 to 1962

**pinprick**—when the examiner actually pricks a patient's skin with a sharp point to determine feeling; part of the evaluation of the central nervous system

**pleura** (ploor'ah)—a serous membrane lining the thoracic or pleural cavity

**prone** (prōn)—lying face downward

**radicular pain** (rah-dĭk'ū-lăr)—pain along an area of distribution of a specific nerve or nerves caused by pressure on the nerve root; pain may be felt in the low back or legs or, in cervical radicular pain, in one or both arms

**rongeur** [Fr.] (ron-zhur')—a surgical instrument used for cutting tough tissue, such as bone

**S1 root**—nerve root exiting from the spinal cord and passing through the vertebra of the *s*acral spine, 1st vertebra

**sacroiliac** (sā"krō-ĭl'ē-ăk)—the sacral and iliac spines—where they join, with associated ligaments

**scaphoid** (skăf'oid)—in physical examination of the abdomen, the abdominal wall has a concave, or sunken, contour

**scoliosis** (skō"lē-ō'sĭs)—a sideways deviation in the normally straight vertical line of the spine (S-shaped spine)

**SICU**—abbreviation for *s*urgical *i*ntensive *c*are *u*nit (sometimes dictated "sic-u")

**spurring**—small projecting outgrowths from any structure; most often pertaining to bony outgrowths

**straight-leg raising** *or* **straight leg raising**—the examiner observes the patient's ability to raise the legs; part of the evaluation of the central nervous system

**subarachnoid space** (sub"ah-răk-noid)—space between the arachnoid membrane and the pia mater, 2 of the layers of membranes that cover the brain and spinal cord

**Tylenol with codeine**—brand name anti-inflammatory pain reliever with narcotic taken for relief of moderate to severe pain

**Vi-Drape**—brand name antibiotic-impregnated transparent plastic sheet used in surgery to cover area surrounding the surgical field

## TABLE CS6-1   THE CRANIAL NERVES

| NUMBER | Name | Function |
| --- | --- | --- |
| I | Olfactory | Sensory: smell |
| II | Optic | Sensory: vision |
| III | Oculomotor | Motor: movement of the eyeball, regulation of the size of the pupil |
| IV | Trochlear | Motor: eye movements |
| V | Trigeminal | Sensory: sensations of head and face, muscle sense<br>Motor: mastication<br>Note: divided into three branches: the ophthalmic branch, the maxillary branch and the mandibular branch |
| VI | Abducens | Motor: movement of the eyeball, particularly abduction |
| VII | Facial | Sensory: taste<br>Motor: facial expressions, secretions of saliva |
| VIII | Vestibulocochlear | Sensory: balance, hearing<br>Note: divided into two branches: the vestibular branch responsible for balance and the cochlear branch responsible for hearing |
| IX | Glossopharyngeal | Sensory: taste<br>Motor: swallowing, secretion of saliva |
| X | Vagus | Sensory: sensation of organs supplied<br>Motor: movement of organs supplied<br>Note: supplies the head, pharynx, bronchus, esophagus, liver and stomach |
| XI | Accessory | Motor: shoulder movement, turning of head, voice production |
| XII | Hypoglossal | Motor: tongue movements |

Source: Rizzo, Donald C. (2007). *Fundamentals of Anatomy & Physiology,* 2nd ed. Clifton Park, NY: Delmar Cengage Learning.

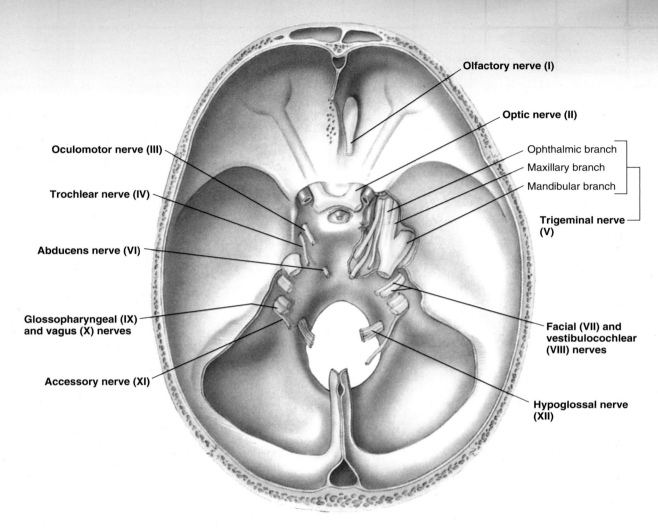

Olfactory nerve (I)

Optic nerve (II)

Ophthalmic branch
Maxillary branch
Mandibular branch

Trigeminal nerve (V)

Oculomotor nerve (III)

Trochlear nerve (IV)

Abducens nerve (VI)

Glossopharyngeal (IX) and vagus (X) nerves

Facial (VII) and vestibulocochlear (VIII) nerves

Accessory nerve (XI)

Hypoglossal nerve (XII)

**Figure CS6-1** The cranial nerves are named by roman numerals or by name, indicating distribution or function. (*Delmar/Cengage Learning*)

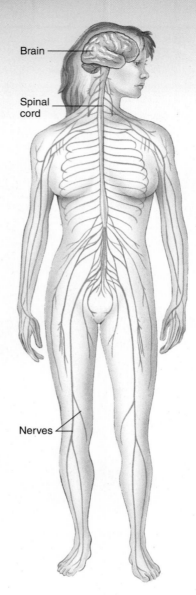

**Figure CS6-2**  Nervous system—brain, spinal cord, nerves. (*Delmar/Cengage Learning*)

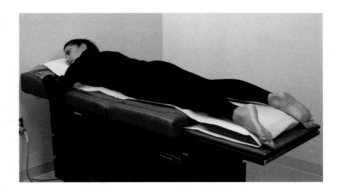

**Figure CS6-3**   Prone position. (*Delmar/Cengage Learning*)

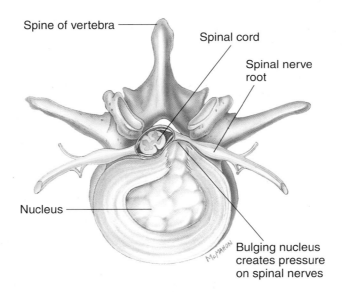

**Figure CS6-4**   Herniated disk. (*Delmar/Cengage Learning*)

# CASE STUDY 7: ORTHOPEDICS/ENDOCRINE SYSTEMS

**Patient Name**

T. J. Moreno

**Address**

10620 SW 72nd Court
Miami FL 33156-5902

**Situation**

Mr. Moreno was involved in an automobile accident that resulted in his left ankle joint being unstable. He was treated conservatively for several months, but conservative treatment failed. The patient was therefore admitted for surgical correction of the left ankle via fusion stabilization of the joint. When the patient's preoperative laboratory work was done, it was discovered that he had previously undiagnosed diabetes mellitus and hypertension. He was referred to a medical doctor for consultation and further treatment of his medical conditions. His ankle was repaired surgically, and he was discharged to the care of his endocrinologist, who entered Mr. Moreno into an Actos and metformin trial for diabetes mellitus.

Review Figure CS7-1, Endocrine system; Figure CS7-2A, Right ankle and foot, lateral view, and B, right ankle and foot, superior view.

**Student Name** _____

**Patient:  T. J. Moreno**

| SEQUENCE OF REPORTS | Date Completed | Grade |
|---|---|---|
| History and Physical Examination | _____ | _____ |
| Consultation | _____ | _____ |
| Diagnostic Imaging Report | _____ | _____ |
| Operative Report | _____ | _____ |
| Discharge Summary | _____ | _____ |

**NOTE**:  Study the glossary for Case Study 7. Enter the date each report is completed in the space provided. When you have transcribed all reports, tear this sheet out and attach it to the front of the reports (in the order listed above); give completed reports to the instructor.

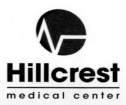

**Hillcrest**
medical center

# GLOSSARY FOR CASE STUDY 7

**A₁c** *or* **A1C** (dictated "A-one-see")—test of overall effectiveness of blood glucose control over a period of time, usually for about the preceding 3 months

**acanthosis nigricans** (ak-ăn-thō'sĭs nī'grĭ-kănz)—velvety, benign growths on the skin of the neck, groin, and axillae; may be associated with insulin resistance, malignancy, or obesity

**Actos** (ak'tōs)—brand name oral antidiabetic agent

**Ancef** (ăn'sĕf)—brand name antibiotic used to treat a wide variety of bacterial infections; used either intramuscularly or intravenously

**arthrodesis** (ăr-thrō-dē'-sis)—surgical fusion of a joint

**arthrosis** (ăr-thrō'-sis)—degenerative joint changes

**calcaneocuboid** (kăl-kā'-nē-ō-kyū'boyd)—relating to the calcaneus (heel bone) and cuboid bone (bone in front of the heel bone)

**cubonavicular** (kyū'bō-nă-vĭk'yū-lăr)—relating to the cuboid bone and the navicular bone (bone on top of the cuboid bone)

**dexamethasone** (dĕk'să-mĕth'ă-sōn)—generic name for anti-inflammatory agent; used to test adrenal function

**dysuria** (dĭs-yū'rē-ă)—difficulty or pain with urination

**equinus** (ē-kwī'nŭs)—abnormal position of the foot in which the toes are lower than the heel, causing toe-walking

**exsanguinated** (ek-săng'gwĭ-nāt'd)—the action or process of having drained or lost circulating blood; made bloodless

**extensor digitorum brevis** (eks-tĕn'sŏr dĭj"-ĭ-tŏr'-ŭm brĕ'vĭs)—muscle of the foot that extends the 2nd through 5th toes

**Glucophage** (glū'kō-făzh)—trade name for antidiabetic medication

**goiter** (goy'tĕr)—chronic enlargement of the thyroid gland, not usually due to malignancy

**hindfoot** (hīnd'foot)—the part of the foot that contains the calcaneus, talus, cuboid, and navicular bones; the back part of the foot

**Humalog** (hū'mă-log)—trade name for antidiabetic medication

**inferior peroneal retinaculum**—a fibrous band that holds in place the tendons of the muscles on the outside of the ankle

**intraneural** (in'tră-nū-răl)—within a nerve

**Lantus** (lăn'tŭs)—brand name for a type of insulin

**lisinopril** (lī-sĭn'ō-prĭl)—generic name of drug used primarily to treat hypertension

**Lortab**—brand name of narcotic used to treat moderate to severe pain

**malalignment** (măl'ă-līn'ment)—displacement of bones out of line in relation to joints

**metatarsal** (met'ă-tar'-săl)—one of the 5 long bones on the top of the foot

**metformin** (met-for'mĭn)—generic name for Glucophage, antidiabetic medication

**occult fracture**—a fracture that is not visible in an x-ray within 24 to 48 hours of trauma or injury but will become visible in x-rays within 3 to 4 weeks, at the time the fracture site is healing or new bone is forming

**osteophyte** (os'tē-ō-fīt")—a bony outgrowth or protuberance

**osteotome** (os'tē-ō-tōm")—an instrument used for cutting bone

**perihardware fracture**—a fracture of the bone around a plate or screws that are already in place

**periosteum** (pĕr"ē-os'tē-ŭm)—the thick, fibrous membrane covering the entire surface of a bone

**polydipsia** (pol"ē-dip'sē-ă)—excessive, prolonged thirst

**polyuria** (pol"ē-yū'rē-ă)—excessive excretion of urine resulting in frequent and profuse urination

**popliteal sciatic block** (pop-li-tē'ăl sī-ăt'ik)—nerve block of the sciatic nerve at the popliteal fossa (back of the knee); used to relieve pain in the lower leg

**posterior tibial tendon**—tendon that starts in the calf, stretches down behind the inside of the ankle, and attaches to bones in the middle of the foot

**S/P**—abbreviation for *status post*

**subtalar** (sŭb-tā'lăr)—below the talus bone

**talonavicular** (tā'lō-nă-vik'yū-lăr)—relating to the talus bone and the navicular bone (both bones are on the top of the ankle)

**Telfa** (tĕl'fa)—brand name for a wound dressing consisting of a thin layer of cotton fibers wrapped in plastic film to keep it from sticking to wounds

**Webril** (web'rĭl)—brand name for cotton material used as absorbent surgical dressing

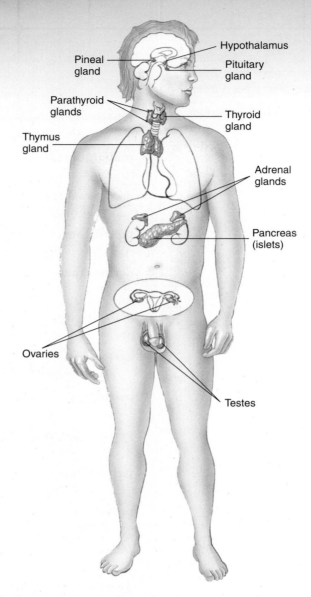

**Figure CS7-1**    Endocrine system. (*Delmar/Cengage Learning*)

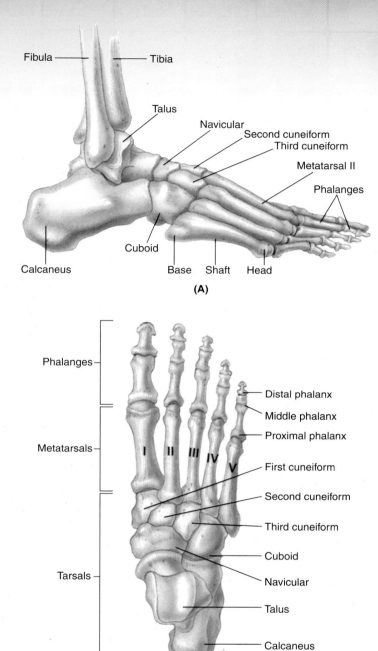

**Figure CS7-2**  (A) Right ankle and foot, lateral view. (B) Right ankle and foot, superior view. (*Delmar/Cengage Learning*)

# CASE STUDY 8: VASCULAR/RENAL SYSTEMS

**Patient Name**

Chapman Robert Kinsey

**Address**

309 North Fifth Street
Miami FL 33133-4038

**Situation**

Mr. Chapman Kinsey is an elderly gentleman with multiple medical problems. The most acute problem at this time is a gangrenous ulcer on his left great toe, and he was admitted to Hillcrest for incision and drainage of this ulcer along with the administration of intravenous antibiotics. The patient was scheduled for an arteriogram, but his admission laboratory work showed him to be in renal failure. His admission was prolonged due to several complications, which ultimately required surgical intervention. After 2 weeks of a difficult admission, the patient was discharged to a skilled nursing facility for further care and rehabilitation.

Review Figure CS8-1, Common sites for peripheral arterial occlusive disease; Figure CS8-2, Circulatory system; and Figure CS8-3, Organs of the urinary system.

**Student Name** _____

**Patient:  Chapman Robert Kinsey**

| SEQUENCE OF REPORTS | Date Completed | Grade |
|---|---|---|
| History and Physical Examination | _____ | _____ |
| Consultation | _____ | _____ |
| Diagnostic Imaging Report 1 | _____ | _____ |
| Diagnostic Imaging Report 2 | _____ | _____ |
| Diagnostic Imaging Report 3 | _____ | _____ |
| Diagnostic Imaging Report 4 | _____ | _____ |
| Operative Report | _____ | _____ |
| Diagnostic Imaging Report 5 | _____ | _____ |
| Diagnostic Imaging Report 6 | _____ | _____ |
| Discharge Summary | _____ | _____ |

**NOTE**:  Study the glossary for Case Study 8. Enter the date each report is completed in the space provided. When you have transcribed all reports, tear this sheet out and attach it to the front of the reports (in the order listed above); give completed reports to the instructor.

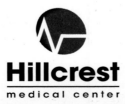

**Hillcrest**
medical center

# Glossary for Case Study 8

**acute renal failure**—sudden loss of kidney function

**anaphylactic shock** (an′ă-fĭ-lak′tĭk)—widespread and very serious allergic reaction; symptoms can include dizziness, swelling of tongue, low blood pressure, and labored breathing

**anastomosis** (ă-nas″tō-mō′sis)—an operative union of 2 structures (blood vessels, nerves)

**anterior tibial artery**—artery that runs from the knee to the ankle on the front of the leg

**aortic bifurcation** (ā-ōr′tic bī′fūr-kā′shun)—the point at which the abdominal aorta branches into the right and left common iliac arteries; this point is usually at about the level of the 4th lumbar vertebra

**Bicitra** (bī-sī′tră)—brand name of medication used to make urine less acidic

**BUN**—abbreviation for *b*lood *u*rea *n*itrogen, a blood test used to evaluate kidney function; each letter is dictated individually

**cardiac silhouette** (kăr′dē-ăk sĭl″oo-ĕt′)—the shadow of the heart as it appears on a chest x-ray

**cardiomegaly** (kar″dē-ō-meg′ă-lē)—enlargement of the heart

**carotid endarterectomy** (ka-rot′id end′ar-ter-ek′tŏ-mē)—surgical removal of material occluding the carotid artery

**CHF**—abbreviation for *c*ongestive *h*eart *f*ailure, a condition in which the heart cannot pump enough blood to the body's other organs

**common iliac artery**—one of the 2 arteries in which the aorta branches at the 4th lumbar vertebra

**COPD**—abbreviation for *c*hronic *o*bstructive *p*ulmonary *d*isease, a progressive condition of the lungs in which the tiny air sacs (alveoli) are damaged or destroyed, making it more difficult to breathe and leading to emphysema and chronic bronchitis; each letter is dictated individually

**C-reactive protein**—blood test that measures inflammation (sometimes dictated CRP)

**creatinine** (krē-ăt′i-nēn, -nĭn)—a blood test that measures kidney function

**diltiazem** (dĭl-tī′ă-zĕm)—generic name for medication used to treat high blood pressure, chest pain, and certain heart rhythm disorders

**dorsalis pedis artery** (dor-săl′is pēd′is)—artery that passes along the top of the foot from the ankle to close to the toes

**echogenic** (ek′ō-jen′ik)—pertaining to a structure or tissue that is able to be imaged on x-ray

**ectatic** (ek-tat′ik)—related to or marked by distension, dilatation, or expansion

**external iliac artery**—one of the 2 branches into which the common iliac artery divides; the common iliac artery is 1 of the branches of the aortic bifurcation

**extruding** (eks-trūd′ing)—the condition of thrusting or pressing out

**furosemide** (fyū-rō′sĕ-mīd)—generic name of medication used to increase urine formation and output (diuretic)

**hallux valgus** (hal′ŭks văl′gŭs)—a drifting of the large toe in the direction of the small toe, with formation of a bump on the inside of the big toe over the metatarsal bone; bunion deformity

**heparin** (hep′ă-rin)—generic name of medication used to treat and prevent blood clots in the veins, arteries, or lungs

**hydronephrosis** (hī′drō-nĕ-frō′sis)—distension of the kidney with urine, caused by backward pressure on the kidney when flow of urine is obstructed

**hyperkalemia** (hī′per-kā-lē′mē-ă, hī′per-kă-lē′mē-ă)—elevated blood level of potassium

**Lanoxin** (lă-nŏk′sĭn)—brand name of medication used to treat congestive heart failure and atrial fibrillation

**metabolic acidosis** (met′ă-bŏl′ik as′i-dō′sis)—a condition of pH imbalance in which the body has accumulated too much acid; can occur as a result of diarrhea or kidney failure

**metatarsophalangeal joint** (met′ă-tar′sō-fă-lăn′jē-ăl)—the joint between the head of the metatarsal and the base of the phalanx of the toe

**Micro-Stick needle**—brand name for needle used to obtain intravenous access

**Mills valvulotome** (văl′vū-lō-tōm′)—brand name for an instrument used to surgically convert a vein into an artery in arterial bypass

**Omni Flush catheter**—a type of catheter used to perform vascular studies

**organomegaly** (ōr′gă-nō-měg′ă-lē)—abnormal enlargement of the abdominal organs

**osteomyelitis** (ŏs′tē-ō-mī′ĕ-lī′tis)—inflammation of the bone marrow and adjacent bone

**paramediastinal contours** (pă'ra-mē'dē-ă-stī'năl)—the structures that appear in the proximity of the middle of the chest cavity as seen on chest x-ray; the heart, aorta, chest portion of the trachea, esophagus, lymph nodes, and thymus gland

**pentoxifylline** (pěn'tŏx-ĭf'ĭ-lēn)—generic name of medication used to improve the symptoms of blood flow problems in the extremities (legs and arms)

**peripheral vascular disease**—refers to disease of blood vessels outside the brain and heart

**posterior tibial artery**—artery that runs from the knee to the ankle on the back side of the leg

**Potts scissors**—brand name for fine-pointed scissors used in vascular surgery

**Prolene** (prō'lēn)—brand name for nonabsorbable suture material used for skin closure

**radio-opaque**—not transparent to x-rays or other forms of radiation

**skilled nursing facility** (abbreviated SNF, sometimes dictated "snif")—nursing home that provides skilled nursing and/or skilled rehabilitation services to patients who need skilled medical care that cannot be provided in a custodial level nursing home or in the patient's home

**superficial femoral artery**—artery that runs along the front of the thigh toward the knee, gradually coursing toward the inside of the knee

**thrombolysis** (throm'bō-lī'sis, throm-bol'i-sis)—dissolving of a thrombus (blood clot)

**tibioperoneal** (tib'ē-ō-per'ō-nē'ăl)—relating to the tibia and fibula

**tortuous** (tōr'chū-ŭs)—having many curves; full of turns and twists

**Zocor** (zō'kor)—brand name for a cholesterol-lowering medication

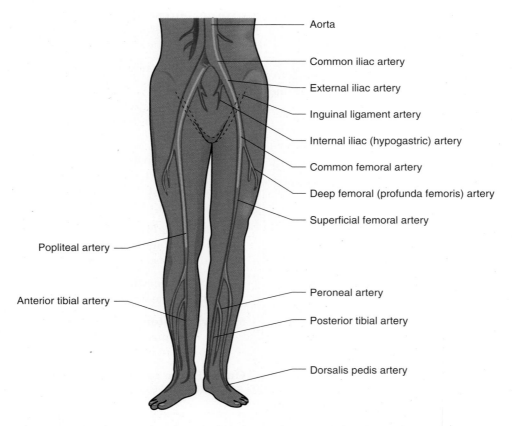

**Figure CS8-1**    Common sites for peripheral arterial occlusive disease. (*Delmar/Cengage Learning*)

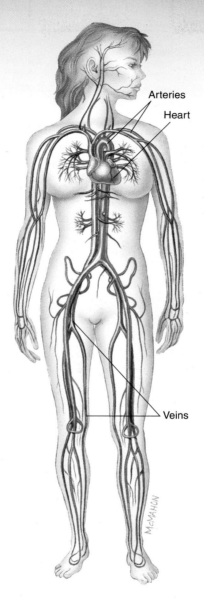

Arteries

Heart

Veins

**Figure CS8-2** Circulatory system. (*Delmar/Cengage Learning*)

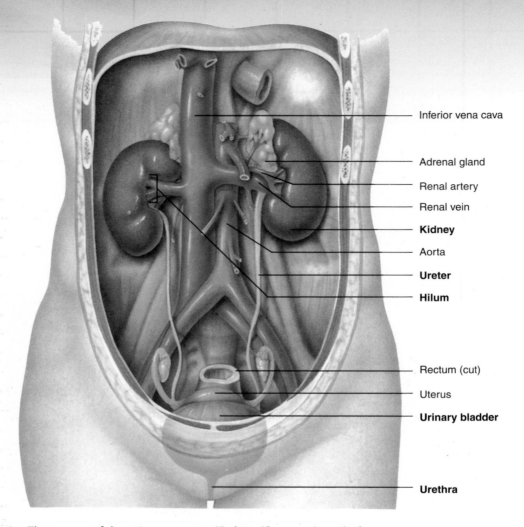

**Figure CS8-3** The organs of the urinary system. (*Delmar/Cengage Learning*)

# CASE STUDY 9: MUSCULOSKELETAL SYSTEM

**Patient Name**

Marilyn Sue Stone

**Address**

9038 SW 45th Terrace
Miami FL 33165-5912

**Situation**

Marilyn Sue Stone is a middle-aged lady who has had multiple hip replacements and revisions of those replacements in the past. She was admitted to the hospital for total right hip replacement revision. Her prior right hip replacement, which had been present for 28 years, was seen on x-ray to be loosened, thus requiring revision. The patient's surgery was accomplished, and x-rays showed a good result. She was discharged to a skilled nursing facility. Physical Therapy will consult on Ms. Stone and develop a plan for her postoperative rehabilitation.

Review Figure CS9-1, Skeletal system; Figure CS9-2, Location of hip fractures; Figure CS9-3, Internal fixation device.

**Student Name** _____

**Patient: Marilyn Sue Stone**

| SEQUENCE OF REPORTS | Date Completed | Grade |
|---|---|---|
| History and Physical Examination | _____ | _____ |
| Diagnostic Imaging Report 1 | _____ | _____ |
| Operative Report | _____ | _____ |
| Pathology Report | _____ | _____ |
| Diagnostic Imaging Report 2 | _____ | _____ |
| Diagnostic Imaging Report 3 | _____ | _____ |
| Discharge Summary | _____ | _____ |

**NOTE**: Study the glossary for Case Study 9. Enter the date each report is completed in the space provided. When you have transcribed all reports, tear this sheet out and attach it to the front of the reports (in the order listed above); give completed reports to the instructor.

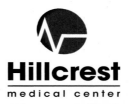

**Hillcrest**
medical center

# GLOSSARY FOR CASE STUDY 9

**abduct** (ab-dukt')—to move away from the middle of the body

**acetabular component** (as'-ĕ-tab'yū-lār)—the part of an artificial hip joint that takes the place of the diseased or injured acetabulum

**acetabulum** (as'-ĕ-tab'yū-lŭm)—a cup-shaped depression at the base of the hip bone into which the ball-shaped head of the femur (thigh bone) fits

**adduct** (ă'dŭkt)—to move toward the middle of the body

**Allegra** (a-lĕ'gra)—brand name of medication used to treat seasonal allergies

**allograft** (al'ō-graft)—a graft of tissue from a donor of the same species but different genetic makeup than the recipient; tissue transplant between 2 humans

**All-Poly cup**—brand name of polyethylene cup used for cemented fixation in total hip replacement

**arthrogryposis** (ar'thrō-gri-pō'sis)—defect of the limbs noted at birth and characterized by severe contractures of multiple joints

**arthroplasty** (ar'thrō-plas'tē)—creation of an artificial joint to correct advanced degenerative arthritis

**autologous** (aw-tol'ŏ-gŭs)—referring to blood or blood components the donor has previously donated and receives at a later time

**Burch-Schneider retention cage**—hip reconstruction cage that screws onto the pelvic bone; allows a prosthesis to be cemented into the cage for total hip arthroplasty

**cancellous bone** (kan-sĕ'lŭs, kan'sĕ-lŭs)—spongy interior layer of bone that protects the bone marrow; also found on edges of rounded bones on arms and legs

**cephalosporin** (sĕf'ă-lō-spōr'ĭn)—generic name for antibiotic

**codeine** (kō'dēn)—generic name for narcotic medication used to treat mild to moderate pain

**congenital** (kŏn-jĕn'ĭ-tăl)—acquired during development in the uterus and not through heredity

**directed packed cells**—packed cells are separated from plasma when blood is donated; directed packed cells is blood that has been donated for a specific person

**dysplastic** (dĭs-plas'tĭk)—pertaining to abnormal tissue development

**external rotation**—rotation away from the center of the body

**femoral canal** (fĕm'ŏ-răl)—in orthopedics, the interior longitudinal cavity of the femur bone

**femoral component**—the part of an artificial hip joint that takes the place of the diseased or injured femoral head

**flex** (fleks)—to bend; to move a joint in such a direction as to approximate the 2 parts it connects

**gluteus medius/minimus group** (glū'tē-ŭs mē'dē-ŭs mĭn'ĭ-mŭs)—muscles situated on the outer surface of the pelvis that abduct the thigh when the limb is extended

**greater trochanter** (trō'kăn-tĕr)—an upper part of the femur to which the gluteus medius and minimus muscles, and others, attach

**hepatitis B core antibody** (hĕp-ă-tī'tis)—first antibody to appear following an acute hepatitis B infection; it will persist, sometimes for years, following resolution of the infection

**internal rotation**—rotation toward the center of the body

**ischium** (is'kē-ŭm, ish'ē-ŭm)—the lower and back part of the hip bone where it joins the pelvis

**IT band**—abbreviation for *ilio*tibial band; the letters are dictated individually

**left lateral decubitus position** (dē-kyū'bĭ-tŭs)—lying down on the left side

**methyl methacrylate** (mĕth'il meth-ă'krĭ-lāt)—a cement used in joint replacement surgery

**musculoskeletal system** (mŭs"kyū-lō-skĕl'ĕ-tăl)—relating to the muscles and to the skeleton

**Nasacort** (nāz'ă-kŏrt)—brand name of nasal spray used to treat seasonal allergies or hay fever

**nulliparous** (nŭl-ip'ă-rŭs)—never having borne a child

**osteolysis** (os'tē-ol'i-sis, os'tē-ō-lī'sis)—softening, absorption, and destruction of bony tissue

**osteotomized** (os'tē-ŏt'ŏ-mīzd)—bone that has been cut, usually by means of a saw or osteotome (cutting instrument)

**pelvic dissociation**—loss of bony continuity through both anterior and posterior columns of the pelvis

**polyethylene** (pŏl'i-eth'i-lēn)—most popular plastic used in the world

**prosthesis** (prŏs-thē'sis)—a fabricated substitute used to assist a damaged or replace a missing body part

**spironolactone** (spī-rō'nō-lăk-tōn)—generic name for medication used to treat fluid retention

**verapamil** (ve-răp'ă-mĭl)—generic name for medication used to treat abnormal heart rhythms, chest pains, and also migraine headaches

**wing of the ilium** (ĭ'-lē-ŭm)—the upper flaring portion of the ilium that looks like a fan; the ilium forms the top two-thirds of the hip bone

**Zoloft** (zō'loft)—brand name for medication used to treat depression and anxiety

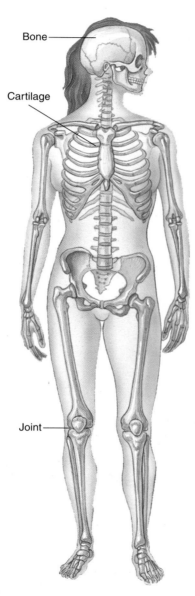

**Figure CS9-1**    Skeletal system. (*Delmar/Cengage Learning*)

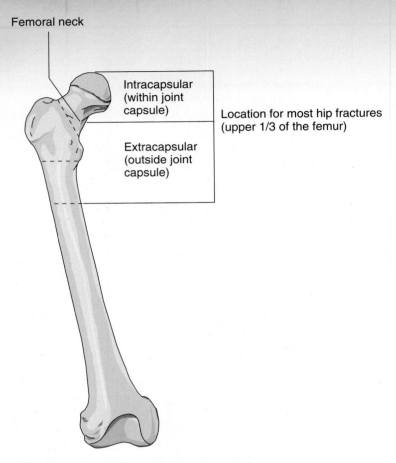

**Figure CS9-2** Location of hip fractures. (*Delmar/Cengage Learning*)

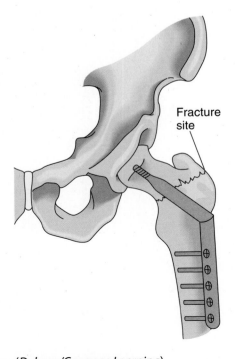

**Figure CS9-3** Internal fixation device. (*Delmar/Cengage Learning*)

# CASE STUDY 10: RESPIRATORY SYSTEM

**Patient Name**

J. Randy Rolen

**Address**

14302 Briarbend
Key Biscayne FL 33149-6747

**Situation**

This patient experienced respiratory distress and was brought by ambulance to Hillcrest emergency room early one morning. The emergency room physician performed chest tube insertion. Serial chest x-rays were performed in the radiology department to determine whether the patient's lung remained expanded. Due to a worsening in the patient's respiratory status, a 2nd procedure had to be performed. After continued complications and significant deterioration in the patient's condition, a pulmonary/thoracic surgeon was requested to assess the patient. He recommended transfer to Forrest General Medical Center for more complicated surgery. The patient was transferred to Forrest General for further evaluation and care.

Review Figure CS10-1, Respiratory system; Figure CS10-2, Emphysema; and Figure CS10-3, Anteroposterior (AP) view of the chest.

**Student Name** _____

**Patient:  J. Randy Rolen**

| SEQUENCE OF REPORTS | Date Completed | Grade |
| --- | --- | --- |
| History and Physical Examination | _____ | _____ |
| Operative Report 1 | _____ | _____ |
| Radiology Report 1 | _____ | _____ |
| Radiology Report 2 | _____ | _____ |
| Operative Report 2 | _____ | _____ |
| Radiology Report 3 | _____ | _____ |
| Consultation | _____ | _____ |
| Discharge Summary | _____ | _____ |

**NOTE**:  Study the glossary for Case Study 10. Enter the date each report is completed in the space provided. When you have transcribed all reports, tear this sheet out and attach it to the front of the reports (in the order listed above); give completed reports to the instructor.

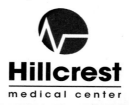

**Hillcrest**
medical center

# GLOSSARY FOR CASE STUDY 10

**ablation** (ăb-lā'shŭn)—separation, detachment, or removal of organ or tissue, especially by surgical means

**anesthetize** (ah-něs'thě-tīz)—to put under the influence of anesthetics—drugs or agents used to abolish the sensation of pain

**aorta** (ā-ŏr'tah)—the main trunk of the arterial system, conveying blood from the heart

**benzoin** (běn'zoin)—a generic topical anesthetic

**Betadine solution** (bā'tă-dīn)—brand name for an antiseptic solution used on the skin

**bronchodilator** (brŏng'kō-dī'lā-tor)—a class of medication that expands the air passages of the lungs

**bronchopleural** (brŏng'kō-ploor'ăl)—pertaining to a bronchus and the pleura

**cannula** (kăn'ū-lă)—a tube for insertion into a duct or cavity

**catheter** (kăth'ě-těr)—a tubular, flexible instrument (metal or rubber) for either withdrawing fluids or introducing fluids into a body cavity or vessel

**ciprofloxacin** (sĭp'rō-flŏx'ă-sin)—generic name for a broad-spectrum antibiotic

**COPD**—abbreviation for *c*hronic *o*bstructive *p*ulmonary *d*isease

**emergent** (ē-měr'gent)—pertaining to an emergency

**emphysema** (ěm'fĭ-sē'mă)—a pathologic accumulation of air in tissues or organs that causes abnormal swelling of body tissues

**Heimlich valve** (hīm'lĭk)—a one-way valve that allows air to flow out of the chest through a chest tube; allows attachment of chest tube apparatus to be carried on the patient's body

**hemithorax** (hěm'ē-thō'raks)—one side of the chest

**hemostat** (hē'mō-stăt)—a small surgical clamp for constricting a blood vessel

**HJR**—abbreviation for *h*epato*j*ugular *r*eflux (a GI term)

**hypertension** (hī'pěr-těn'shŭn)—persistently high arterial blood pressure

**ichthyosis** (ĭk'thē-ō'sis)—dryness and fishlike scaling of the skin

**intercostal** (in'těr-kos'tăl)—between the ribs

**loculate** (lŏk'ū-lāt)—divided into cavities (loculi)

**loculus** (pl. loculi) (lŏk'ū-lŭs)—a small space or cavity

**marked**—noticeable; to an extreme

**PCO₂ or PCO2**—*p*artial pressure (or tension) of carbon dioxide or $CO_2$ (lab test done on blood gas studies)

**percutaneous** (pěr'kū-tā'nē-ŭs)—performed through the skin

**pH**—hydrogen ion concentration in urine, blood, and other body fluids (neutral = 7.00; more than 7.00 is alkaline; less than 7.00 is acidic). NOTE: Should always be written with lowercase p and capitalized H, even at the beginning of sentence.

**Pleur-evac system** (suction or tube) (ploor'ē-văk)—thoracic drainage system to evacuate air and/or fluid from the chest cavity

**pleurodesis** (ploo'-rō-dē-sis)—the production of adhesions between the parietal and the visceral pleura

**pneumothorax** (nū'mō-thōr'aks)—the presence of free air or gas in the pleural cavity

**PO₂ or PO2**—*p*artial pressure (tension) of oxygen or $O_2$ (a blood gas term)

**portable chest**—medical jargon pertaining to the equipment used and the process of obtaining a chest x-ray outside of the radiology department; e.g., at the patient's bedside

**Proventil** (prō-věn-til)—trade name of a bronchodilator medication

**Pseudomonas aeruginosa** (soo'dō-mō'năs ě-rū'jĭn-ō'sa)—the type of bacterial species of the genus, and the only one pathogenic for humans, made up of microorganisms that produce the blue-green pigment that give the color to "blue pus" observed in certain suppurative infections

**radiograph** (rā'dē-ō-grăf)—film produced by radiography, commonly called an x-ray

**resolution**—the subsidence or disappearance of a pathologic condition

**Rocephin** (rō-cěf'in)—trade name for antibiotic medication

**sclerotherapy** (sklě'rō-thěr'ah-pē)—treatment involving the injection of a hardening solution into vessels or tissues

**stat**—abbreviation for [L.] statim (immediately)

**Streptococcus** (strep'tō-kŏk'ŭs)—bacteria growing in chains found in human mouth and intestine; sometimes they can cause disease

**subtherapeutic** (sub'thĕr'ah-pū'tik)—a less than therapeutic level, usually referring to the blood level of a particular drug or medication

**Theo-Dur** (thē'ō-dŭr)—trade name for a bronchodilator

**theophylline** (thē-ŏf'ĭ-lĭn)—generic name for a smooth muscle relaxant, used chiefly for its bronchodilator effect

**thoracic** (thō-răs'ĭk)—pertaining to the chest

**thoracostomy** (thō'rah-kŏs'tō-mē)—surgical creation of an opening in the thorax (chest wall) for the purpose of drainage

**thoracotomy** (thō'rah-kŏt'ō-mē)—surgical incision into the thorax

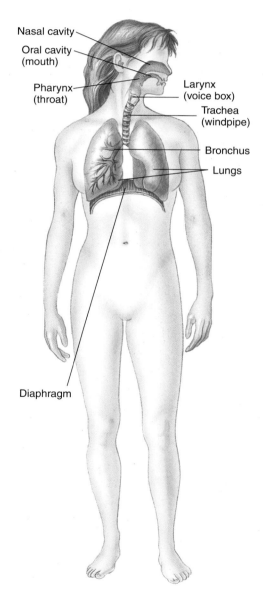

**Figure CS10-1**   Respiratory system. (*Delmar/Cengage Learning*)

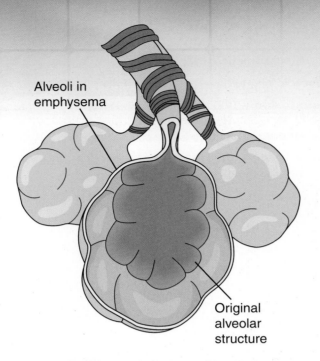

**Figure CS10-2**    Emphysema. (*Delmar/Cengage Learning*)

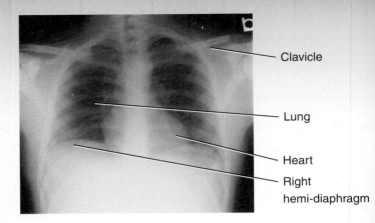

**Figure CS10-3**    Anteroposterior (AP) view of the chest. (*Delmar/Cengage Learning*)

# SECTION 5

## QUALI-CARE CLINIC

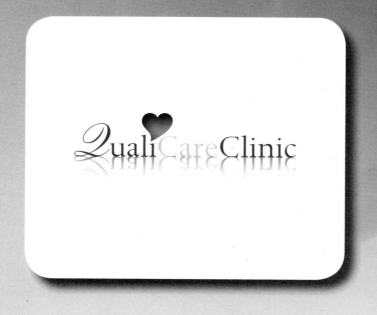

# WELCOME TO QUALI-CARE CLINIC

You will be transcribing outpatient medical reports for Quali-Care Clinic, a medical facility housed in a free-standing office building adjacent to Hillcrest Medical Center and containing the offices of physicians and health care providers from different medical specialties. Those in the specialties of Family Practice and Internal Medicine act as primary care physicians (PCPs) who see their patients on a regular basis, paying close attention to their over-all well-being and referring them to specialists or to Hillcrest Medical Center for further evaluation and treatment as necessary. (*NB*: PCPs for female patients include Gynecology and Obstetrics.)

You will be transcribing 25 outpatient reports that relate to these medical specialty areas. These reports demonstrate variations in style, format, and content common to the dictating habits of the originators of medical records—habits usually learned while in medical school. Model Report Forms include a model HPIP report (history, physical, impression, plan) and a model SOAP note (subjective, objective, assessment, plan). These two formats or variations thereof are the mainstay of physicians' outpatient medical record (chart) on each patient. The SOAP format is less formal and is generally used in doctors' chart notes. Each physician personalizes a format using a preferred style. Correspondence is introduced in these reports, which is one way PCPs and consultants communicate with each other. See Model Report Form 10 for an example.

Included in a medical record would be patient demographic information, the next of kin, what to do in case of emergency, laboratory and x-ray results, and vital signs written in at each visit. The doctor may dictate chart notes after each patient visit or telephone call to or from the patient *or* these notes may be handwritten. Elderly or very ill patients or families may be counseled regarding a living will, a directive to physicians, or otherwise be asked to indicate their wishes should a terminal situation exist. This may be referred to as "DNR" status or a "no code" status, which means do not resuscitate (DNR) should cardiac or respiratory failure occur, and do not allow hospital or emergency personnel to institute lifesaving measures (like a "Code Blue"). There are many variations in this type of planning, but patients and their families have the right and the responsibility to state their wishes and to have them honored.

When a patient is referred to a specialist, special examinations or procedures, both invasive and noninvasive, may occur. If all attempts to improve a patient's health fail using outpatient measures, then inpatient treatment must follow. This involves admission to a hospital, perhaps Hillcrest, a transplant facility, burn center, or a rehabilitation unit.

In summary, outpatient care is done on the following levels:
- Telephone calls and/or letters to the PCP
- Scheduled appointments with the PCP
- Requests for laboratory tests and x-rays for diagnostic purposes
- Referral to a specialist (or consultant) for further evaluation and treatment
- Treatment in the specialist's (or consultant's) office with more advanced, noninvasive procedures
- Invasive procedures that may include surgery
- Transfer to Hillcrest Medical Center, if necessary, for further evaluation and treatment
- Aftercare to include physical therapy, occupational therapy, nursing home care—either skilled (short term) or custodial (long term)—with appropriate followup by the original PCP or a hospitalist (physician whose job is exclusively attending to patients in hospitals and nursing homes and communicating with the PCP)

Extensive records are kept at each level of patient care, and this involves dictation and transcription. Remember, *legally*, what was not written down or transcribed was not done. MTs create records that are vital to patient care and are legal documents subject to subpoena. They create a medical history that is the basis for reimbursement from third-party payers (insurance companies), for research purposes, and for risk management purposes (documenting medical errors).

We hope that transcribing the outpatient reports proves to be a valuable learning experience.

Sincerely,

*Jeannette Rachel Soler*

Jeannette Rachel Soler, CMT, RHIA
Director, Health Information Management Department

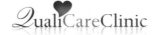

# QUALI-CARE CLINIC OUTPATIENT REPORT LOG

### QualiCareClinic

**Student Name:** _____

*Attach this form (or a copy) to your transcribed work; give to Instructor for grading.*

| QC Report No./Patient Name/Report Type | Grade | Date Completed |
|---|---|---|
| QC 1a&b   Murray R. Abell/Consult & Echocardiogram (Cardiology) | _____ | _____ |
| QC 2   Richard Cates/Operative Procedure (Genitourinary) | _____ | _____ |
| QC 3   Leslie Michael Smith/Operative Report (Orthopedics) | _____ | _____ |
| QC 4   Ursula Emma Wagner/Surgical Pathology Report (Breast) | _____ | _____ |
| QC 5   Craig S. Duran/Emergency Dept Treatment Record (Pediatrics) | _____ | _____ |
| QC 6   Wilhelm Heidelberg/Interventional Radiology Report (Vascular) | _____ | _____ |
| QC 7   Jack P. Strong/Spine Clinic HPIP Note (Orthopedics) | _____ | _____ |
| QC 8   Brian Albert/Radiology Report (Orthopedics) | _____ | _____ |
| QC 9   Yuan S. Kao/Clinic SOAP Note (Vascular) | _____ | _____ |
| QC 10   Paul G. Catrou/Surgical Procedure (Orthopedics) | _____ | _____ |
| QC 11   Debbie Dolle Russell/Operative Report (Plastic Surgery) | _____ | _____ |
| QC 12   Betsy H. Bennett/Colonoscopy Procedure (Gastroenterology) | _____ | _____ |
| QC 13   Mary Fisher Lipscomb/Clinic HPIP Note (Internal Medicine) | _____ | _____ |
| QC 14   Ruby Kay Bell/Operative Report (Neurosurgery) | _____ | _____ |
| QC 15   Sherman L. Kermit/Operative Report (Urology) | _____ | _____ |
| QC 16   Suzanne S. Mira/Radiology Report (Orthopedics/Neurology) | _____ | _____ |
| QC 17   Grace Pereira/Clinic Note (Pediatric Neurology) | _____ | _____ |
| QC 18   Janet Marie Bruner/Operative Report (Obstetrics) | _____ | _____ |
| QC 19   Eduardo J. Yunis/Operative Report (Orthopedics) | _____ | _____ |
| QC 20   Merle W. Delmer/Clinic Note (Vascular) | _____ | _____ |
| QC 21   Savannah Crumrine/Operative Report (Dental Surgery) | _____ | _____ |
| QC 22   Thomas J. Gill/Operative Report (Orthopedics) | _____ | _____ |
| QC 23   Ramzi S. Cotran/Consult (Orthopedics) | _____ | _____ |
| QC 24   Barbara Christine Anello/Psychological Eval (Psychology) | _____ | _____ |
| QC 25a&b   James H. Helland/Letter & Consult (Cardiology) | _____ | _____ |

# OUTPATIENT REPORTS

This section contains a brief explanation of each patient's reason for receiving outpatient medical care at Quali-Care Clinic. A glossary of medical terms found in each report is included along with illustrations.

## REPORTS 1A&B: CARDIOLOGY CONSULT AND ECHOCARDIOGRAM

Murray R. Abell is an elderly patient with multiple medical problems who was recently diagnosed with congestive heart failure. He was referred to a cardiologist at the Quali-Care Clinic for a consult and an echocardiogram in order to determine a proper course to follow medically. See Figure QC1-1, Echocardiography; Figure QC1-2, Emphysema; Figure QC1-3, The Quest Exercise Stress System.

## GLOSSARY

| Word | Phonetic Pronunciation | Definition |
| --- | --- | --- |
| 2-D echo | | medical jargon for two-dimensional echocardiogram, a test that uses sound waves to create a moving picture of the heart |
| aortic root | (ā-ōr'tĭk) | the portion of the aorta that is attached to the heart |
| aortic valve | (ā-ōr'tĭk) | one of the 4 heart valves; it is between the left ventricle and aorta |
| atrial fibrillation | (ā'trē-ăl fĭb-rĭ-lā'shŭn) | when the normal rhythmic contractions of the atria (chambers of the heart) are replaced by rapid, irregular twitching of the muscular wall |
| Atrovent | (ă'trō-vĕnt) | brand name of medication used to prevent bronchospasm in people with bronchitis, emphysema, or chronic obstructive pulmonary disease (COPD) |
| bruits | (brū'ēz) | sounds or murmurs heard on auscultation, especially abnormal ones (sing. bruit) |
| carotids | (kă-rŏt'ĭds) | the arteries of the neck |
| color Doppler | (dŏp'ler) | technique that uses standard ultrasound methods to produce a picture of a blood vessel; the computer converts the Doppler sounds into colors that are overlaid on the image of the blood vessel to represent the direction and speed of the blood flow |
| congestive heart failure | (kon-jĕs'tĭv) | a condition in which the heart cannot pump enough blood to the body's other organs |
| Coumadin | (kū'mă-dĭn) | medication used to prevent blood clots in veins and arteries (brand name) |
| cusp | (kŭsp) | a cup-like, passive soft tissue structure that is part of the structure of a heart valve; opens during pumping and closes at other times, thus preventing backward blood flow |

(Continued)

# GLOSSARY

| Word | Phonetic Pronunciation | Definition |
|---|---|---|
| diltiazem | (dĭl-tī′ă-zĕm) | generic name for medication used to treat high blood pressure, chest pain, and certain heart rhythm disorders |
| dyspnea | (disp′nē-ah) | shortness of breath |
| emphysema | (ĕm′fĭ-sē′mă) | a pathologic accumulation of air in tissues or organs, which causes abnormal swelling of body tissues |
| fundi | (fŭn′dī) | the retinal arteries and veins, which can be seen by shining a light into the eye; usually dictated in the plural form (sing. fundus) |
| gradient | (grā′dē-ĕnt) | a measurement of the blood flow across the aortic valve |
| Lanoxin | (lă-nŏk′sĭn) | brand name of medication used to treat congestive heart failure and atrial fibrillation |
| Lasix | (lā′siks) | used to treat fluid retention in people with congestive heart failure, liver disease, or a kidney disorder (brand name) |
| left atrium | (ā′trē-ūm) | one of 4 chambers of the heart; it receives blood from the lungs and pumps it to the left ventricle |
| left ventricle | (ven′trĭ-kĕl) | one of 4 chambers of the heart; it receives blood from the left atrium and pumps it to the aorta |
| mitral valve | (mī′trăl) | one of the 4 heart valves; it is between the left atrium and left ventricle |
| M-mode echocardiogram | | single-dimension images that allow accurate measurement of the heart chambers |
| myocardial infarction | (mī″ō-kăr′dē-ăl ĭn-fărk′shŭn) | injury or necrosis of the heart muscle due to lack of blood supply to the area (heart attack) |
| niacin | (nī′ă-sĭn) | used to lower cholesterol and triglycerides (generic medication) |
| Pulmicort | (pŭl′mĭ-kŏrt) | brand name medication; used to prevent asthma attacks |
| right ventricle | (ven′trĭ-kĕl) | one of 4 chambers of the heart; it receives blood from the right atrium and pumps it to the lungs |
| Singulair | (sing′ū-lār) | brand name medication used to prevent asthma attacks in adults and children as young as 12 months old |
| thrombi | (throm′bī) | blood clots (sing. thrombus) |
| tricuspid (valve) | (trī-kŭs′pĭd) | one of the 4 heart valves; it is between the right atrium and right ventricle |
| warfarin | (wōr′fă-rin) | anticoagulant; generic name for Coumadin |

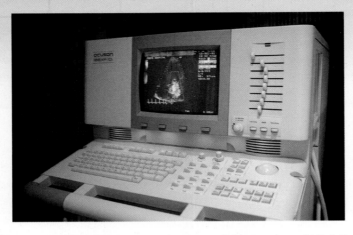

**Figure QC1-1** Echocardiograph. (*Source: Photo by Marcia Butterfield. Courtesy of W. A. Foote Memorial Hospital, Jackson, MI.*)

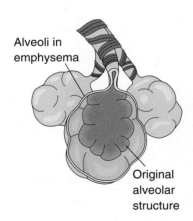

Alveoli in emphysema

Original alveolar structure

**Figure QC1-2** Emphysema. (*Delmar/Cengage Learning*)

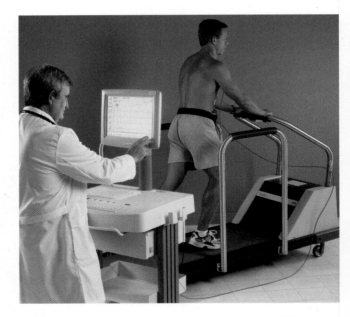

**Figure QC1-3** The Quest Exercise Stress System (*Courtesy of Quinton Cardiology, Inc.*)

# REPORT 2: OPERATIVE PROCEDURE

Richard Cates is a 53-year-old man with prostate cancer. After a complete workup that showed his disease to be localized, he was referred to a urologist for laparoscopic prostatectomy. This procedure will involve removal of the entire prostate gland in an attempt to cure the patient of cancer. See Figure QC2-1, The male reproductive system; Figure QC2-2, Supine position.

## GLOSSARY

| Word | Phonetic Pronunciation | Definition |
|---|---|---|
| aseptic technique | (ā-sĕp'tĭk) | a set of specific procedures performed under carefully controlled conditions to minimize contamination by bacteria |
| cephalad | (sĕf'ă-lad) | in a direction toward the head |
| Denonvilliers fascia | (dĕ-nŏn-vē-āz) | a membranous partition that separates the prostate and bladder from the rectum |
| dorsal venous complex | (vē'nŭs) | a network of large veins that runs along the anterior (toward the front of the body) surface of the prostate |
| Endo Catch bag | | a bag used in laparoscopic surgeries to remove the resected specimen (see laparoscopic prostatectomy) |
| endopelvic fascia | | containing elastin, collagen, and smooth muscle that helps support the structures of the lower pelvis |
| indigo carmine | (ĭn'di-go kar'-mīn) (kar'mēn) | a blue dye administered by injection for measurement of kidney function |
| infraumbilical incision | (ĭn'fră-ŭm-bĭl'ĭ-kăl) | a vertical incision made just below and extending into the umbilicus (navel or belly button) |
| laparoscopic prostatectomy | (lap'a-rō-skŏp'ic pros'ta-tĕk'tō-mē) | removal of the prostate through 4 to 5 small incisions in the abdomen through which instrumentation is inserted; the prostate is removed through one of these incisions with a retrieval bag (see Endo Catch bag) |
| Lapra-Ty | | suture clip applied to 1 strand of suture material to act as a knot |
| peritoneum | (per"ĭ-tō-nē'um) | the serous membrane lining the abdominal walls and investing the viscera |
| prostate | (prŏs'tāt) | a gland in the male surrounding the beginning of the urethra; produces a secretion that is the fluid part of semen |
| puboprostatic ligaments | (pū'bō-pros-tă'tĭk) | three strands of pelvic fascia that support the prostate |
| retrovesical space | (rĕt'rō-vĕs'ĭ-kăl) | space behind the bladder |
| seminal vesicles | (sĕm'ĭ-nĕl vĕs'ĭ-kĕlz) | structures in the male about 2 inches long, located behind the bladder; the seminal vesicles contribute fluid to the ejaculate |
| space of Retzius | (rĕt'zē-ŭs) | the space occurring between the pubic symphysis (the piece of cartilage joining the 2 halves of the pelvic bone) and the bladder; named after Anders Retzius, a Swedish professor of anatomy |

(Continued)

## GLOSSARY

| Word | Phonetic Pronunciation | Definition |
| --- | --- | --- |
| trocar | (trō′kar) | a blunt instrument used to enter the abdominal cavity; used for insufflation and introduction of laparoscope |
| ureteral orifices | (yū-rē′tĕr-ăl or′ĭ-fĭs-ĭs) | the 2 openings of the 2 ureters in the bladder |
| urethra | (yū-rē′thră) | the tube leading from the bladder through which urine leaves the body |
| vasa deferentia | (dĕf-er-ĕn′chēa) | the tubes connecting the testes with the urethra; 1 tube connects each testis to the urethra and carries sperm during ejaculation (sing. vas deferens) |

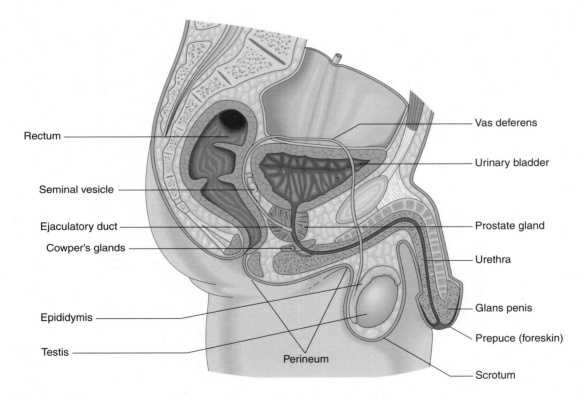

**Figure QC2-1**    The male reproductive system. (*Delmar/Cengage Learning*)

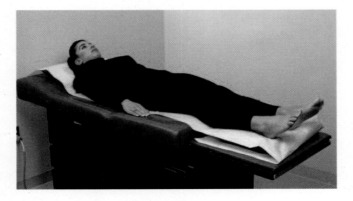

**Figure QC2-2**    Supine position. (*Delmar/Cengage Learning*)

# REPORT 3: OPERATIVE REPORT

Leslie Michael Smith is a young man who, while on active duty, suffered injuries to his right leg from an improvised explosive device (IED). He was treated in theater, then in Germany, and he has been back in the United States undergoing further treatment for his injuries. Today he has undergone surgical irrigation and debridement of his wounds. The wounds must be debrided on an ongoing basis to keep them clean and free of infection. Cultures of the wounds are taken routinely to check for the growth of bacteria. See Figure QC3-1, Superficial muscles of the leg; Figure QC3-2, Epidermal and dermal layers of the skin.

## GLOSSARY

| Word | Phonetic Pronunciation | Definition |
|---|---|---|
| delayed primary closure | | the approach of cleaning the wound, leaving the wound open under a moist dressing for approximately 4 to 5 days, and then suturing the wound if there is no evidence of infection |
| extubated | (ĕks'tū-bā'ted) | after surgery, removed the tube through which anesthesia was administered |
| GETA | | abbreviation for *general endotracheal tube anesthesia*; each letter is pronounced individually |
| irrigation and debridement | (dē-brēd'ment) | the procedure of using a balanced salt solution to flush out an infected wound, then surgically removing any dead tissue |
| left lateral decubitus position | (dē-kyū'bĭ-tŭs) | lying down on the left side |
| recovery room | | room where patients are taken for close monitoring after surgery |
| wound V.A.C. | | a system that applies suction to a wound dressing to remove fluids and infectious material, helps draw together wound edges, and promotes wound healing; dictated as the word "vac" for vacuum-assisted closure (trade name) |

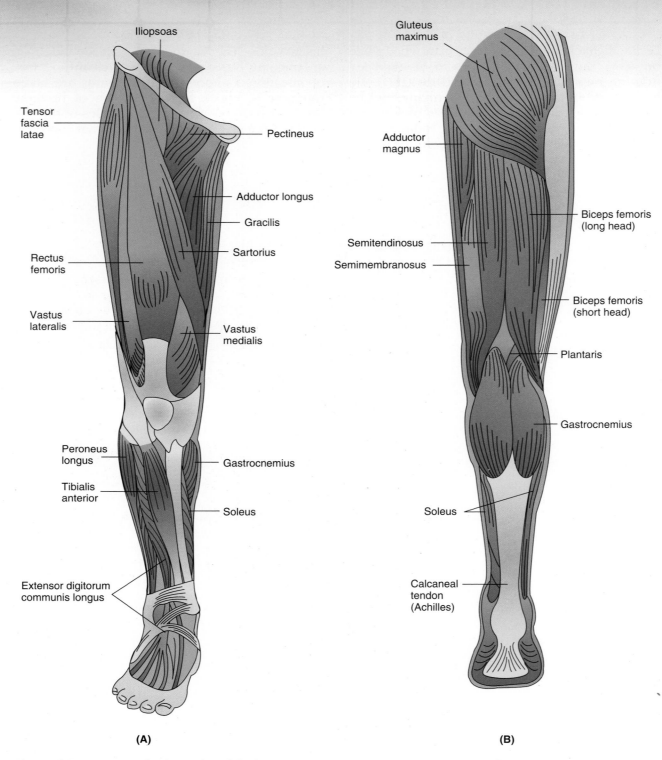

**(A)**

**(B)**

**Figure QC3-1**     Superficial muscles of the leg: (A) anterior view; (B) posterior view. (*Delmar/Cengage Learning*)

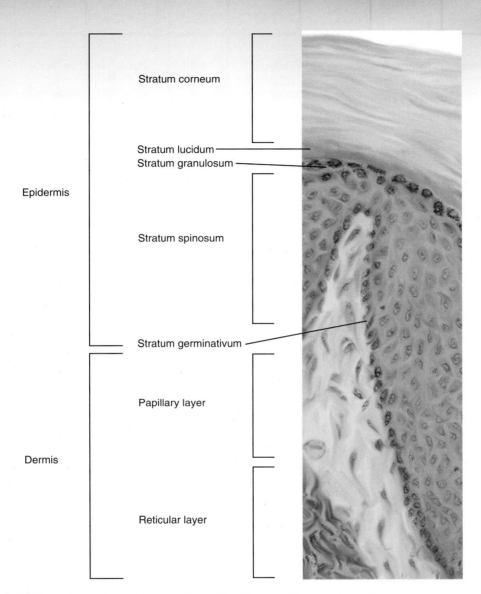

Stratum corneum

Stratum lucidum

Stratum granulosum

Epidermis

Stratum spinosum

Stratum germinativum

Dermis

Papillary layer

Reticular layer

**Figure QC3-2**    Epidermal and dermal layers of the skin. (*Delmar/Cengage Learning*)

# REPORT 4: SURGICAL PATHOLOGY REPORT

On a routine mammogram, Ursula Emma Wagner was found to have a suspicious lump in her right breast. This lump was removed at surgery via needle biopsy, and the specimen was sent to Pathology for a definitive diagnosis. See Figure QC4-1, Mammography, two views.

## GLOSSARY

| Word | Phonetic Pronunciation | Definition |
|------|------------------------|------------|
| adipose | (ăd'ĭ-pōs) | denoting fat |
| carcinoma in situ | (sī'too) | cancer that involves only the site where it began |
| cytologic atypia | (sī'tō-lŏj-ĭk ā-tĭp'ē-ah) | the abnormal characteristics of cancer cells that can be seen microscopically |
| ductal epithelial hyperplasia | (dŭk'tal ep'ĭ-thē'lē-al hī-pĕr-plā'zhē-ă) | increase in the number of epithelial cells in breast tissue; not associated with increased risk of malignancy |
| fibrofatty | (fī'brō-fat'ē) | relating to or pertaining to both fibrous and fatty structures |
| foci | (fō'sī) | localized areas of disease (sing. focus) |
| microcalcifications | (mī'krō-kăl'sĭ-fi-kā'shuns) | tiny bits of calcium that may show up in clusters on a mammogram |
| mucinous | (myū'sĭ-nŭs) | containing mucus |
| spec board | (spĕk) | medical jargon for "specimen board," on which tissue removed at surgery is sent to Pathology for processing |

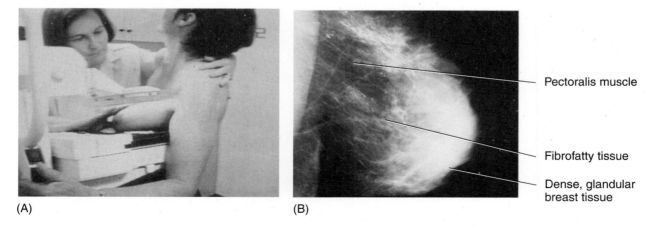

(A)  (B)

**Figure QC4-1**    Mammography, two views: (A) positioning for Cleopatra view; (B) Cleopatra view radiograph. (*Delmar/Cengage Learning*)

# REPORT 5: EMERGENCY DEPARTMENT TREATMENT RECORD

Craig S. Duran is a pediatric cancer patient undergoing chemotherapy, and he has developed a fever. His mother contacted the hematologist on call who advised her to take Craig to the Quali-Care Clinic ER right away. The ER physician gave Craig a complete examination, including laboratory testing, and it was determined that the patient required admission to Hillcrest for further evaluation and care. His hematologist was kept informed of the situation. See Figure QC5-1, Test tube with major components of blood; Figure QC5-2, The life span and function of blood cells; Figure QC5-3, Reagent strip in urine sample.

## GLOSSARY

| Word | Phonetic Pronunciation | Definition |
|---|---|---|
| **Broviac catheter** | (brō'vē-ăk) | a type of long-term catheter used for administration of medication and to draw blood |
| **ceftazidime** | (cĕf-tăz'ĭ-dēm) | an antibiotic (generic name) |
| **conjunctival injection** | (kŏn'jŭnk-tī'văl) | nonuniform redness of the conjunctiva, the clear membrane that covers the white part of the eyeball and the inside of the eyelids |
| **ecchymoses** | (ĕk"ĭ-mō'sēz) | purplish patches on the skin caused by blood passing from a vessel into the tissues (sing. ecchymosis) |
| **Ewing sarcoma** | (ū'wing) | cancer that occurs primarily in the bone or soft tissue; usually found in children or young adults |
| **lethargic** | (lĕ-thar'jĭk) | drowsy, sluggish |
| **listless** | | lack of interest, energy, or spirit |
| **lymphadenopathy** | (lĭm'făd-ĕ-nop'ă-thē) | enlargement of lymph nodes, which may indicate infection |
| **neutropenia** | (nū'trō-pē'nē-ă) | decrease in number of neutrophils, white blood cells that fight infection |
| **normocephalic** | (nōr"mō-sĭ-fal'ik) | having a head of medium length |
| **Zofran** | (zō'frăn) | brand name of medication given to prevent nausea and vomiting caused by surgery or cancer medicines |

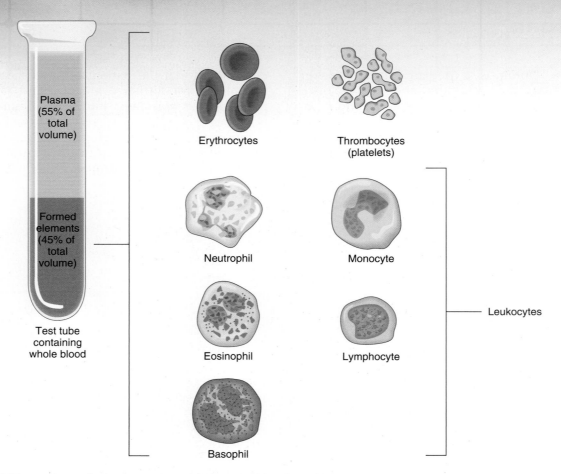

**Figure QC5-1**    Test tube with major components of blood. (*Delmar/Cengage Learning*)

| Blood cell | Life span in blood | Function |
|---|---|---|
| Erythrocyte | 120 days | $O_2$ and $CO_2$ transport |
| Neutrophil | 7–12 hours | Immune defenses |
| Eosinophil | Unknown | Defense against parasites |
| Basophil | Unknown | Inflammatory response |
| Monocyte | 3 days–years | Immune surveillance (precursor of tissue macrophage) |
| B Lymphocyte | Unknown | Antibody production (precursor of plasma cells) |
| T Lymphocyte | Unknown | Cellular immune response |
| Platelets | 7–8 days | Blood clotting |

**Figure QC5-2**    The life span and functions of blood cells. (*Delmar/Cengage Learning*)

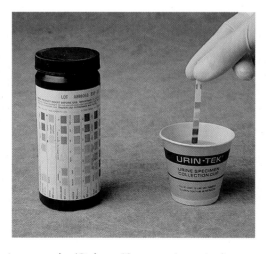

**Figure QC5-3**    Reagent strip in urine sample. (*Delmar/Cengage Learning*)

# REPORT 6: INTERVENTIONAL RADIOLOGY REPORT

This elderly German patient, Wilhelm Heidelberg, is receiving an interventional radiologic procedure today (arteriography) because of significant narrowing of his vein after having had a femoropopliteal vein bypass graft in the past. It is important to keep his vein open, and he requires immediate intervention. See Figure QC6-1, Major arteries of the systemic circulation; Figure QC6-2, Major veins of the body.

## GLOSSARY

| Word | Phonetic Pronunciation | Definition |
|---|---|---|
| aborted | | terminated a procedure prematurely |
| antegrade | (an'tĕ-grade) | in the direction of normal movement, as in blood flow |
| anterior tibial artery | | artery that runs from the knee to the ankle on the front of the leg |
| arteriography | (ăr-tēr'ē-og'ră-fē) | demonstration of an artery or arteries by x-ray imaging after injection of a contrast medium |
| Demerol | (dĕm'er-all) | trade name for meperidine hydrochloride, a drug to sedate and relieve pain |
| duplex | (dū'pleks) | performing 2 functions |
| femoropopliteal | (fem'ŏ-rō-pop-lĭ-tē'al) | pertaining to the femoral artery and the popliteal artery in the leg |
| fluoroscopy | (flōr-os'kŏ-pē) | examination of the tissues and deep structures of the body using the fluoroscope, an instrument used to obtain real-time images |
| gadolinium | (găd'ō-lĭn'ē-ŭm) | material used as contrast media for magnetic resonance imaging |
| Glide catheter | | specialized catheter used for venous pressure monitoring, blood sampling, and administration of drugs and fluids |
| Glidewire | | a wire with a special coating containing a lubricant, making it easy to insert into blood vessels; the wire also has a tip that can be seen on x-ray |
| peroneal artery | (per'ō-nē-ăl) | artery that runs deeply on the back outside of the leg |
| posterior tibial artery | | artery that runs from the knee to the ankle down the middle on the back side of the leg |
| profunda femoris artery | (prō-fŭn'dă fĕm'ŏr-is) | a branch of the femoral artery that travels down the thigh, closer to the femur than the femoral artery |
| retrograde | | moving backward |
| reversed greater saphenous vein | | the saphenous vein (in the leg) that is used as a bypass from one artery to another, usually for arteries in the heart |
| stenosis | (ste-nō'sis) | a stricture of any canal or orifice |

(Continued)

# GLOSSARY

| Word | Phonetic Pronunciation | Definition |
| --- | --- | --- |
| **Sterling balloon** | | device used to stretch the wall of an artery that has become narrowed |
| **transluminal** | (trans-lū′mĭ-năl) | passing or occurring across a lumen (interior) as of a blood vessel |
| **Visipaque** | (vĭz′ĭ-pāk) | contrast agent commonly used during coronary arteriography, particularly within individuals with renal dysfunction, as it is believed to be less toxic to the kidneys than other contrast agents |
| **waist** | | the narrowed portion of a vessel during inflation of a balloon to try to expand the vessel; the balloon expands on both sides of the narrowed portion, thus making the narrowed portion look like a person's waist |

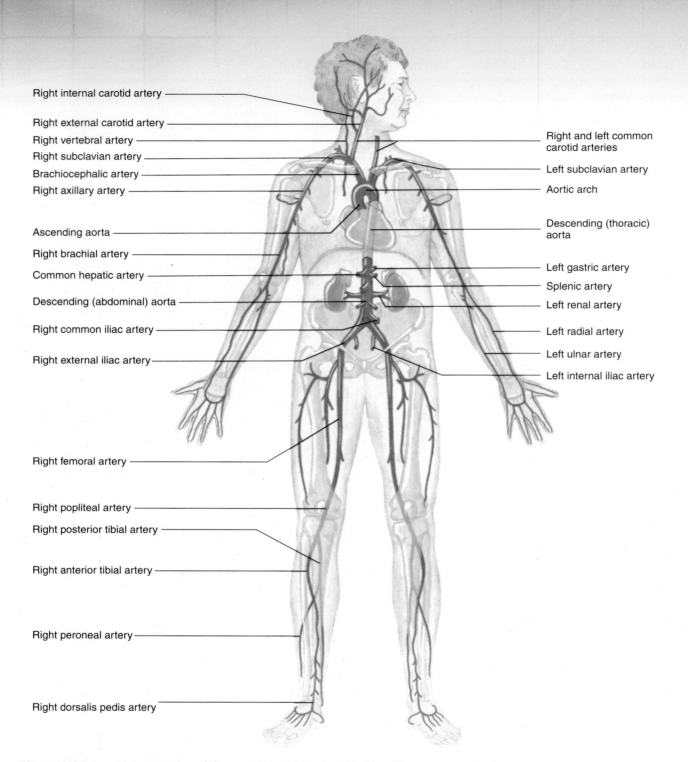

Right internal carotid artery

Right external carotid artery

Right vertebral artery

Right subclavian artery

Brachiocephalic artery

Right axillary artery

Ascending aorta

Right brachial artery

Common hepatic artery

Descending (abdominal) aorta

Right common iliac artery

Right external iliac artery

Right femoral artery

Right popliteal artery

Right posterior tibial artery

Right anterior tibial artery

Right peroneal artery

Right dorsalis pedis artery

Right and left common carotid arteries

Left subclavian artery

Aortic arch

Descending (thoracic) aorta

Left gastric artery

Splenic artery

Left renal artery

Left radial artery

Left ulnar artery

Left internal iliac artery

**Figure QC6-1**    Major arteries of the systemic circulation. (*Delmar/Cengage Learning*)

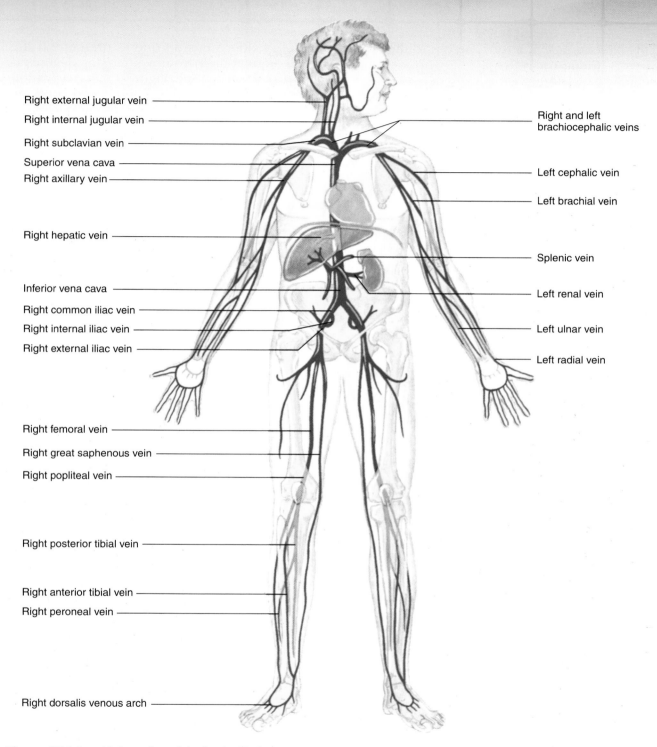

Right external jugular vein

Right internal jugular vein

Right subclavian vein

Superior vena cava

Right axillary vein

Right hepatic vein

Inferior vena cava

Right common iliac vein

Right internal iliac vein

Right external iliac vein

Right femoral vein

Right great saphenous vein

Right popliteal vein

Right posterior tibial vein

Right anterior tibial vein

Right peroneal vein

Right dorsalis venous arch

Right and left brachiocephalic veins

Left cephalic vein

Left brachial vein

Splenic vein

Left renal vein

Left ulnar vein

Left radial vein

**Figure QC6-2**     Major veins of the body. (*Delmar/Cengage Learning*)

# REPORT 7: SPINE CLINIC HPIP NOTE

This patient, Jack P. Strong, comes to the Spine Surgery Clinic today for a followup visit after having had surgery for cauda equina syndrome. This syndrome can result in pain in the sacral region of the back, a lack of feeling in the buttocks and thigh, and a disturbance in bowel/bladder function due to pressure in the cauda equina area from a tumor or degenerative disk disease. See Figure QC7-1, Location of compression of lumbar and sacral roots by herniated disks; Figure QC7-2, Straight-leg raising test.

## GLOSSARY

| Word | Phonetic Pronunciation | Definition |
|------|------------------------|------------|
| cauda equina syndrome | (kaw'dă ē-kwĭ'nă) | involvement, often on one side or the other, of multiple roots making up the cauda equina (L2-S3 roots) manifested by low back pain, numbness in the groin or area of contact if sitting on a saddle, and bowel and bladder disturbances |
| disk herniation | | rupture or slipping out of place of the disk in between 2 vertebrae |
| EHL | | *extensor hallucis longus*—a thin muscle that functions to extend the big toe, lift the foot up, and assist with foot inversion |
| gastrocsoleus complex | (găs'trŏk-sō'lē-ŭs) | the muscles of the calf, the gastrocnemius and the soleus; the complex is connected to the foot through the Achilles tendon |
| proprioception | (prō'prē-ō-sep'shun) | the awareness of the position of one's body |
| straight-leg raise | | test performed by having the patient lie flat on a bed and, with the leg straight, the patient should raise their foot off the bed and hold it in the air; test performed to determine whether a patient with low back pain has a disk herniation |

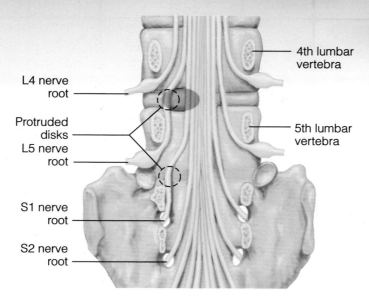

4th lumbar
vertebra

L4 nerve
root

Protruded
disks

5th lumbar
vertebra

L5 nerve
root

S1 nerve
root

S2 nerve
root

**Figure QC7-1**    Location of compression of lumbar and sacral roots by herniated disks. (*Delmar/Cengage Learning*)

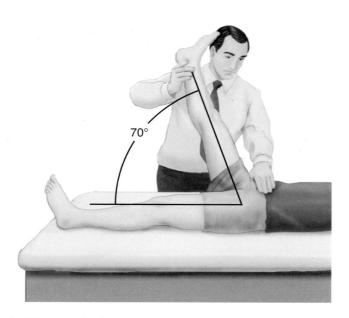

70°

**Figure QC7-2**    Straight-leg raising test. (*Delmar/Cengage Learning*)

# REPORT 8: RADIOLOGY REPORT

Brian Albert is a 67-year-old male with history of back pain. His PCP ordered a series of x-rays to diagnose his pain. The films showed degenerative disk disease, moderate to severe, and he will report back to his PCP for diagnosis and treatment recommendations. See Figure QC8-1, Human skeleton: (A) anterior and (B) posterior views.

## GLOSSARY

| Word | Phonetic Pronunciation | Definition |
|------|------------------------|------------|
| anterolisthesis | (ăn′tĕr-ō-lĭs-thē′sis) | the upper vertebral body is positioned abnormally compared to the vertebral body below it; it is slipped forward on the one below |
| degenerative disk disease | | refers to wear changes in the individual disks of the spine in any part of the spine |
| L2-3 | | lumbar spine; denotes disk space between the 2nd and 3rd lumbar vertebrae |
| L3-4 | | lumbar spine; denotes disk space between the 3rd and 4th lumbar vertebrae |
| L4-5 | | lumbar spine; denotes disk space between the 4th and 5th lumbar vertebrae |
| L5-S1 | | lumbar spine and sacral spine; denotes space between 5th lumbar vertebra and 1st sacral vertebra |
| levoscoliosis | (lē′vō-skō′lē-ō′sis) | a curve in the spine that points to the left |
| osteophyte | (os′tē-ō-fīt′) | a bony outgrowth or protuberance |
| vertebral body | (vĕr′tĕ-brăl) (vĕr-tē′brăl) | main portion of each of the bones of the spine; bears about 80% of the load while standing and provides an attachment for the disks between the vertebrae |

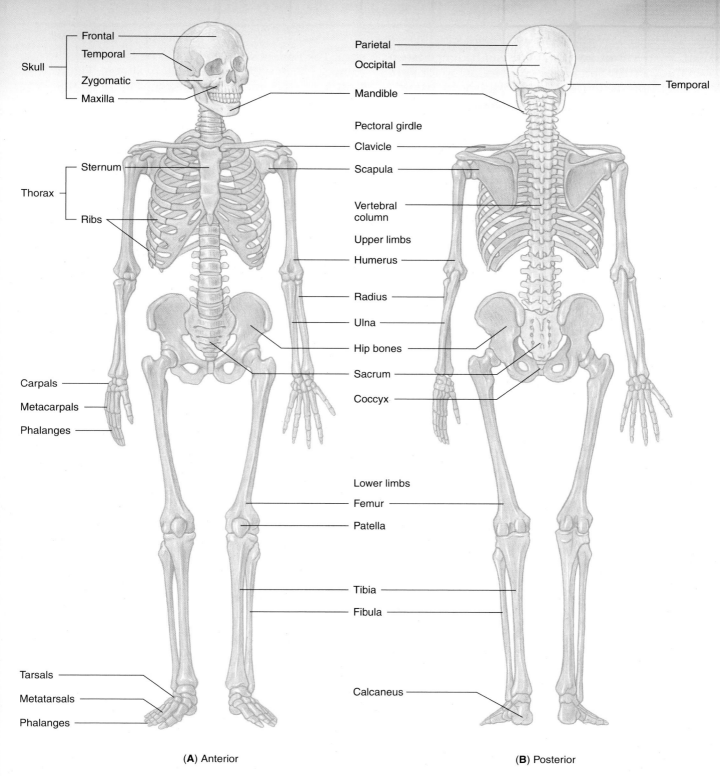

**Figure QC8-1**     Human skeleton: (A) anterior and (B) posterior views. (*Delmar/Cengage Learning*)

# REPORT 9: VASCULAR SURGERY CLINIC SOAP NOTE

Mr. Yuan S. Kao, an elderly Korean patient, is seen in the Vascular Surgery Clinic in followup for right calf claudication. He also has had heart palpitations. Today the physician performed a duplex scan. The patient will continue to be treated medically. See Figure QC9-1, Circulatory system; Figure QC9-2, Carotid artery duplex scan; Figure QC9-3, Doppler ultrasound.

## GLOSSARY

| Word | Phonetic Pronunciation | Definition |
|------|------------------------|------------|
| 12-point ROS | | a review of systems that includes 12 systems of the body; dictated twelve-point R O S, each letter individually |
| beta blocker | | a class of drugs used primarily for the management of cardiac rhythm disorders |
| carotid upstrokes | (kă-rŏt'ĭd) | the pulse that can be felt in the carotid arteries when the heart is contracting |
| claudication | (klaw'dĭ-kā'shŭn) | limping |
| metoprolol | (mĕ-tō'prō-lŏl) | generic name for medication used to treat high blood pressure, heart pain, abnormal rhythms of the heart, and some neurologic conditions |
| palpitations | (păl″pĭ-tā'shŭns) | rapid or irregular heartbeats; primarily used in the plural form |
| Pletal | (plē'tăl) | used to treat symptoms of claudication (brand name) |

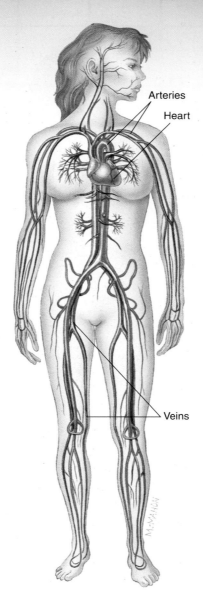

**Figure QC9-1**    Circulatory system. (*Delmar/Cengage Learning*)

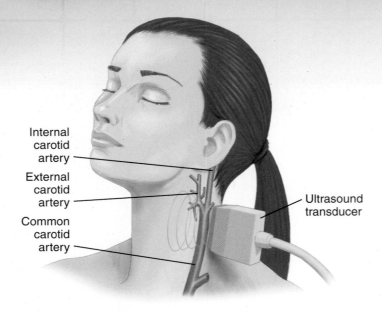

Internal carotid artery

External carotid artery

Common carotid artery

Ultrasound transducer

**Figure QC9-2** Carotid artery duplex scan. (*Delmar/Cengage Learning*)

**How the Doppler probe works**

To recorder

Transducer

Emitter crystal

Receiver crystal

Skin and muscle tissue

Blood vessel

Blood flow

RBCs

**Figure QC9-3** Doppler ultrasound. (*Delmar/Cengage Learning*)

# REPORT 10: SURGICAL PROCEDURE

Paul G. Catrou, 37 years old, is being treated surgically for a broken arm sustained when patient jumped from a second-story building. The patient was treated and stabilized by the Psychiatry Team for suicidal ideations prior to his surgery. See Figure QC10-1, Bones of the upper extremity.

## GLOSSARY

| Word | Phonetic Pronunciation | Definition |
|---|---|---|
| anconeus | (ang-kō′nē-ŭs) | small muscle on the back of the elbow joint |
| Bovie cautery | (bō′vē kaw′tĕr-ē) | brand name of a machine used to close small blood vessels with heat |
| callus | (kăl′ŭs) | a mass of tissue that forms at a fracture site that ultimately becomes bone |
| capitulum | (kă-pit′yū-lŭm) | a small head or rounded articular end of a bone |
| comminution | (kŏm′ĭ-nū′shŭn) | a breaking into several pieces, particularly when describing a fracture |
| coronoid | (kōr′ŏ-noyd) | part of the ulna that meets the humerus to form the elbow joint |
| curette *or* curet | (kū-rĕt′) | spoon-shaped surgical instrument for removing tissue from a cavity wall or other bodily surface |
| ECU | | *extensor carpi ulnaris*—muscle that extends the wrist |
| exsanguinated | (ek-săng′gwĭ-nāt′d) | the action or process of having drained or lost circulating blood; made bloodless |
| external fixator | (fik-să′tŏr, fik′să-tŏr) | device with screws that are inserted into a broken bone and come through the skin |
| FCR | | *flexor carpi radialis*—muscle of the forearm that flexes and abducts the hand |
| FPL | | *flexor pollicis longus*—muscle of the forearm that flexes the thumb |
| fracture | | a bone fracture is a condition in which a bone is cracked or broken |
| general anesthesia | (an′es-thē′zē-ă) | loss of ability to perceive pain with loss of consciousness produced by intravenous or inhalation anesthetic agents |
| Kocher approach | (kō′kĕr) | approach to the humerus for open reduction, internal fixation |
| lateral epicondyle | (ĕp′ĭ-kon′dīl) | outside elbow bone |
| NSS | | abbreviation for *normal saline solution* |
| open reduction, internal fixation | | open reduction is open surgery to set bones; internal fixation involves the use of plates, screws, or a rod |
| ORIF | | abbreviation for *open reduction, internal fixation*; the letters are dictated individually |

(Continued)

## GLOSSARY

| Word | Phonetic Pronunciation | Definition |
|------|------------------------|------------|
| **pronator quadratus** | (quad-rā′tŭs) | muscle of forearm that pronates forearm |
| **radius** | | the shorter of the 2 bones of the forearm |
| **rongeur [Fr.]** | (ron-zhur′) | a surgical instrument used for cutting tough tissue, such as bone |
| **suicidal ideation** | (ĭ′dē-ā′shŭn) | thoughts of killing oneself |
| **trochlea** | (trok′lē-ă) | in the humerus, a depression where it meets the ulna to form the elbow joint |

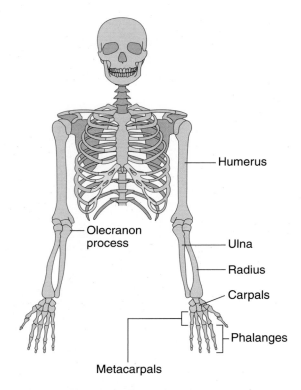

**Figure QC10-1** Bones of the upper extremity. (*Delmar/Cengage Learning*)

# REPORT 11: OPERATIVE REPORT

Debbie Dolle Russell, a 42-year-old Caucasian female, is being treated surgically for bilateral breast atrophy, requiring augmentation, plus the removal of excess abdominal skin and fat after childbirth. See Figure QC11-1, Structures of the breast: (A) anterior and (B) sagittal views.

## GLOSSARY

| Word | Phonetic Pronunciation | Definition |
|---|---|---|
| abdominoplasty | (ab-dom'ĭ-nō-plas-tē) | an operation performed on the abdominal wall for cosmetic purposes |
| breast augmentation | (awg'měn-tā'shun) | the process of enlarging the breasts, often by insertion of an implant |
| cefazolin | (sef'ă-zō'lin) | an antibiotic (generic name) |
| crystalloid | (kris'tăl-oyd') | a hydration solution containing only electrolytes |
| inframammary fold | (in'fră-mam'ă-rē) | the natural boundary under the breast where the breast meets the chest wall |
| mons pubis | (mŏns pū'bĭs) | a rounded, fleshy protuberance situated over the pubic bone that becomes covered with hair during puberty |
| pectoralis | (pěk'tōr-ă-lis) | one of the muscles on the chest wall |
| postpartum | (pōst-păr'tŭm) | after childbirth |
| scopolamine | (skō-pol'ă-mēn) | generic name for medication used to prevent motion sickness |
| tumescent | (tū-mes'ěnt) | anesthesia used for liposuction with a very dilute local anesthetic |
| umbilicus | (ŭm-bil'ĭ-kŭs, ŭm-bi-lī'kŭs) | pit in the abdominal wall marking the point where the umbilical cord entered the fetus; navel; belly button |

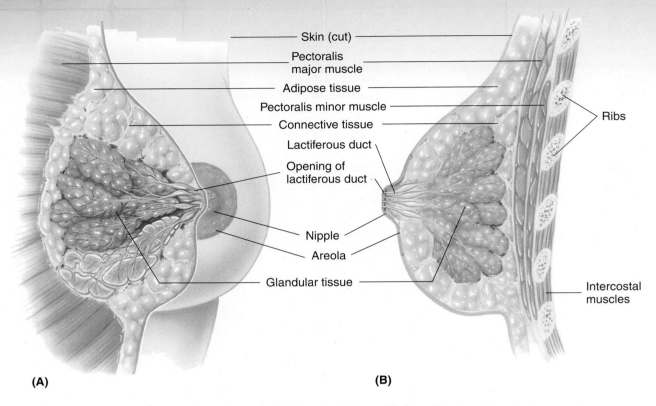

**Figure QC11-1**    Structures of the breast: (A) anterior and (B) sagittal views. (*Delmar/Cengage Learning*)

# REPORT 12: COLONOSCOPY PROCEDURE NOTE

Betsy H. Bennett, 67 years old, presented to the Endoscopy Center for an elective colonoscopy to be done as an outpatient. The patient has a family history of colon cancer, and she had been advised by her PCP to have a screening colonoscopy every 5 years. See Figure QC12-1, A colonoscope is used to examine the bowel.

## GLOSSARY

| Word | Phonetic Pronunciation | Definition |
|---|---|---|
| appendiceal orifice | (ă-pen′dĭ-sēl) | seen on colonoscopy, an indentation indicating the location of the appendix |
| colitis | (kō-lī′tis) | inflammation of the colon |
| colonoscopy | (kō″lon-os′kŏ-pē) | examination by means of a flexible, elongated scope that permits visual examination of the colon |
| Demerol | (dĕm′er-all) | trade name for meperidine hydrochloride, a drug to sedate and relieve pain |
| diverticula | (dī′vĕr-tik′yū-lă) | pouches or sacs opening from a tubular organ, such as bowel or bladder (sing. diverticulum) |
| internal hemorrhoids | | hemorrhoids located inside the anus |
| polyps | (pŏl′ĭps) | small growths that project outward from the normal surface level; may be cancerous, foci of inflammation, or degenerative lesions |
| pulse oximetry | (ok-sim′ĕ-trē) | procedure using a device on the fingertip or earlobe to measure oxygen saturation by fluctuations of light absorption |
| Versed | (vĕr′-sĕd, vĕr-sĕd′) | trade name for a drug given intravenously either before or during surgery to produce sedation and amnesia |

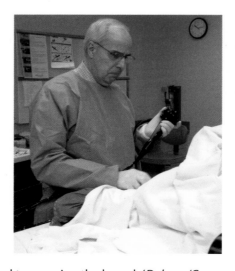

**Figure QC12-1**  A colonoscope is used to examine the bowel. (*Delmar/Cengage Learning*)

# REPORT 13: INTERNAL MEDICINE CLINIC HPIP NOTE

Mary Fisher Lipscomb, 63 years old, is a cancer patient who presents to the Internal Medicine Clinic in followup for bloating. Her doctor referred her to the Endoscopy Center for an esophagogastroduodenoscopy (EGD), which should provide a definitive diagnosis. See Figure QC13-1, Thoracic and abdominopelvic cavities of the body.

## GLOSSARY

| Word | Phonetic Pronunciation | Definition |
|---|---|---|
| bilateral mastectomies | (mas-tĕk′tŏ-mēz) | removal of both breasts |
| differential diagnosis | | the process of weighing the symptoms of one disease against those of other diseases, possibly accounting for a patient's illness |
| early satiety | (să-tī′ĕ-tē) | feeling full after eating less than normal or feeling full sooner than normal |
| EGD | | esophagogastroduodenoscopy; diagnostic procedure examining the lining of the stomach, esophagus, and upper small bowel with a camera |
| empiric | (em-pĭr-ik) | treatment based on experience, usually without adequate data to support its use |
| epigastric | (ep′ĭ-găs′trik) | relating to the epigastrium, the upper central region of the abdomen |
| flatus | (flā′tŭs) | gas or air in the gastrointestinal tract that may be expelled through the anus |
| globus sensation | (glŏ′bŭs) | the sensation of a lump in the throat |
| Murphy sign | | a positive Murphy sign is usually seen in acute inflammation of the gallbladder |
| noncontrast CT | | a CT scan performed without contrast media given |
| osteopenia | (os′tē-ō-pē′nē-ă) | decreased density of bone |
| prokinetic agent | (prō-kĭ-net′ik) | drug that increases the movement of ingested material through the gastrointestinal tract |
| Protonix | (prō-tŏn′iks) | brand name of medication used to treat symptoms of acid reflux and other conditions involving excess stomach acid |
| regurgitation | (rē-gŭr′ji-tā′shun) | a return of small amounts of gas or food from the stomach |
| stools | | discharging of the bowels |
| total abdominal hysterectomy | (hĭs′ter-ek′tŏ-mē) | surgical procedure of removal of the uterus and cervix |

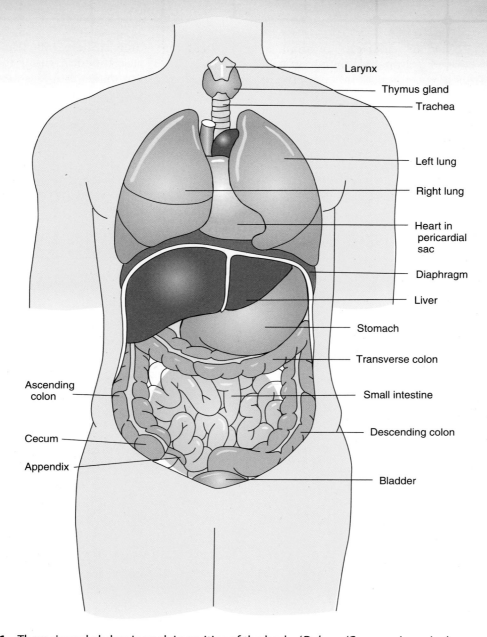

Larynx

Thymus gland

Trachea

Left lung

Right lung

Heart in
 pericardial
 sac

Diaphragm

Liver

Stomach

Transverse colon

Small intestine

Descending colon

Bladder

Ascending
colon

Cecum

Appendix

**Figure QC13-1** Thoracic and abdominopelvic cavities of the body. (*Delmar/Cengage Learning*)

# REPORT 14: OPERATIVE REPORT

Ruby Kay Bell, 67 years old, was brought in by EMS as a Level I trauma following a rollover motor vehicle accident. She underwent physical exam and an extensive radiology workup and was diagnosed as having an incomplete spinal cord injury. The patient was started on a steroid protocol and taken for emergent surgical intervention. After surgery, Ms. Bell continued to have no motor function distal to the triceps in her upper extremities, but she kept her lower extremity motor function. She will be transferred to a skilled nursing facility. See Figure QC14-1, Spine; Figure QC14-2, Bones of lower extremities.

## GLOSSARY

| Word | Phonetic Pronunciation | Definition |
|---|---|---|
| anterior cervical diskectomy and fusion | (dĭs-kĕk'tō-mē) | removal of an intervertebral disk in the neck through an incision in the front of the neck (anterior), then placement of bone graft after the disk has been removed (fusion) |
| Aspen cervical collar | | a brace that is worn after neck surgery to immobilize the neck |
| diskectomy | (dĭs-kĕk'tō-mē) | removal of an intervertebral disk |
| internal carotid artery | | major artery of the head and neck that helps supply blood to the brain |
| internal jugular vein | (jŭg'ū-lar) | the 2 internal jugular veins collect blood from the brain, the superficial parts of the face, and the neck and carry it to the heart |
| Metzenbaum scissors | (mĕt'sēn-bŏm) | lightly built, curved scissors with blunt-pointed, narrow blades |
| platysma | (plă-tĭz'mă) | facial muscle in neck region; depresses lower lip, increases diameter of neck, as seen in intense breathing while running |
| posterior longitudinal ligament | (pōs-tēr'ē-or lŏn-jĭ-tū'dĭ-năl) | one of the 3 more important ligaments of the spine, it runs up and down behind the spine and inside the spinal canal |
| prevertebral fascia | (prē'vĕr-tē'brăl fash'ē-a) | the part of the cervical fascia that covers the bodies of the cervical vertebrae and the muscles attaching to them |
| subluxation | (sŭb'lŭk-sā'shun) | one or more of the bones of the spine move out of position and create pressure on or irritate spinal nerves |

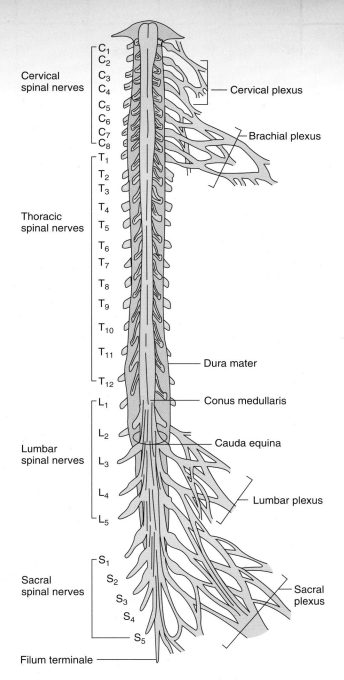

**Figure QC14-1** Spine. (*Delmar/Cengage Learning*)

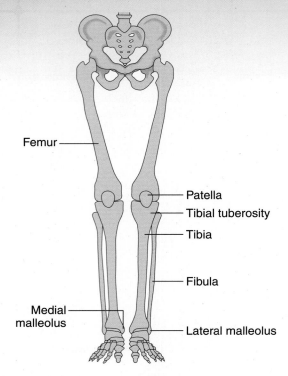

**Figure QC14-2** Bones of the lower extremities. (*Delmar/Cengage Learning*)

# Report 15: Operative Report

Sherman L. Kermit, a 38-year-old black male combat engineer, is seen in the Ambulatory Surgery Center because of bilateral nephrolithiasis (kidney stones). This is not the first episode for him, and he requires repeat surgery with replacement of bilateral double-J stents. See Figure QC15-1, Internal anatomy of a kidney.

## GLOSSARY

| Word | Phonetic Pronunciation | Definition |
|---|---|---|
| calyces | (kal'ĭ-sēz) | funnel-shaped hollows in the pelvis of the kidney through which urine passes to the ureter (sing. calyx) |
| cystoscopy | (sis-tos'kŏ-pē) | inspection of the interior of the bladder by means of a cystoscope |
| lithotripsy | (lith'ō-trip'sē) | the crushing of a stone in the kidney, ureter, or bladder by mechanical force, laser, or sound energy |
| nephrolithiasis | (nĕf'rō-li-thī'ă-sis) | presence of renal stones |
| PACU | | *postan*esthesia *c*are *u*nit; sometimes dictated "pack-u," or the individual letters may be pronounced |
| pyeloscopy | (pī'ĕ-los'kŏ-pē) | endoscopic or fluoroscopic observation of the pelvis and calyces of the kidney |
| retrograde pyelogram | (pī'ĕ-lō-gram) | a urologic procedure in which the physician injects contrast into the ureter in order to visualize the ureter and the kidney; the flow of contrast is opposite the usual flow of urine, hence the use of the word retrograde |
| ureter | (yū'rĕ-ter, yū-rē'tĕr) | one of the tubes that takes urine from the kidney to the bladder; there are normally 2 ureters, 1 connecting each kidney to the bladder |
| ureteroscopy | (yū-rē'ter-os'kŏ-pē) | examination of the upper urinary tract, usually performed with an endoscope that is passed through the urethra, bladder, and directly into the ureter |
| urethra | (yū-rē'thră) | the canal leading from the bladder, discharging the urine externally |

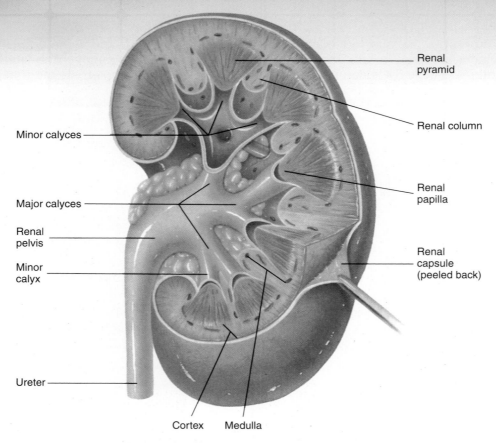

**Figure QC15-1** Internal anatomy of a kidney. (*Delmar/Cengage Learning*)

# REPORT 16: RADIOLOGY REPORT

This middle-aged Caucasian patient, Suzanne S. Mira, has complained of ongoing back pain. She is scheduled for a lumbar spine x-ray and reports to the Quali-Care Radiology Department for this procedure. See Figure QC16-1, Divisions of the back.

## GLOSSARY

| Word | Phonetic Pronunciation | Definition |
|---|---|---|
| L1-2 | | lumbar spine; denotes disk space between the 1st and 2nd lumbar vertebrae |
| lumbar lordosis | (lŭm'bar lōr-dō'sis) | the normal curved segment of the lower back; secondary curvature acquired as one learns to walk |
| osteoporosis | (os'tē-ō-pō-rō'sis) | reduction in quantity of bone leading to increased susceptibility to fractures |
| sciatica | (sī-at'ĭ-kă) | pain in the lower back and hip radiating down the back of the thigh into the lower leg, caused by a herniated lumbar disk compressing a nerve root, most commonly the L5 or S1 root |
| senescent | (sē-něs'ěnt) | growing old |
| spondylolisthesis | (spon'dĭ-lō-lis-thē'sis) | forward movement of the body of 1 of the lower lumbar vertebrae onto the vertebra below it or onto the sacrum |

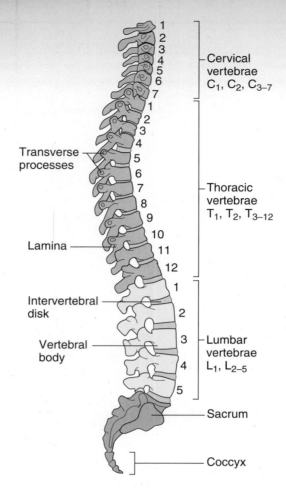

**Figure QC16-1** Divisions of the back. (*Delmar/Cengage Learning*)

# REPORT 17: PEDIATRIC NEUROLOGY CLINIC NOTE

Grace Pereira, a 7-year-old Portuguese child, has been diagnosed with severe behavior problems, including ADHD, bipolar disorder, and borderline intellectual disability. Her mother has brought her to the Pediatric Neurology Clinic for a routine followup visit. Their doctor performed a complete physical exam, reviewed Grace's x-rays and laboratory test results, and provided a plan of action for the child. See Table QC17-1, DSM-IV-TR Multiaxial Classification System; Figure QC17-1, The Draw-A-Person (DAP) test.

## GLOSSARY

| Word | Phonetic Pronunciation | Definition |
|------|------------------------|------------|
| ADHD | | abbreviation for *a*ttention *d*eficit *h*yperactivity *d*isorder |
| articulation | (ar-tik′ū-lā′shun) | in speech, the act or manner of producing a speech sound |
| bipolar disorder | (bī-pō′lăr) | brain disorder that causes unusual mood swings from overly "high" and irritable to sad and hopeless |
| demyelinating process | (dē-mī′ĕ-lin-ā′ting) | process of the loss of myelin, the white matter coating the nerves, helping them to conduct impulses; seen in some diseases, such as multiple sclerosis |
| encephalopathy | (en-sef′ă-lŏp′ă-thē) | any of various diseases of the brain |
| FISH study | (pronounced "fish") | *f*luorescence *in situ h*ybridization—laboratory technique used to detect structural chromosome abnormalities |
| hydrocephalus | (hī′drō-sef′ă-ŭs) | a condition of excessive cerebrospinal fluid in the brain, resulting in enlargement of the cranium |
| hyperopia | (hī′pĕr-ō′pē-ă) | farsightedness |
| MR spectroscopy | (spek-tros′kŏ-pē) | allows noninvasive exploration of the molecular composition of tissue |
| Neurontin | (nyū-rŏn′tĭn) | brand name of medication used to treat seizures and also to treat nerve pain |
| TORCH titer | (pronounced "torch") | test that measures the level of an infant's antibodies against 5 groups of chronic infections: *t*oxoplasmosis, *o*ther infections, *r*ubella, *c*ytomegalovirus (CMV), and *h*erpes simplex virus |
| velocardiofacial syndrome | (vē′lō-kăr′dē-ō-fā′shul) | genetic syndrome with nasal speech, abnormal facial features, and cardiac abnormalities |

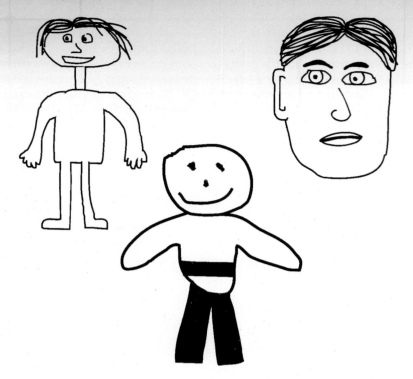

**Figure QC17-1** The Draw-A-Person (DAP) test. (*Source: Jones, Betty Davis (2008).* Comprehensive Medical Terminology, *3rd ed. Clifton Park, NY: Delmar Cengage Learning.*)

## TABLE QC17-1 DSM-IV-TR MULTIAXIAL CLASSIFICATION SYSTEM

**AXIS I**
Major Mental Disorders
Developmental Disorders and Learning Disabilites

**AXIS II**
Personality Disorders
Mental Retardation

**AXIS III**
General Medical Conditions

**AXIS IV**
Psychosocial and Environmental Problems

**AXIS V**
Global Assessment of Functioning

*Source:* Jones, Betty Davis. (2008). *Comprehensive Medical Terminology,* 3rd ed. Clifton Park, NY: Delmar Cengage Learning.

# REPORT 18: OPERATIVE REPORT

Janet Marie Bruner, a 23-year-old Caucasian lady who is pregnant at 36 weeks 6 days, presents to the Obstetrics Clinic with severe preeclampsia and a non-reassuring fetal heart tracing. The patient is rushed to the delivery room and prepared for an emergent cesarean section. See Figure QC18-1, Position of fetus prior to labor; Figure QC18-2, Fetoscope used to hear fetal heartbeat; Figure QC18-3, Doppler.

## GLOSSARY

| Word | Phonetic Pronunciation | Definition |
| --- | --- | --- |
| Ancef | (ăn'sĕf) | an antibiotic (brand name) |
| Apgar | (ăp'gar) | evaluation of a newborn infant's physical status by assigning numerical values (0-2) to each of 5 criteria: heart rate, respiratory effort, muscle tone, response to stimulation, and skin color; a score of 8 to 10 indicates the best possible condition; named for Virginia Apgar, anesthesiologist |
| bradycardia | (brād'ē-kăr'dē-ă) | slow heartbeat |
| cul-de-sac | (from the French) (kŭl'-duh-săk) | a blind pouch |
| hysterotomy | (hĭs'ter-ot'ŏ-mē) | incision of the uterus |
| Pfannenstiel skin incision | (făn'ĕn-stēĕl") | abdominal incision across the abdomen curved in a "smile" at the bikini line; named for Dr. Hermann Johann Pfannenstiel, a German gynecologist |
| placenta | (plă-sen'tă) | the organ of metabolic interchange between the fetus and the mother |
| preeclampsia | (prē'ē-klamp'sē-ă) | in pregnancy, development of hypertension with protein in the urine or edema, or both; usually occurs after the 20th week of pregnancy |
| supine position | (sū-pīn') | lying face upward |

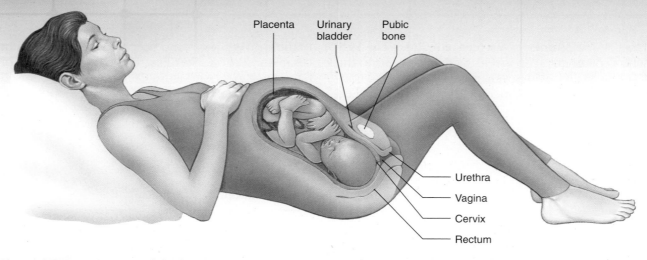

**Figure QC18-1** Position of the fetus prior to labor. (*Delmar/Cengage Learning*)

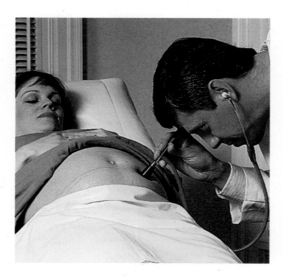

**Figure QC18-2** Fetoscope used to hear fetal heartbeat. (*Delmar/Cengage Learning*)

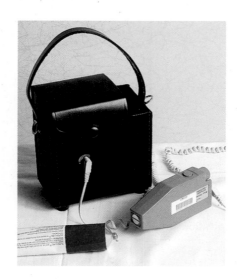

**Figure QC18-3** Doppler. (*Delmar/Cengage Learning*)

# REPORT 19: OPERATIVE REPORT

Eduardo J. Yunis, a young Hispanic man, was involved in a motorcycle accident, suffering a left radius fracture and some facial injuries. He also complained of left knee pain. The patient was taken to surgery where he had repair of his broken left arm by Orthopedics and repair of his facial injuries by Oromaxillofacial Surgery. Orthopedics examined his left knee during the procedure, and he will be put into a hinged knee brace postoperatively. See Figure QC19-1, Knee; Figure QC19-2, Right radius and ulna: (A) anterior view, (B) posterior view; Figure QC19-3, Superficial versus deep veins in development of phlebitis and thrombus.

## GLOSSARY

| Word | Phonetic Pronunciation | Definition |
|---|---|---|
| brachioradialis | (brā′kē-ō-rā′dē-ă′lis) | muscle in the forearm that flexes elbow and assists in returning the pronated or supinated limb to neutral position |
| Esmarch | (ĕs′mark) | a broad, flat, rubber bandage used as a tourniquet during surgery |
| FluoroScan | (flōr′ō-scan) | brand name for x-ray device |
| interdigitation | (in′ter-dĭj′i-tā′shun) | the mutual interlocking of toothed or tonguelike processes |
| pronation | (prō-nā′shun) | rotation of the forearm such that the palm is downward |
| pronator teres | (prō-nā′tor tēr′ēz) | muscle in the forearm that, along with pronator quadratus, serves to pronate the forearm (turn the palm downward) |
| radial artery | | artery that passes along the radial side of the forearm |
| superficial radial nerve | | a branch of the radial nerve that provides sensation to the back of the hand, including the web of skin between the thumb and index finger |
| supination | (sū′pi-nā′shun) | rotation of the forearm such that the palm is upward |

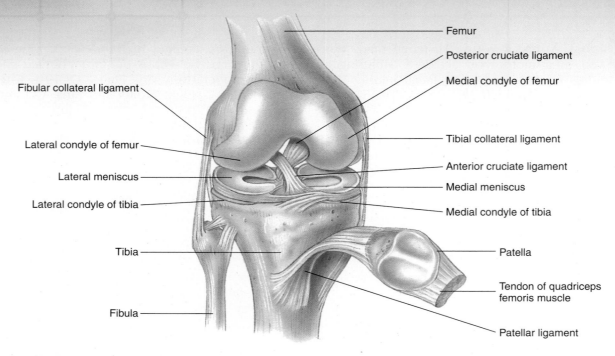

**Figure QC19-1** Knee. (*Delmar/Cengage Learning*)

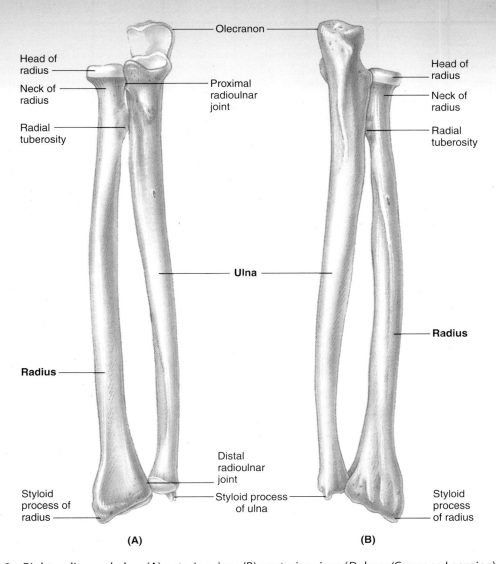

**Figure QC19-2** Right radius and ulna: (A) anterior view, (B) posterior view. (*Delmar/Cengage Learning*)

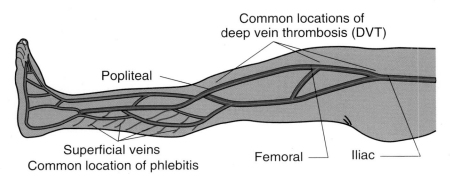

**Figure QC19-3** Superficial versus deep veins in development of phlebitis and thrombus. (*Delmar/Cengage Learning*)

# REPORT 20: VASCULAR SURGERY CLINIC NOTE

Merle W. Delmer is an elderly Caucasian male patient of the Vascular Surgery Clinic who has been treated in the past. He presents today in routine followup for peripheral vascular disease (PVD). He is given a complete physical examination, a review of his recent x-ray data, and a complete assessment/plan that includes possible further surgical treatment. See Figure QC20-1, Common sites for peripheral arterial occlusive disease.

## GLOSSARY

| Word | Phonetic Pronunciation | Definition |
|------|------------------------|------------|
| ABIs | | ankle-brachial indices—measurement of blood pressure in the ankle and in the arm; normally the blood pressures should be about equal, but if the blood pressure in the ankle is lower than in the arm, this may indicate arterial disease in the legs |
| aortobifemoral bypass | (ā-ŏr'tō-bī-fem'ŏr-ăl) | bypass of clogged arteries in the lower abdomen and upper legs using a graft |
| Dilantin | (dī-lăn'tĭn) | brand name of medication used to control seizures |
| fem-fem bypass | | medical jargon for femorofemoral bypass, a procedure in which blood flow is diverted around a blocked portion of the femoral artery by using a vascular graft to bypass the blocked portion of the artery |
| fem-pop bypass | | medical jargon for femoropopliteal bypass, a procedure in which blood flow is diverted from a point above a blocked femoral artery and connected to the popliteal artery at a point below the blockage |
| fraught | (frŏt) | filled with a specified element or elements; charged |
| Hunter canal | | the space in the thigh through which the femoral vessels pass |
| Nembutal | (nem'bū-tăl) | barbiturate medication used prior to anesthesia, used as a sedative, used for insomnia, and used as an anticonvulsant (brand name) |
| SFA | | superficial femoral artery—artery that runs along the front of the thigh toward the knee, gradually coursing toward the inside of the knee |

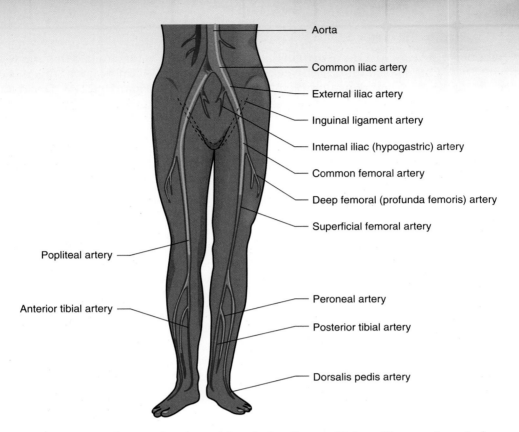

- Aorta
- Common iliac artery
- External iliac artery
- Inguinal ligament artery
- Internal iliac (hypogastric) artery
- Common femoral artery
- Deep femoral (profunda femoris) artery
- Superficial femoral artery
- Popliteal artery
- Anterior tibial artery
- Peroneal artery
- Posterior tibial artery
- Dorsalis pedis artery

**Figure QC20-1**   Common sites for peripheral arterial occlusive disease. (*Delmar/Cengage Learning*)

# REPORT 21: OPERATIVE REPORT

Savannah Crumrine, a 5-year-old Caucasian child, presented to the Quali-Care Dental Clinic last week for a complete exam that revealed dental problems requiring a full-mouth dental rehabilitation. Because of her age, it was determined that she would have to be treated in the Ambulatory Surgery Center under anesthesia. See Figure QC21-1, Deciduous and permanent teeth; Figure QC21-2, Layers of a tooth.

## GLOSSARY

| Word | Phonetic Pronunciation | Definition |
|---|---|---|
| ActCel gauze | | brand name of a type of gauze made from chemically treated cellulose; when placed in a wound, it facilitates the clotting process and converts to a gel that dissolves into glucose and saline over a 1- to 2-week period. |
| amalgam restoration | (ă-măl′gam) | a tooth cement composed of an alloy of mercury with another metal that is solid or liquid at room temperature that is used to restore the missing portion of a tooth |
| caries | (kăr′-ēz) | the formation of cavities in the teeth by the action of bacteria; decay |
| composite | (kŏm-pŏs′ĭt) | a material utilized in dental bonding technique, such as filling cavities or for cosmetic purposes |
| dental prophylaxis | (prō-fĭ-lăck′sĭs) | the removal of bacterial plaque, stains, food debris, and calculus from the roots and crowns of the teeth (teeth cleaning) |
| dental rehabilitation | | extensive dental restoration involving the rebuilding of natural teeth, filling in spaces where teeth are missing, and establishing the conditions that allow each tooth to function in harmony with the occlusion (bite) |
| facial surface | | the surface of a tooth that faces the inside of the cheek or lips |
| facial composite shade C-3 | | composite material placed on the surface of the tooth that faces the inside of the cheek or lips; shade C-3 is the color of the composite material used to match the existing tooth or teeth |
| halogen light | (hăl′ō-jĕn) | a light used by dentists to set or "cure" dental composite; the setting or curing process is activated by a specific wavelength range (color) of light |
| Ketac cement | (kē′tăk) | brand name for a type of cement used for lining the cavity of a tooth that has been removed |
| lingual surface | (ling′gwăl) | the surface of a tooth that faces the tongue |
| nasoendotracheal intubation | (nā′zō-en′dō-trā′kē-ăl) | insertion of a tube through the nostril into the trachea for purposes of general anesthetic instead of through the mouth into the trachea; done for oral surgical procedures |

(Continued)

## GLOSSARY

| Word | Phonetic Pronunciation | Definition |
|------|------------------------|------------|
| **nitrous oxide** | (nī'trŭs ŏx'īd) | gas used in dentistry for anesthetic and analgesic effects |
| **occlusal surface** | (ŏ-klū'zal) | the surface of a tooth that contacts an opposing surface of a tooth in the opposing jaw |
| **rubber dam isolation** | | the technique of isolating a tooth or group of teeth from its environment; a rubber dam is a thin, rectangular square of latex or silicone that is clamped to the tooth or teeth, and the tooth stands out from the rubber dam through a hole made with a hole punch, thus permitting a dry operative field |
| **sevoflurane** | (sē-vō-flū'rān) | a general anesthetic agent |
| **stainless steel crown** | | top of a tooth made out of stainless steel; used for restoring molars in children and adults |
| **throat pack** | | a sponge placed in the throat to absorb saliva and fluids during oral procedures; 1 side has an impervious layer to prevent the flow of fluids through it |

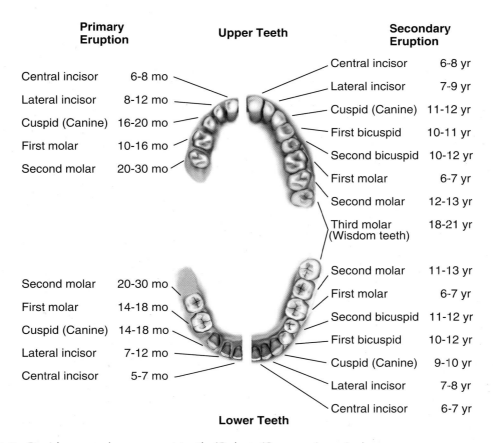

**Figure QC21-1**   Deciduous and permanent teeth. (*Delmar/Cengage Learning*)

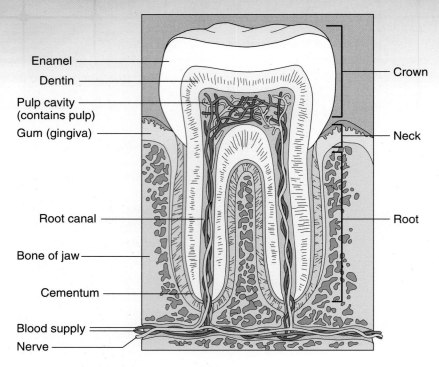

Enamel

Dentin

Pulp cavity
(contains pulp)

Gum (gingiva)

Root canal

Bone of jaw

Cementum

Blood supply

Nerve

Crown

Neck

Root

**Figure QC21-2**   Layers of a tooth. (*Delmar/Cengage Learning*)

# REPORT 22: OPERATIVE REPORT

Thomas J. Gill is a 32-year-old Caucasian male who has suffered from shoulder pain for several months, being unable to lift his arm above his head. Conservative treatment has failed, and he is scheduled for surgical repair of his anterior labral tear today. See Figure QC22-1, Rotator cuff tear; Figure QC22-2, Scapula; Figure QC22-3, Muscles that move the arm and fingers: (A) anterior and (B) posterior views.

## GLOSSARY

| Word | Phonetic Pronunciation | Definition |
|---|---|---|
| **acromion** | (ă-krō-mē-on) | bony prominence at the top of the shoulder blade that forms the point of the shoulder |
| **clavicle** | (klăv′ĭ-kĕl) | collar bone |
| **coracoid** | (kōr′ă-koyd) | a small fingerlike projection from the scapula that serves to stabilize the shoulder joint |
| **EBIce** | | cold therapy system with adjustable settings (trade name); dictated as letters E B, then Ice, altogether |
| **exacerbate** | (ĕg-zăs′ĕr-bāt″) | to worsen or make more severe |
| **glenohumeral joint** | (glē′nō-hyū′mĕr-ăl, glĕn′ō-) | the ball-and-socket joint between the head of the humerus and the glenoid cavity of the scapula |
| **interscalene block** | (ĭn′tĕr-skā′lēn) | regional anesthetic used for shoulder, arm, and elbow surgery. |
| **labrum** | (lā′brŭm) | cuff of cartilage that encircles the shoulder socket (glenoid) to make the socket deeper |
| **rotator cuff** | | composed of the tendons of the 4 muscles surrounding the glenohumeral joint (supraspinatus, infraspinatus, subscapularis, and teres minor) |
| **SLAP lesion** | (pronounced "slap") | superior *l*abrum, *a*nterior to *p*osterior—a type of labral tear seen in overhead-throwing athletes, such as tennis players and baseball players; the torn labrum is at the top of the shoulder socket |
| **subscapularis** | (sŭb-skap′yū-lā′ris) | one of the 4 muscles that surround the glenohumeral joint; the muscles are attached to the scapula |
| **supraspinatus** | (sū′pră-spī-nā′tus) | one of the 4 muscles that surround the glenohumeral joint; the muscles are attached to the scapula |
| **Xeroform** | (zē′rō-form) | nonadherent petrolatum gauze that conforms to body contours; for use on open wounds, minor burns, surgical incisions (trade name) |

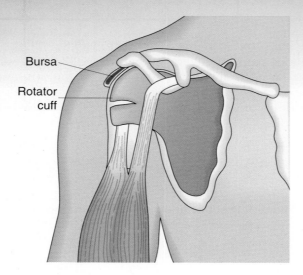

**Figure QC22-1**    Rotator cuff tear. (*Delmar/Cengage Learning*)

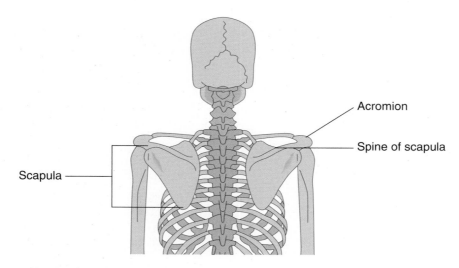

**Figure QC22-2**    Scapula. (*Delmar/Cengage Learning*)

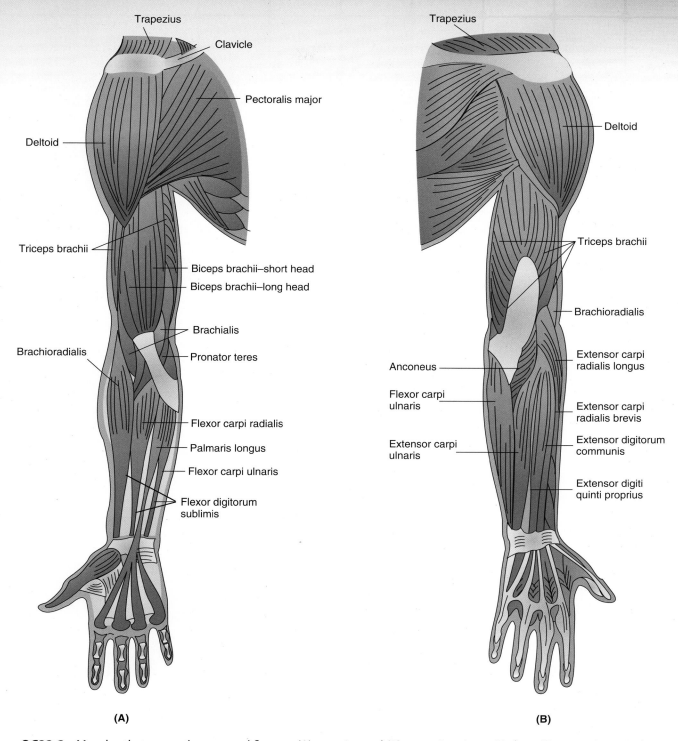

**Figure QC22-3** Muscles that move the arm and fingers: (A) anterior and (B) posterior views. (*Delmar/Cengage Learning*)

# REPORT 23: ORTHOPEDICS CONSULT

This 2-year-old Lebanese boy, Ramzi S. Cotran, was seen by his pediatrician because of an injury to his right middle finger with infection of the nail bed. Orthopedics was called for a consult today because of possible paronychia. See Figure QC23-1, Structure of the nail; Figure QC23-2, Paronychia; Figure QC23-3, Before and after circumcision.

## GLOSSARY

| Word | Phonetic Pronunciation | Definition |
|------|------------------------|------------|
| capillary refill | (kăp′i-lār-ē) | the rate at which blood refills empty capillaries (tiny blood vessels); measured by pressing a fingernail until it turns white, then releasing and taking note of how long the nail takes to return to normal color |
| erythema | (ĕr″ĭ-thē′mah) | redness of the skin produced by abnormal accumulation of blood |
| nail bed | | the part of the nail under the nail plate |
| paronychia | (par′ō-nik′ē-ă) | infection of the nail fold surrounding the nail plate |
| phalanx | (fā′langks, fă-langks′) | one of the long bones of the digits, 14 in number for each hand or foot |
| purulence | (pyūr′ū-lĕns, pyūr′ŭ-lĕns) | the condition of containing or forming pus |

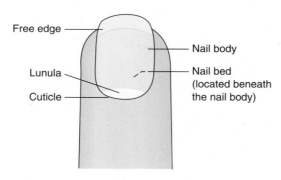

**Figure QC23-1**   Structure of the nail. (*Delmar/Cengage Learning*)

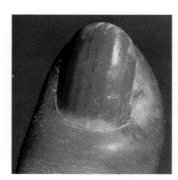

**Figure QC23-2**   Paronychia. (*Delmar/Cengage Learning*)

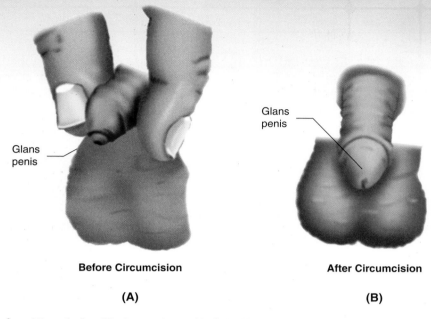

Glans
penis

Glans
penis

**Before Circumcision**

**After Circumcision**

**(A)**

**(B)**

**Figure QC23-3** Before (A) and after (B) circumcision. (*Delmar/Cengage Learning*)

# REPORT 24: PSYCHOLOGICAL/INTELLECTUAL EVALUATION

Barbara Christine Anello is a 14-year-old Italian girl who is undergoing psychological/intellectual evaluation by a psychologist because of continuing difficulties in school. She is new to the area and seems to be having a hard time with her school work and generally fitting in. See Figure QC24-1, Lonely, isolated child; Figure QC24-2, Patient receiving outside counseling.

## GLOSSARY

| Word | Phonetic Pronunciation | Definition |
|---|---|---|
| Achenbach Youth Self Report | (ŏk'en-bŏk) | an assessment test for violent behavior; youths rate themselves |
| animated | (ăn'ĭ-mā-tĕd) | full of vigor and spirit; lively |
| industrious | (ĭn-dŭs'trē-ŭs) | constantly, regularly, or habitually active or occupied |
| passive | | tending not to take an active or dominant part |
| Wechsler Intelligence Scale for Children-III (WISC-III) | (wĕks'ler) | an intelligence test for children age 6 to 16 that can be completed without reading or writing |
| Woodcock-Johnson Psychoeducational Battery (WJPB) | | useful for measuring cognitive ability for people age 2 years and older; contains 21 different subtests and measures 7 broad intellectual abilities including visual process, processing speed, long-term retrieval, short-term memory, auditory processing, comprehension knowledge, and fluid reasoning |

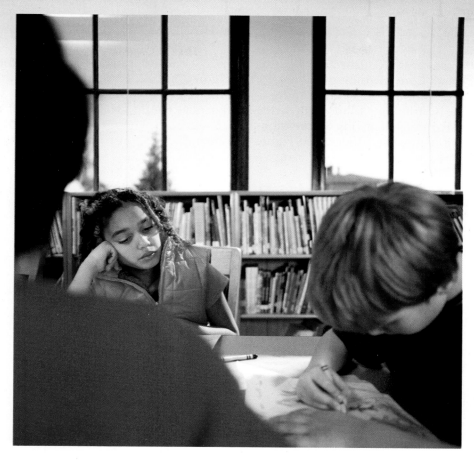

**Figure QC24-1**    Lonely, isolated child. (*Source: © Getty Images/Photodisc.*)

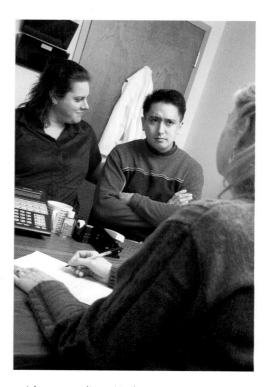

**Figure QC24-2**    Patient receiving outside counseling. (*Delmar/Cengage Learning*)

# Report 25a&b: Correspondence and Cardiology Consult

James H. Helland, an elderly Caucasian male, was referred to the Quali-Care Cardiology Clinic for evaluation of his cardiopulmonary and endocrinology status. The Cardiology Clinic sent a letter and an extensive consult giving impressions and recommendations for the patient. See Figure QC25-1, Standard chest lead placements for EKG; Figure QC25-2, Marked edema of the lower legs, ankles, and part of the feet due to venous insufficiency; Figure QC25-3, The CPAP mask applies pressure to keep the airway open while the patient sleeps, preventing sleep apnea.

## GLOSSARY

| Word | Phonetic Pronunciation | Definition |
| --- | --- | --- |
| ACE inhibitor | (pronounced "ace") | angiotensin-converting enzyme—class of medications used primarily to treat hypertension |
| antecedent | (an'tĭ-sē'dent) | a preceding event, condition, or cause |
| atherosclerotic vascular disease | (ath'er-ō-skler-ŏt'ĭk) | the progressive narrowing and hardening of arteries over time |
| habitus | (hăb'ĭ-tŭs) | the physical characteristics of a person |
| cor pulmonale | (kor pŭl-mō'năl-ē) | alteration in the structure and function of the right ventricle of the heart caused by a primary disorder of the respiratory system |
| dobutamine echocardiogram | (dō-bū'tă-mēn) | study performed after the patient is given dobutamine (drug that makes the heart work harder) to assess the heart muscle under stress |
| lung apices | (ā'pi-sēz) | the tops of the lungs |
| obstructive sleep apnea | (ăp'nē-ă) | sleep disorder characterized by pauses in breathing during sleep; caused by obstruction of the airway |
| orthopnea | (ōr-thop'nē-ă) | discomfort in breathing that is brought on by lying flat |
| PND | | paroxysmal nocturnal dyspnea—a sensation of shortness of breath that awakens the patient from sleep |
| P-R interval | | one of the parts of an electrocardiogram tracing that shows electrical heart activity |
| presyncope | (prē-sĭn'kō-pē) | lightheadedness |
| Q-T interval | | one of the parts of an electrocardiogram tracing that shows electrical heart activity |
| reactive airway disease or reactive airways disease | | a general term that does not indicate a specific diagnosis; can be used to indicate a history of coughing, wheezing, or shortness of breath of unknown cause |
| syncope | (sĭn'kō-pē) | loss of consciousness; fainting |

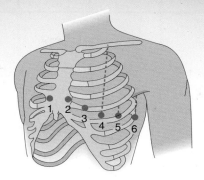

**Figure QC25-1** Standard chest lead placements for EKG. (*Delmar/Cengage Learning*)

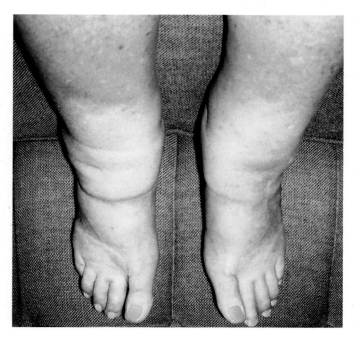

**Figure QC25-2** Marked edema of the lower legs, ankles, and part of the feet due to venous insufficiency. (*Delmar/ Cengage Learning*)

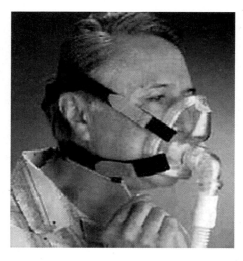

**Figure QC25-3** The CPAP mask applies pressure to keep the airway open while the patient sleeps, preventing sleep apnea. (*Delmar/Cengage Learning*)

# SECTION 6

## EXPAND YOUR KNOWLEDGE

# CROSSWORD PUZZLE:
## CASE 1 GLOSSARY

STUDENT _____

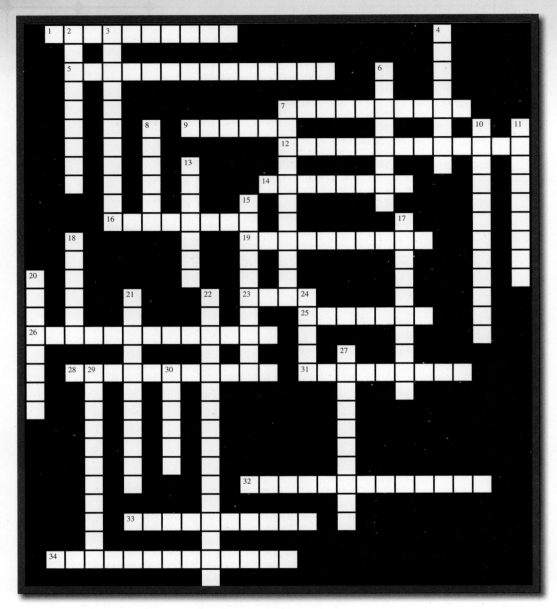

# ACROSS

1. pain in a joint
5. across or through the abdominal wall
7. the serous membrane lining the abdominal walls and investing the viscera
9. supportive layer of thin connective tissue within the muscles and/or organs of the body
12. absorbable catgut suture material
14. performed using both hands
16. perceptible by touch
19. one thousandth of a liter
23. to cut or separate, as at surgery
25. trade name for meperidine hydrochloride
26. also called oviduct or uterine tube
28. layers that enclose a uterine tube, which are composed of the broad ligament of the uterus

and are located above the mesovarium
31. fibrous bands or structures by which body parts abnormally adhere, as in wound healing
32. a cyst containing a tuft of hairs, usually found at the base of the spine
33. physical, chemical, or microscopic analysis of urine
34. surgical removal of a uterine tube

# DOWN

2. instrument used to hold wound edges and/or tissues apart during surgery
3. medical tool used to grasp and manipulate tissue
4. instrument used to spread open a passage or cavity for ease in its examination
6. nearest the trunk or point of origin, said of part of a limb, artery, or nerve
7. cloths used to pack off the tissues and aid in hemostasis during surgery
8. trade name for an absorbable suture made of multifilament braided material

10. beneath the skin
11. blood in the urine
13. acute infectious disease caused by the toxin of the bacterium Clostridium tetani
15. carries oxygen from the lungs to the tissues and carbon dioxide from the tissues to the lungs
17. the volume percentage of erythrocytes in whole blood
18. situated away from the center of the body, or from the point of origin
20. antibiotic against gram-negative bacteria, trade name
21. to bring close together or into apposition

22. a pregnancy in which the fertilized ovum becomes implanted on tissue outside of the uterine cavity
24. abnormal accumulation of fluid in the intercellular tissue spaces of the body, resulting in swelling
27. describes blood with no Rh antigen
29. within the vagina
30. appendages or adjunct parts; in gynecology, used to describe the tubes and ovaries

# CROSSWORD PUZZLE:
## CASE 2 GLOSSARY

STUDENT _____

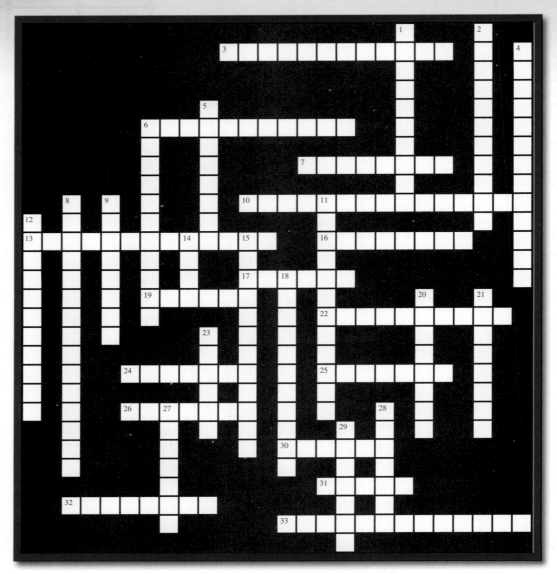

# ACROSS

3. the act of listening for sounds within the body
6. examination by means of a flexible, elongated scope which permits visual examination of the colon
7. tensing of muscles in response to touch
10. near the appendix
13. removal of the right or left side of the colon

16. a spreading inflammatory reaction to infection that can form multiple pus pockets
17. lying face upward
19. entirely, in the whole
22. enveloping membrane of the body, including skin, hair, and nails
24. to spread out in all directions from a center
25. large areas of sustained outward motion of the chest felt when performing a heart examination

26. when the abdomen is pressed, then released, more pain is felt upon release than when it is applied
30. vomiting
31. used to describe the closed end of the large intestine
32. a condition of thickening and widening of the fingers and toes with abnormally curved nails
33. pain in the lower abdomen or inside of thigh when the hip is flexed and internally rotated

# DOWN

1. stretching or enlarging an opening of a hollow structure
2. air or gas removed from a cavity or chamber of the body
4. related to the liver and bile ducts
5. chemical substances introduced in radiography to increase the difference between different tissues or between abnormal and normal tissues

6. a hydration solution containing only electrolytes
8. enlargement of lymph nodes, which may indicate infection
9. dead, as in dead tissue
11. infection or inflammation of the vermiform appendix
12. enlargement of the thyroid gland
14. a soft mass formed when a liquid (blood or lymph) thickens
15. fold of tissue attaching the appendix to the small bowel
18. the two arterial pulses able to be felt in the foot

20. containing, consisting of, or forming pus
21. Diminished appetite; aversion to food
23. gas or air in the gastrointestinal tract passed through the anus
27. a topical skin protectant
28. an abnormal passage between 2 organs in the body or between an organ and the outside of the body
29. bony

# CROSSWORD PUZZLE:
## CASE 3 GLOSSARY

STUDENT _____

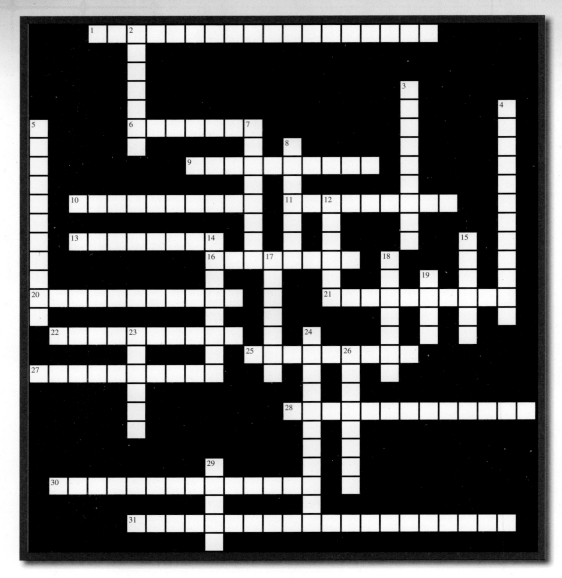

# ACROSS

1. rapid, irregular contractions of the atria
6. pertaining to deficient oxygenation of the tissues
9. the insertion of a tube into a body canal or hollow organ
10. toxins in the blood, formerly called "blood poisoning"
11. supplementary
13. medical jargon meaning a patient's heartbeat and/or respirations have ceased, calling for immediate CPR
16. the presence of a fungal growth in the blood stream
20. within or into a vein
21. inflammation of the air sacs in the lung
22. the lidlike cartilaginous structure that folds back over the larynx during swallowing
25. occurring on both sides
27. swelling of blood vessels due to engorgement with blood
28. within the bronchi or bronchial tubes
30. the record obtained by using ultrasound to bounce back ultrasonic waves from the heart
31. injury or necrosis of the heart muscle due to lack of blood supply to the area

# DOWN

2. sounds with a musical pitch (heard on auscultation) in bronchial tubes due to inflammation, spasm of muscle, or presence of mucus
3. pertaining to the lungs
4. a medical specialist in diagnosing and treating kidney disease
5. abnormally decreased motor function or activity
7. trade name for warfarin sodium
8. a vague feeling of bodily discomfort
12. a downward and backward projection of the lowest tracheal cartilage, forming a ridge between the openings of the right and left main bronchi
14. the escape of fluid into a body part or tissue
15. material coughed up from the lower respiratory tract
17. the vocal apparatus of the larynx consisting of several structures that form the supporting structures of the vocal cords
18. pertaining to the serous membrane that covers the lungs and lining of the thoracic cavity
19. an abnormal air-filled or fluid-filled sac
23. any abnormality involving an organ or tissue due to a disease process or injury
24. pertaining to the functional elements of an organ
26. cause or origin of a disease or disorder
29. pertaining to the depression, notch, or opening where the vessels and nerves enter an organ

# CROSSWORD PUZZLE:
## CASE 4 GLOSSARY

STUDENT _____

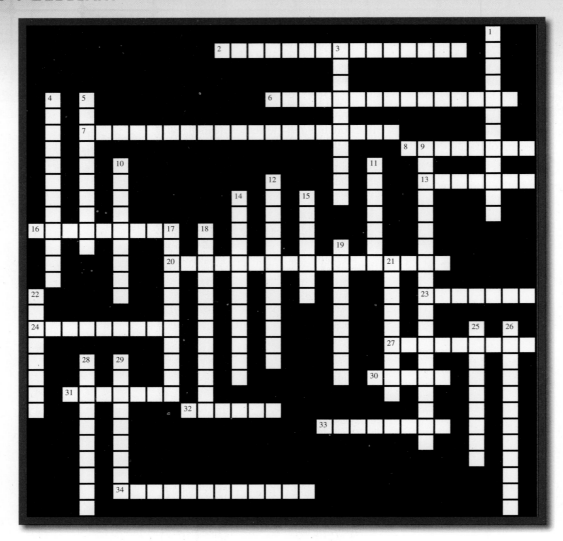

# ACROSS

2. a group of steroids (or lip-ids) used clinically in immune suppression or in hormonal replacement
6. dehydrated state
7. any break or rupture of bone due to compression, e.g., the bones of the spine
8. redness of the skin produced by abnormal accumulation of blood

13. any fluid that has escaped from blood vessels and deposited in tissues
16. a B complex vitamin necessary for normal production of red blood cells
20. abnormally increased coloration
23. (adj.) widely distributed, not concentrated
24. difficulty swallowing
27. inflammation of the joints
30. to intensify suddenly

31. a strictly regulated plan of therapy, diet, exercise, or other activity designed to achieve a certain goal
32. roof of the mouth
33. humpback
34. a laboratory test to determine the level of all proteins in the serum

# DOWN

1. generic name for chemotherapy drug; used also in treatment of rheumatoid arthritis
3. inflammation of the oral mucosa, the mucous membranes of the mouth
4. decreased bone mass leading to pathologic fractures
5. a purplish patch on the skin caused by blood passing from a vessel into the tissues
9. chronic systemic, painful joint disease that can result in deformities

10. estrogen produced by the ovaries; used as hormone replacement therapy
11. the pale pink tissues of the oral mucosa
12. causing weakness or a lack of strength
14. generic name of drug used in chemotherapy
15. a necessary protein substance produced in the liver
17. condition resulting from either excessive loss of or inadequate intake of water
18. decreased reflexes
19. inflammation of the intestine, particularly the small intestine

21. applied to the skin
22. trade name for topically applied gel, which has anti-inflammatory properties
25. splitting of the skin; can include painful ulcerations
26. indentations when a finger is pressed on the skin; occurs when excessive fluid is in the tissues
28. generic name for a type of steroid used as an anti-inflammatory agent
29. at rest; inactive

# CROSSWORD PUZZLE:
## CASE 5 GLOSSARY

STUDENT _____

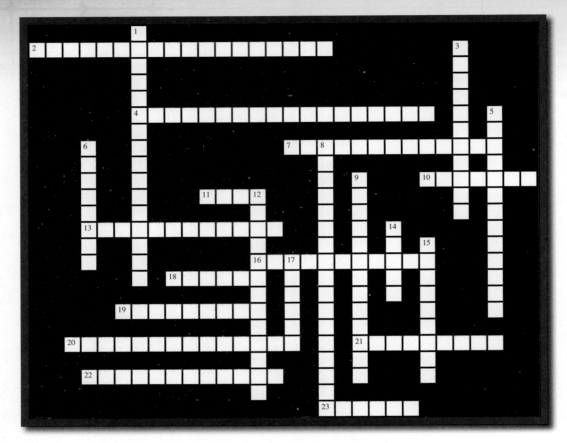

# ACROSS

2. inability to coordinate and carry out facial and lip movements on command, such as whistling or winking
4. thoughts about killing another person
7. involuntary contractions, or twitching, of groups of muscle fibers
10. test performed for balance
11. rudely abrupt; blunt; brief; gruff
13. an antibiotic
16. inclined to act on impulse rather than thought
18. prescription medicine used to treat symptoms of overactive bladder
19. x-ray contrast medium for use in computerized tomography (CT)
20. arthritis characterized by erosion of the articular cartilage
21. a nonsteroidal anti-inflammatory agent

22. removal of the uterus
23. implies a silent ill humor and refusal to be sociable

# DOWN

1. substitution of an incorrect sound (e.g., tree for free) or related word (e.g., chair for bed)
3. condition characterized by neck stiffness, headache, and other symptoms of meningeal irritation but without meningitis
5. on stepping forward, placing the heel of the foot in front against the toe of the foot in back
6. the progressive loss of cognitive and intellectual functions without impairment of perception or consciousness
8. thoughts of killing oneself
9. harsh or musical abnormal sounds in the artery of the neck

produced by turbulent blood flow
12. removal of the entire tonsil
14. a gradual movement, as from an original position; dictated in neurologic exam
15. an emotional state characterized by anxiety, depression, or unease
17. conception and planning of a motor act in response to an environmental demand

# CROSSWORD PUZZLE:
## CASE 6 GLOSSARY

STUDENT _____

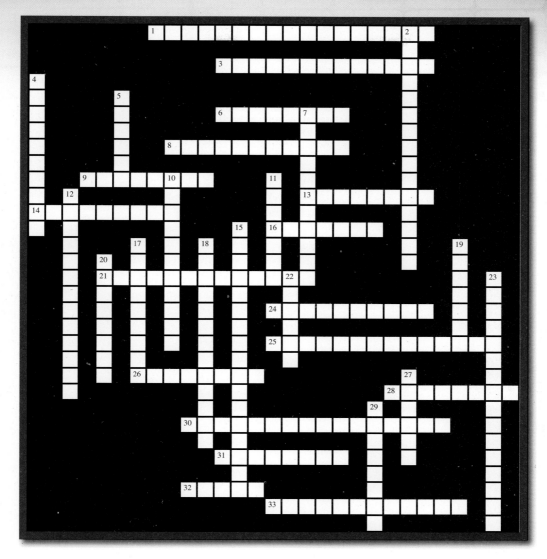

# ACROSS

1. space between the arachnoid membrane and the pia mater
3. rupture of the intervertebral disk cartilage, allowing contents to protrude through it, putting pressure on the spinal nerve roots; can cause pain
6. a smear of cells taken from the vagina or cervix to be studied for evidence of cancer
8. crowding or clustering together
9. a powerful disinfectant gas, used in water as a fluid to preserve tissue removed at surgery for pathologic evaluation
13. when the examiner pricks a patient's skin with a sharp point to determine feeling
14. the record produced by an x-ray of the spinal cord obtained after injection of dye into the spinal canal
16. trade name for a drug used to treat muscle spasms
21. surgical equipment in which a patient is placed for back surgery; trade name
24. walking
25. located between 2 adjoining vertebrae
26. small projecting outgrowths from any structure; most often used with bony outgrowths
28. bruised
30. band of yellow elastic tissue that assists in maintaining or regaining the erect position between 2 adjoining vertebrae
31. made up of separate and distinct parts or defined by lesions that do not become unified
32. lying face downward
33. periodically stopping and starting again at separated intervals

# DOWN

2. delivery of a fetus by making an incision in the abdominal wall and uterus
4. removal of an intervertebral disk
5. low area, trough, or groove
7. drug used as a vasoconstrictor, cardiac stimulant, and bronchodilator; generic name
10. pertaining to the lumbar region of the spine and the sacrum
11. less sharp; dull
12. trade name for absorbable, sterile gelatin sponge

15. main area or center of deterioration
17. a sideways deviation in the normally straight vertical line of the spine
18. pain along an area of distribution of a specific nerve or nerves caused by pressure on the nerve root; pain may be felt in the low back or legs or in 1 or both arms
19. a surgical instrument used for cutting tough tissue, such as bone
20. in physical examination of the abdomen, the abdominal wall has a concave, or sunken, contour

22. part of the back of the bony arch of each vertebra
23. the inward displacement of the nipple below the level of the surrounding breast tissue
27. having a surface that is rounded and somewhat elevated
29. trade name for drug used to treat muscle spasm

# CROSSWORD PUZZLE:
## CASE 7 GLOSSARY

STUDENT _____

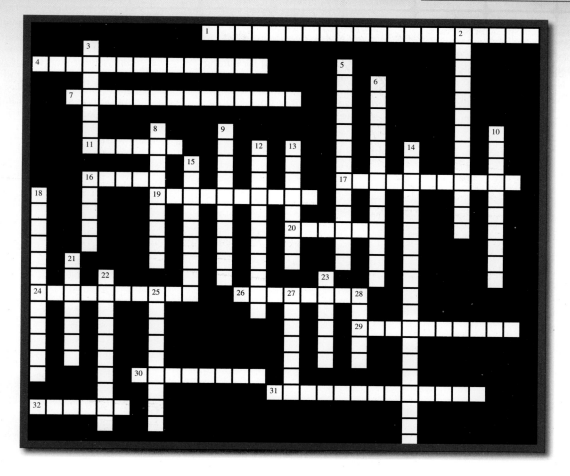

## ACROSS

1. a fracture of the bone around a plate or screws that are already in place
4. a fracture that is not visible in an x-ray within 24 to 48 hours of trauma or injury but will become visible in x-rays within 3 to 4 weeks
7. relating to the calcaneus and cuboid bone
11. chronic enlargement of the thyroid gland
16. antibiotic used to treat a wide variety of bacterial infections; used intramuscularly or intravenously
17. within a nerve
19. a bony outgrowth or protuberance
20. a type of insulin
24. brand name oral antidiabetic medication
26. the back part of the foot
29. generic name of drug used to treat primarily hypertension
30. excessive excretion of urine resulting in frequent and profuse urination
31. relating to the talus bone and the navicular bone
32. brand name for cotton material used as absorbent surgical dressing

# DOWN

2. relating to the cuboid bone and the navicular bone
3. brand name oral antidiabetic medication
5. made bloodless
6. anti-inflammatory agent; used to test adrenal function
8. generic name for Glucophage
9. the thick, fibrous membrane covering the entire surface of a bone

10. one of the 5 long bones on the top of the foot
12. surgical fusion of a joint
13. below the talus bone
14. velvety, benign growths on the skin of the neck, groin, and axillae
15. an instrument used for cutting bone
16. oral antidiabetic agent
18. displacement of bones out of line in relation to joints

21. abnormal position of the foot in which the toes are lower than the heel, causing toe-walking
22. excessive, prolonged thirst
23. brand name of narcotic used to treat moderate to severe pain
25. degenerative joint changes
27. difficulty or pain in urination
28. brand name for a wound dressing consisting of thin layer of cotton fibers wrapped in plastic film to keep it from sticking to wounds

# CROSSWORD PUZZLE:
## CASE 8 GLOSSARY

STUDENT _____

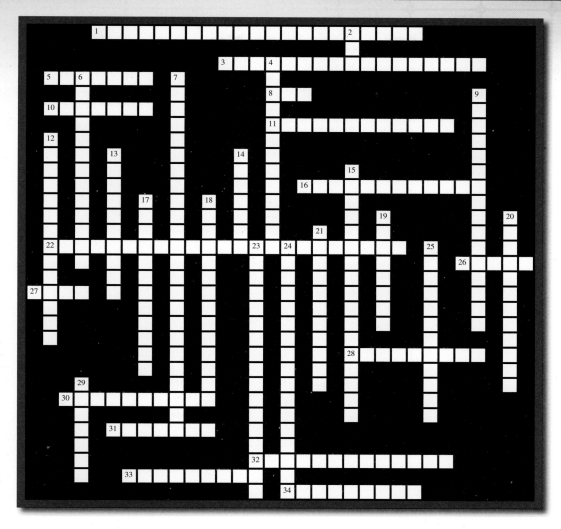

# ACROSS

1. surgical removal of material occluding the carotid artery
3. the point at which the abdominal aorta branches into the right and left common iliac arteries
5. generic name of medication used to treat and prevent blood clots
8. abbreviation for blood urea nitrogen, a blood test used to evaluate kidney function
10. related to or marked by distension, dilatation, or expansion
11. abnormal enlargement of the abdominal organs
16. elevated blood level of potassium
22. the structures that appear in the proximity of the middle of the chest cavity as seen on chest x-ray
26. brand name for a cholesterol-lowering medication
27. abbreviation for chronic obstructive pulmonary disease
28. generic name for medication used to treat high blood pressure, chest pain, and certain heart rhythm disorders
30. a blood test that measures kidney function
31. brand name of medication used to make urine less acidic
32. inflammation of the bone marrow and adjacent bone
33. pertaining to a structure or tissue that is able to be imaged on x-ray
34. the condition of thrusting or pressing out

# DOWN

2.  abbreviation for congestive heart failure
4.  relating to the tibia and fibula
6.  fine-pointed scissors used in vascular surgery
7.  the joint between the head of the metatarsal and the base of the phalanx of the toe
9.  brand name for an instrument used to surgically convert a vein into an artery in arterial bypass
12. distension of the kidney with urine, caused by backward pressure on the kidney when flow of urine is obstructed

13. generic name of medication used to increase urine formation and output (diuretic)
14. brand name of medication used to treat congestive heart failure and atrial fibrillation
15. a condition of pH imbalance in which the body has accumulated too much acid
17. enlargement of the heart
18. generic name of medication used to help improve the symptoms of blood flow problems in the legs and arms
19. having many curves; full of turns and twists
20. dissolving of a thrombus
21. an operative union of 2 structures

23. widespread and very serious allergic reaction
24. the shadow of the heart as it appears on a chest x-ray
25. a drifting of the large toe in the direction of the small toe, with formation of a bump on the inside of the big toe over the metatarsal bone
29. brand name for nonabsorbable suture material used for skin closure

# CROSSWORD PUZZLE:
## CASE 9 GLOSSARY

STUDENT _____

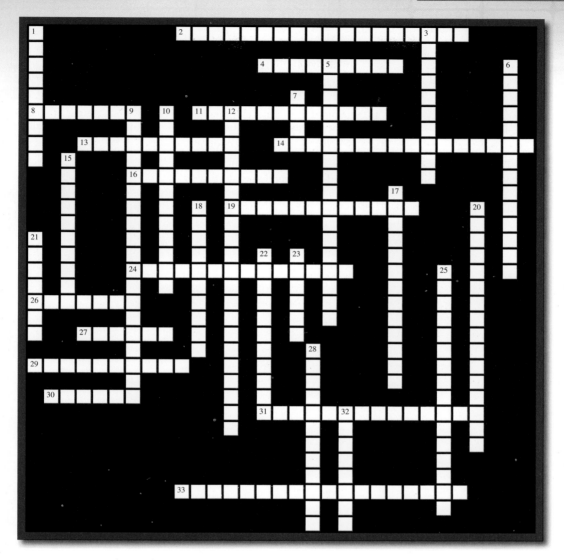

# ACROSS

2. a cement used in joint replacement surgery
4. tissue transplant between 2 humans
8. brand name of medication taken to treat seasonal allergies
11. in orthopedics, the interior longitudinal cavity of the femur bone
13. softening, absorption, and destruction of bony tissue
14. rotation away from the center of the body
16. a cup-shaped depression at the base of the hip bone into which the ball-shaped head of the femur (thigh bone) fits
19. bone that has been cut
24. spongy interior layer of bone that protects the bone marrow
26. the lower and back part of the hip bone where it joins the pelvis
27. brand name for medication used to treat depression and anxiety
29. a fabricated substitute used to assist a damaged or replace a missing body part
30. to move toward the middle of the body
31. generic name for medication that treats fluid retention
33. loss of bony continuity through both anterior and posterior columns of the pelvis

# DOWN

1. generic name for medication used to treat abnormal heart rhythms, chest pains, and also migraine headaches
3. referring to blood or blood components the donor has previously donated and receives at a later time
5. an upper part of the femur to which the gluteus medius and minimus muscles, and others, attach
6. defect of the limbs characterized by severe contractures of multiple joints noted at birth

7. to bend
9. the part of an artificial hip joint that takes the place of the diseased or injured acetabulum
10. most popular plastic used in the world
12. relating to the muscles and to the skeleton
15. pertaining to abnormal tissue development
17. generic name for antibiotic
18. acquired during development in the uterus and not through heredity
20. the part of an artificial hip joint that takes the place of the diseased or injured femoral head

21. generic name for narcotic medication used to treat mild to moderate pain
22. never having borne a child
23. to move away from the middle of the body
25. rotation toward the center of the body
28. creation of an artificial joint to correct advanced degenerative arthritis
32. brand name of nasal spray used to treat seasonal allergies or hay fever

# CROSSWORD PUZZLE:
## CASE 10 GLOSSARY

STUDENT _____

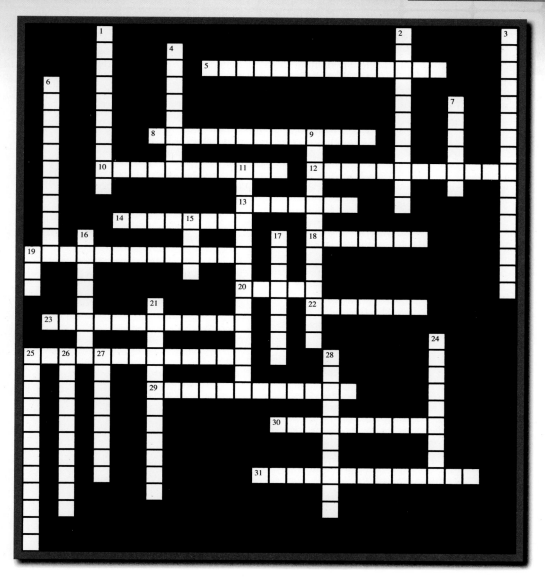

# ACROSS

5. a medication that expands the air passages of the lungs
8. bacteria growing in chains found in human mouth and intestine
10. the production of adhesions between the parietal and the visceral pleura
12. performed through the skin
13. a topical anesthetic, generic name
14. a small surgical clamp for constricting a blood vessel
18. a small space or cavity
19. a 1-way valve that allows air to flow out of the chest through a chest tube
20. the main trunk of the arterial system, conveying blood from the heart
22. a tube for insertion into a duct or cavity
23. a smooth muscle relaxant, used chiefly for its bronchodilator effect
25. medical jargon pertaining to the equipment used and the process of obtaining a chest x-ray outside of the radiology department
29. surgical creation of an opening in the chest wall for the purpose of drainage
30. dryness and fishlike scaling of the skin
31. treatment involving the injection of a hardening solution into vessels or tissues

# DOWN

1. film produced by radiography, commonly called an x-ray
2. between the ribs
3. brand name for an antiseptic solution used on the skin
4. a tubular, flexible instrument for either withdrawing fluids or introducing fluids into a body cavity or vessel
6. to put under the influence of drugs or agents used to abolish the sensation of pain

7. noticeable; to an extreme
9. generic name for a broad-spectrum antibiotic
11. a less than therapeutic level, usually referring to the blood level of a medication
15. abbreviation for immediately
16. pertaining to an emergency
17. pertaining to the chest
19. hepatojugular reflux
21. persistently high arterial blood pressure
24. a pathologic accumulation of air in tissues or organs that causes

abnormal swelling of body tissues
25. the presence of free air or gas in the pleural cavity
26. the subsidence or disappearance of a pathologic condition
27. separation, detachment, or removal of organ or tissue, especially by surgical means
28. one side of the chest

# CROSSWORD PUZZLE:
## QUALI-CARE GLOSSARIES 1–4

STUDENT _____

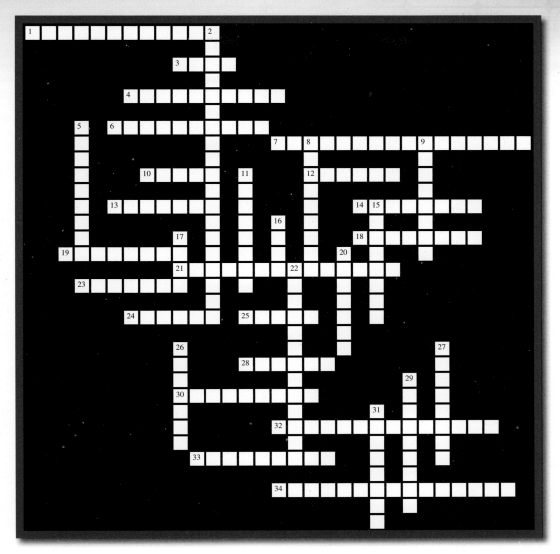

# ACROSS

1. room where patients are taken for close monitoring after surgery
3. localized areas of disease
4. the serous membrane lining the abdominal walls and investing the viscera
6. relating to or pertaining to both fibrous and fatty structures
7. a set of specific procedures performed under carefully controlled conditions to minimize contamination by bacteria

10. the retinal arteries and veins that can be seen by shining a light into the eye
12. a blunt instrument used to enter the abdominal cavity
13. blood clots
14. generic name for Coumadin
18. a measurement of the blood flow across the aortic valve
19. a gland in the male surrounding the beginning of the urethra
21. one of the 4 heart valves; it is between the right atrium and right ventricle
23. the tube leading from the bladder through which urine leaves the body

24. sounds or murmurs heard on auscultation, especially abnormal ones
25. treats fluid retention in people with congestive heart failure, liver disease, or a kidney disorder (brand name)
28. used to lower cholesterol and triglycerides
30. brand name; used to prevent asthma attacks
32. one of 4 chambers of the heart; it receives blood from the right atrium and pumps it to the lungs
33. a pathologic accumulation of air in tissues or organs, which

causes abnormal swelling of body tissues

34. structures in the male about 2 inches long, located behind the bladder

# DOWN

2. tiny bits of calcium that may show up in clusters on a mammogram
5. brand name of medication used to prevent asthma attacks in adults and children

8. after surgery, removed the tube through which anesthesia was administered
9. medication used to prevent blood clots (brand name)
11. containing mucus
15. brand name of medication used to prevent bronchospasm
16. a cuplike, passive soft tissue structure that is part of the structure of a heart valve
17. general endotracheal tube anesthesia

20. brand name of medication used to treat congestive heart failure and atrial fibrillation
22. a blue dye used for measurement of kidney function
26. shortness of breath
27. the arteries of the neck
29. generic name for medication used to treat high blood pressure, chest pain, and certain heart rhythm disorders
31. in a direction toward the head

# CROSSWORD PUZZLE:
## QUALI-CARE GLOSSARIES 5–9

STUDENT _____

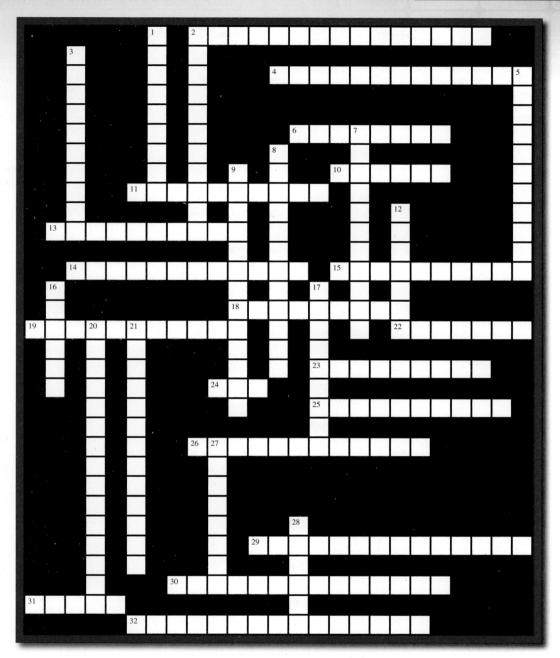

# ACROSS

2.  pertaining to the femoral artery and the popliteal artery in the leg
4.  having a head of medium length
6.  a stricture of any canal or orifice
10. performing 2 functions
11. generic name for medication used to treat high blood pressure, heart pain, abnormal rhythms of the heart, and some neurologic conditions
13. a bony outgrowth or protuberance
14. passing or occurring across a lumen (interior) as of a blood vessel
15. moving backward
18. a wire with a special coating containing a lubricant making it easy to insert into blood vessels
19. a class of drugs used primarily for the management of cardiac rhythm disorders
22. trade name for meperidine hydrochloride
23. in the direction of normal movement, as in blood flow
24. a thin muscle that functions to extend the big toe, lift the

foot up, and assist with foot inversion

25. material used as contrast media for magnetic resonance imaging
26. limping
29. the awareness of the position of one's body
30. rupture or slipping out of place of the disk in between 2 vertebrae
31. the narrowed portion of a vessel during inflation of a balloon to try to expand the vessel
32. enlargement of lymph nodes, which may indicate infection

# Down

1. contrast agent used during coronary arteriography, particularly in individuals with renal dysfunction
2. examination of the tissues and deep structures of the body using an instrument to obtain real-time images
3. purplish patches on the skin caused by blood passing from a vessel into the tissues
5. generic name for antibiotic
7. decrease in number of neutrophils
8. rapid or irregular heartbeats

9. demonstration of an artery or arteries by x-ray imaging after injection of a contrast medium
12. terminated a procedure prematurely
16. used to treat symptoms of claudication (brand name)
17. drowsy, sluggish
20. the upper vertebral body is abnormally slipped forward on the one below
21. a curve in the spine that points to the left
27. lack of interest, energy, or spirit
28. medication given to prevent nausea and vomiting caused by surgery or cancer medicines

# CROSSWORD PUZZLE:
## QUALI-CARE GLOSSARIES 10–12

STUDENT _____

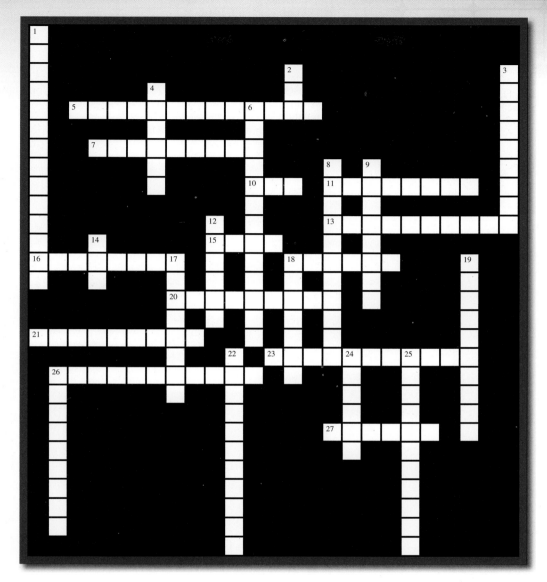

# ACROSS

5. procedure using a device on the fingertip or earlobe to measure oxygen saturation by fluctuations of light absorption
7. a rounded, fleshy protuberance situated over the pubic bone that becomes covered with hair during puberty
10. normal saline solution
11. part of the ulna that meets the humerus to form the elbow joint
13. one of the muscles on the chest wall
15. open reduction, internal fixation
16. in the humerus, a depression where it meets the ulna to form the elbow joint
18. a mass of tissue that forms at a fracture site that ultimately becomes bone
20. a small head or rounded articular end of a bone
21. a very dilute local anesthetic used for liposuction
23. pouches or sacs opening from a tubular organ, such as bowel or bladder
26. a breaking into several pieces, particularly when describing a fracture
27. spoon-shaped surgical instrument for removing tissue from a cavity wall or other bodily surface

# DOWN

1. an operation performed on the abdominal wall for cosmetic purposes
2. muscle of the forearm that flexes and abducts the hand
3. navel; belly button
4. trade name for a drug given intravenously either before or during surgery to produce sedation and amnesia
6. made bloodless
8. generic name for medication used to prevent motion sickness
9. condition in which a bone is cracked or broken
12. small growths that project outward from the normal surface level
14. muscle that extends the wrist
17. small muscle on the back of the elbow joint
18. inflammation of the colon
19. after childbirth
22. examination by means of a flexible, elongated scope that permits visual examination of the colon
24. the shorter of the 2 bones of the forearm
25. a hydration solution containing only electrolytes
26. generic name for antibiotic

# CROSSWORD PUZZLE:
## QUALI-CARE GLOSSARIES 13–17

STUDENT _____

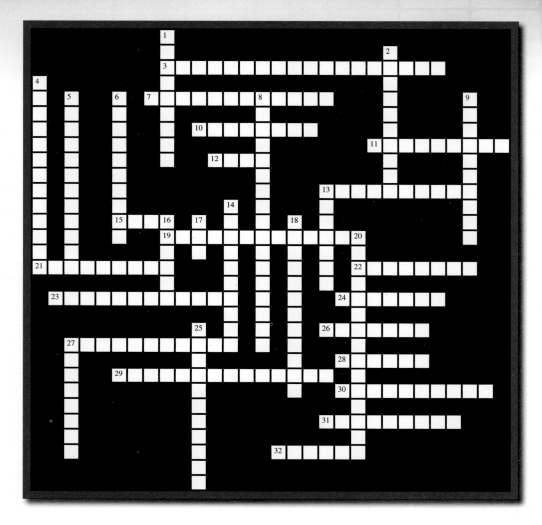

# ACROSS

3. the part of the cervical fascia that covers the bodies of the cervical vertebrae and the muscles attaching to them
7. examination of the upper urinary tract, usually performed with an endoscope
10. brand name of medication used to treat symptoms of acid reflux
11. brand name of medication used to treat seizures and also to treat nerve pain
12. attention deficit hyperactivity disorder
13. relating to the epigastrium
15. postanesthesia care unit
19. a return of small amounts of gas or food from the stomach
21. growing old
22. facial muscle in neck region; depresses lower lip, increases diameter of neck
23. reduction in quantity of bone
24. the canal leading from the bladder, discharging the urine externally
26. funnel-shaped hollows in the pelvis of the kidney through which urine passes to the ureter
27. one or more of the bones of the spine move out of position and create pressure on or irritate spinal nerves
28. discharging of the bowels
29. any of various diseases of the brain
30. removal of an intervertebral disk
31. laboratory technique used to detect structural chromosome abnormalities
32. gas or air in the gastrointestinal tract that may be expelled through the anus

# DOWN

1. farsightedness
2. decreased density of bone
4. a condition of excessive cerebrospinal fluid in the brain, resulting in enlargement of the cranium
5. the act or manner of producing a speech sound
6. endoscopic or fluoroscopic observation of the pelvis and calyces of the kidney
8. forward movement of the body of 1 of the lower lumbar vertebrae onto the vertebra below it or onto the sacrum

9. inspection of the interior of the bladder by means of a scope

13. treatment based on experience, usually without adequate data to support its use

14. a positive sign usually seen in acute inflammation of the gallbladder

16. one of the tubes that takes urine from the kidney to the bladder

17. esophagogastroduodenoscopy

18. feeling full after eating less than normal or feeling full sooner than normal

20. presence of renal stones

25. the crushing of a stone in the kidney, ureter, or bladder by mechanical force, laser, or sound energy

27. pain in the lower back and hip radiating down the back of the thigh into the lower leg caused by a herniated lumbar disk compressing a nerve root

# CROSSWORD PUZZLE:
## QUALI-CARE GLOSSARIES 18–21

STUDENT _____

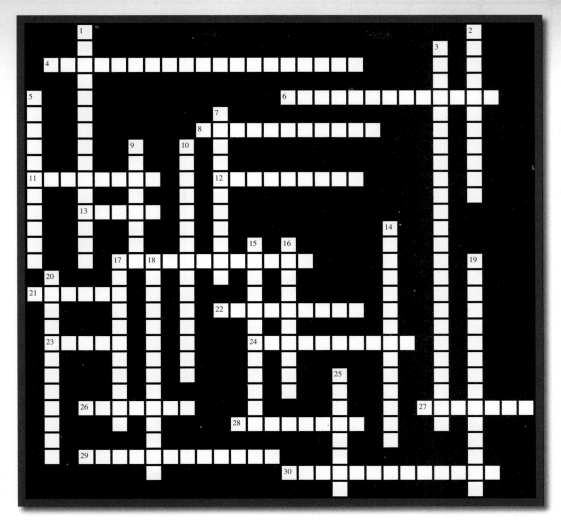

# ACROSS

4. top of a tooth used for restoring molars in children and adults
6. muscle in the forearm that, along with pronator quadratus, serves to pronate the forearm
8. a general anesthetic agent
11. a blind pouch
12. a material utilized in dental bonding technique, such as filling cavities or for cosmetic purposes
13. brand name for antibiotic
17. a light used by dentists to set or "cure" dental composite
21. the formation of cavities in the teeth by the action of bacteria; decay

22. rotation of the forearm such that the palm is downward
23. evaluation of a newborn infant's physical status by assigning numerical values (0-2) to each of 5 criteria
24. rotation of the forearm such that the palm is upward
26. a broad, flat, rubber bandage used as a tourniquet during surgery
27. filled with a specified element or elements; charged
28. barbiturate medication used prior to anesthesia, used as a sedative, used for insomnia, and used as an anticonvulsant (brand name)
29. in pregnancy, development of hypertension with protein in the urine or edema, or both

30. the surface of a tooth that faces the inside of the cheek or lips

# DOWN

1. muscle in the forearm that flexes elbow and assists in returning the pronated or supinated limb to neutral position
2. the space in the thigh through which the femoral vessels pass
3. vessel that runs along the front of the thigh toward the knee, gradually coursing toward the inside of the knee
5. slow heartbeat

7. brand name for a type of cement used for lining a cavity of a tooth that has been removed
9. the organ of metabolic interchange between the fetus and the mother
10. the mutual interlocking of toothed or tonguelike processes
14. lying face upward

15. gas used in dentistry for anesthetic and analgesic effects
16. a sponge placed in the throat to absorb saliva and fluids during oral procedures
17. incision of the uterus
18. the surface of a tooth that faces the tongue

19. the surface of a tooth that contacts an opposing surface of a tooth in the opposing jaw
20. vessel that passes along the radial side of the forearm
25. brand name of medication used to control seizures

# CROSSWORD PUZZLE:
## QUALI-CARE GLOSSARIES 22–25

STUDENT _____

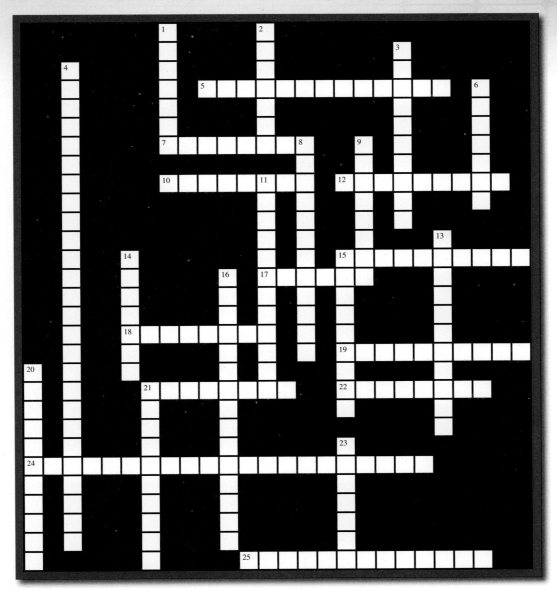

# ACROSS

5. one of the 4 muscles that surround the glenohumeral joint
7. redness of the skin produced by abnormal accumulation of blood
10. collar bone
12. discomfort in breathing that is brought on by lying flat
15. lightheadedness
17. cuff of cartilage that encircles the shoulder socket to make the socket deeper
18. bony prominence at the top of the shoulder blade that forms the point of the shoulder
19. to worsen or make more severe
21. full of vigor and spirit; lively
22. a small fingerlike projection from the scapula that serves to stabilize the shoulder joint
24. sleep disorder characterized by pauses in breathing during sleep
25. one of the 4 muscles that surround the glenohumeral joint

# DOWN

1. loss of consciousness; fainting
2. tending not to take an active or dominant part
3. infection of the nail fold surrounding the nail plate
4. a sensation of shortness of breath that awakens the patient from sleep
6. the part of the nail under the nail plate

8. class of medications used primarily to treat hypertension

9. nonadherent petrolatum gauze that conforms to body contours (trade name)

11. alteration in the structure and function of the right ventricle of the heart caused by a primary disorder of the respiratory system

13. constantly, regularly, or habitually active or occupied

14. one of the long bones of the digits, 14 in number for each hand or foot

15. the condition of containing or forming pus

16. the rate at which blood refills empty tiny blood vessels

20. composed of the tendons of the 4 muscles surrounding the glenohumeral joint

21. a preceding event, condition, or cause

23. the physical characteristics of a person

# CROSSWORD PUZZLE:
## PREFIXES, SUFFIXES, AND COMBINING FORMS

STUDENT _____

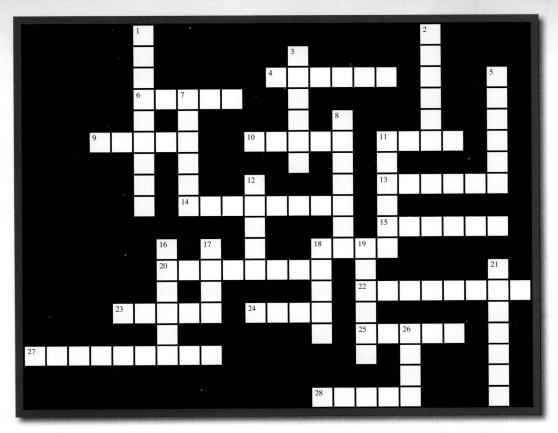

# ACROSS

4. femur (thigh bone)
6. fast, rapid
9. slow
10. tooth
11. middle
13. woman, female
14. narrowing, stricture
15. side
18. study of
20. suture
22. lack of strength
23. beyond, excess
24. on both sides
25. above, excessive
27. brain
28. above, over

# DOWN

1. eye
2. vomiting
3. jejunum (portion of the small intestine)
5. kidney
7. irrigation, washing
8. movement
11. enlargement
12. below, inferior
16. against, opposite
17. urination, urine
18. separation, destruction
19. process of recording
21. internal organs
26. near, beside

# PROOFREADING EXERCISE 1

STUDENT _____ (25 ERRORS)

**DEATG SUMMARY**

**Patient Name**: Teiko Sun

**Patient ID**: 469011

**Admitted**: 08/17/----

**Deceased**: 08/20/---- at 4:30 p.m.

**Consultations**: None.

**Procedures**: Proctoscopy.

This 75-year-old Asian femail patient was admitted through the ER with a cute massive rectal blooding of unknown origin, possibly diverticulitis; congestive heart failure in mild exacerbation; chromic renal failure, worsening since the day before admission, with dehidrition; and cronic atrial fribillation.

Emergency proctoscopy was done in the GI suite immediately after leaving the ER, which reveal only clodded blood without a source for the bleeding. Colonoscopy was scheduled but then later canceled do to pour bowel preparation and extreem weakness on the part of the patient.

A nuclear-tagged red blunt cell bleeding study was preformed in order to localise the bleeding cite in case of the necessity of emergency bowel surgery, but this proved to show no specific source of the bleeding. The bleeding apparently stopped spontaneously. Homoglobin and hemocrat descended to a nadir of 11.9 and 33.7, respectfully, the day after admission.

The patient's chronic renal flailure worsened steadily with increasing creatinine and BON and decreasing $CO2$. At the request of the family no hemodialysis was dun. Her chronic renal failure worsened further, and eventually he died at 4:30 p.m., 3 days after admission.

_____
Sangita Mehtapur, MD

SM:xx
D:08/20/----
T:08/23/----

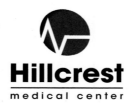

**Hillcrest**
medical center

# PROOFREADING EXERCISE 2

STUDENT _____ (30 ERRORS)

**HISTORY AND PHYSICAL EXAMINATION**

**Patient Name**: Patrick Platt

**Patient ID**: 771033

**Room No.**: 560

**Date of Admission**: 08/30/----

**Admitting Physician**: William Payne, MD

**Admitting Diagnosis**: Rule out fracture of left arm.

CHIEF COMPLAINT: Pain and swelling, left upper arm.

HISTORY OF PRESENT ILLNESS: The patient is an elderly female who fell
four days prior to admission. He noted immediate pain and swelling in the area just
below his left elbow. He presented to the emergency roomf or treatment.

PAST HISTORY: Past illness includes Whooping cough as a child. Tonsillectomy in
the past. No known allergies to medications.

FAMILY HISTORY: No hereditary disorders noted. Mother and father are deceased.
Two brothers are alive and well. One sister has adult-set diabetes mellitus.

SOCIAL HISTORY: The married and has two children. His wife does not work
outside the home.

PHYSICAL EXAMINATION: GENERAL: The patient is a well-developed, well
nourished male who appears to be in moderate distress with pain and swelling in the
upper left arm. Vital sign: Blood pressure 140/90, temperature 98.3 degrees
Fahrenheit, pulse 97, respiration 18.

HEENT: Head normal, no lesions. Eyes, arcus senilis,both eyes. Ears, impacted
cerumen, left ear. Nose, clear. Mouth, dentures fit well, no lesions.

NECK: Normal range of motion in all directs.

(Continued)

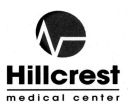

**Hillcrest**
medical center

## HISTORY AND PHYSICAL EXAMINATION

Patient Name:  Patrick Platt
Patient ID:  771033
Date of Admission:  08/30/----
Page 2

INTEGUMENTARY:  Psoriatic lesion, right thigh, approximately 1 mL in diameter.

CHEST:  Clear breath sounds bilaterally. No rales or rhonchi noted.

HEART:  Normal sinus rhythm. There is a holosystolic murmur. No friction rubs noted.

ABDOMEN:  Normal bowl sounds. Liver, kidneys, and spleen are normal to palpitation.

GENITALIA:  Tests normally descended bilaterally.

RECTAL:  Prostrate 2+ and benign.

EXTREMITIES:  Pain and swelling noted above the left elbow, other upper extremities normal. No cyanosis or clubbing. The legs demonstrate 2+ pitting edema to the knees.

NEUROLOGIC:  Cranial nerves II through XII intact, Memory intact, Sensation intact to light tough.

ASSESSMENT AND PLAN:  The patient was sent for plain film of the **left** arm, which revealed a fractured of the left humorous. The fracture was reduce in the emergency room. X-ray revealed anatomic alignment.

He was released to home with a perscription for a nonsteroidal anti-inflammatory and instructions to elevate his arm. He will be follow in the office in three days.

PROGNOSIS:  Good.

_____
William Payne, MD

WM:xx
D:08/30/----
T:09/01/----

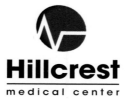

**Hillcrest**
medical center

# PROOFREADING EXERCISE 3

**CONSULTATION**

**Patient Name**:  David Moore

**Patient ID**:  246011

**Consultant**:  Carl M. Martin, MD, Gastroenterology

**Requesting Physician**:  Donald Burns, MD, Family Medicine

**Date of Consult**:  03/15/----

**Reason for Consultation**:  Please evaluate GI distress.

I was ask to see this 23 year old male in consultation because of unremitting nausea, diarrhoea, vomitting, abdominal pain, dizziness, and low-grade fever. The patient has a poor appetite but report no weight loss. He has noted some postprandial cramping, midepigastric pain, and unremitting diarrhoea but no blood in the stols. He states he is "better" but he still has some dizziness.

Initial treatment consisted of IV fluids and control of eletrolites. Thereafter, the patient was progressedto clear fluids and soft diet. He has done well on this regiment; however, his dizziness has persisted. Fever has resolve.

On admission, the patients' lab data revealed CBC with hematocrit of 42, hemoglobin 25, with differential of neutrophils 52%, bands 9%, lymphocytes 25%, monocytes 5%, basophils none. Serum electrolytes were normal. Potassium was low at 3.3, BUN-to-creatinine ration was normal. Glucase was within normal range. Stool studies was normal. Urinalysis within normal limit except for 8 to 10 WBCs. Specific gravy was 1.025.

On exam, I find the patient to be lethargic and uncomfortable with mild nausea and dizziness. He prefers to keep his eyes closed. On examination of the throat, I find no nystagmus. There is paller to the skin, and he seems cool to the touch. Upon standing by the bedside, the patient is unsteady. Although he resists to walking, when he attempts to walk, his gate is halting, and he tends to fall to the left side. Abdomen is flat and nontender. Bowel sounds are WNL. Rectal deferred.

(Continued)

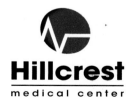

**Hillcrest**
medical center

CONSULTATION

Patient Name: David Moore
Patient ID: 246011
Date of Consult: 03/15/----
Page 2

RECOMMENDATIONS: I think we should continue low-key treat of this elderly gentlemen. Because of the symptoms of dizziness on admission, we may want to consider a CT scan to rule out a intracerebral bleed or subdural hematoma. My opinion at this time is that we are dealing with a resolving about of gastritis.

Thank you for asking me to see this patient. I will be glad to follow him with you throughout his hospitle stay.

_____

Carl M. Martin, MD

CMM:xx
D:03/15/----
T:03/16/----

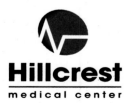

# Proofreading Exercise 4

STUDENT _____ (21 errors)

**DISCHARGE SUMMARY**

**Patinet Name**:  Jack Richardson

**Patient ID**:  157900

**Admitted:**  07/04/----

**Discharged**:  07/16/----

**Consultations**:  None.

**Procedures**:  Open reduction, internal fixation of fractures.

**Complications**:  None.

**Admitting Diagnosis**:  Multiple trauma from motor vehicle accident, brought in through emergency room.

HISTORY:  The patient is a 31-year-old caucasian male which was involved in a MVA approximate 2 hours prior to admission. On admission he was noted to have an unstable pelvis and a traumatic laceration through the left perineum, indicative of an open fracture. The patient also had a left femoral head dislocation. X-rays of the left foot and ankle revealed a severely comminuted fracture, left angle. Patient was admitted ot general surgery service to rule out intra-abdominal injury.

HOSPITAL COARSE:  The day following admittion, patient underwent open reduction, internal fixation of his fractured pelvis and ankle fractured. He did well following surgery and was ambulating on postoperative day 2. He began rehabilitation in the physical therapy department and will continue physiotherapy followed discharge. He remain afebrile throught his hospital stay. On discharge, all wounds were healing without complication and were clean and dry. There were no sighs of infection. A short leg caste was applied to the left leg prior to discharge.

DISCHARGE MEDICATIONS:  Tylenol No, 3 one p.o. q.4-6 h.

DISCHARGE INSTRUCTIONS:  Patient is to be scene in the orthopaedic clinic in 1 week for would check and x-rays of the pelvis and left ankle. He will be seen in general surgery service in 2 weeks. Activities as tolerant, elevate the leg, call if he has any problems prior to his followup visit.

(Continued)

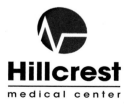

**Hillcrest**
medical center

DISCHARGE SUMMARY

Patinet Name:  Jack Richardson
Patient ID:  157900
Discharged:  07/16/----
Page 2


DISCHARGE DIAGNOSES
1. Comminuded fracture, left ankle.
2. Fractured pelvis.


_____

Ping Wu, MD

PW:xx
D:08/02/----
T:08/03/----

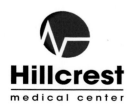

# PROOFREADING EXERCISE 5

STUDENT _____   (20 ERRORS)

**DISCHARGE SUMMARY**

**Patient Name**:  Hank Babcock

**Patient ID**:  652277

**Admitted**:  01/14/----

**Discharged**:  01/18/----

**Consultations**:  Dr. Jose Medina, MD, Surgeon

**Procedures**:  Appendectomy.

**Complications**:  Nine.

**Admitting Diagnosis**:  Rule out acute appendicitis.

This is a 45-year-old black man seen in my office on January 14 with the onset of acute abdominal pain at 10 am that day. He was admitted directly to the hospital with a diagnoses of probable acute appendicitis.

DIAGNOSTIC DATA:  Serm amylase was normal at 64. Cultures of peritoneal fluid at the time of discharged showed no growth. CDC performed as a followup on January 16 showed a white account of 12,400 (decreased from 21,000 on January 14). Hemoglobin to day is 12 (decreased from 15.5 on January 14). Preop diagnostic data was performed in the office prior to admission. The reminder of the values were within the reference range for our facility.

HOSPITAL COURSE:  The patient was admitted, and surgical consultatin was obtained from Dr. Medina. The patient was taken to surgery the evening of admission where acute appendicitis with a small perforation was find. Pathology conformed acute appendicitis. The patient convalecsed without difficulties, although he did have a low-grade fever of 99.9°F until January 17.

He was discharged on the following medication:  Darvocet-N 100 one q.6 h. p.r.n. pain and Keflex 500 mg p.o. q.6 h. for 3 days. Diet and activities at the time of discharge is as tolerated.

DISCHARGE DIAGNOSIS:  Acute suppurative appendicitis.

(Continued)

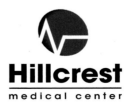

**Hillcrest**
medical center

DISCHARGE SUMMARY

Patient Name:  Hank Babcock
Patient ID:  652277
Discharge Date:  01/18/----
Page 2

DISPOSITION:  He will be seen by Dr. Medina in five days. He will be seen in my office in six weeks to be evaluated four possible hypercholesterolemia and possible hypothyroidism.

_____

Ruth Ellis, MD

RE:xx
D:01/20/----
T:01/22/----

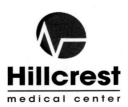

# PROOFREADING EXERCISE 6

**RADIOLOGY REPORT**

**Patient Name**: Wayne Masten

**Patient ID**: 709911

**X-Ray No.**: 11-81938

**Admitting Physician**: Hannah Sommers, MD

**Procedure**: PA and lateral chest.

**Date of Exam**: 12/21/----

CLINICAL INFORMATION: Weakness, lethargy. Rule out AIDS, Pneumocystis pneumonia. Patient has difficulty breathin and has been unable to gain wait. No IV drug abuse but she admits to promisecuity. Old films are unavailable for comparison.

Findings of underling COPD are noted. The heart sized appears normal. The pulmonary vessels, where they can be evaluated, appear unremarkable. Their is no evidence of plural effusion.

Extensive interstitial infiltrates are presnet throughout both lungs. The findings are most consistant with diffused bilateral interstitial pneumonia. I presume we are dealing predominately with interstitial fibrosis. The lung sare hyperinflated, and there are emphysematous changes in both upper lobe, more prominent on the right.

IMPRESSION
1. COPD with bullous emphysema.
2. Sever diffuse interstitial lung disease, most likely interstitial fibrosis.
3. Pneumocystis carinii pneumonia should be considered in the differential diagnosis.

_____

Anne J. Tulsa, MD

ATJ:xx
D:12/11/----
T:12/21/----

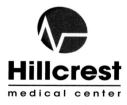

**Hillcrest**
medical center

# PROOFREADING EXERCISE 7

STUDENT _____  (19 ERRORS)

**CONSULTATION**

**Patient Name**:  Victor Peterson

**Patient ID**:  973577

**Consultant**:  Mary Wells, MD, Gastroenterology Services

**Requesting Physician**:  Erik Lunderman, MD, Pulmonary/Respiratory Services

**Date of Consult**:  10/16/----

**Reason for Consultation**:  Please evaluate RUQ abdominal pain.

HISTORY:  This patient, a 58-year-old male, been seen at the request of his pulmonary/respiratory physician on Friday, October 16, has been admitted to the hospital for elective thorocotomy and decortication for suspected mesothelioma. The patient has a long history of asbestos expo sure, having difficulty with shoulder and arm pain, with the diagnosis of mesothelioma. Two days ago he developed right upper quadrant abdominal pain. The patient has never experienced this type of dyscomfort; he has had no history of acid peptic disease, no known cholelithiasis. He denies fever, chills, hemituria, disurea, or frequency.

PHYSICAL EXAMINATION being done at this time is limited to the abdomin where bowel sounds are present and normal. There are no discreet mass felt. There is fullness in the right upper quadrant, and the patient does exhibit some minimal tenderness to palpation in the right upper quadrant. The patient has being a febrile. Ultrasound of the gall bladder does show cholelithiasis with a borderling common duct.

DISCUSSION:  At the present time the patient is known to have stones. I suspect his discomfort is from either an episodes of cholecystitis nor choledocholithiasis. I would suspect that livor function studies may be helpful in suggesting the presents of choledocholithiasis. We will make arrangements for the LFTs and possible sphincterotomy.

IMPRESSION
1. Status post resection of mesothelioma.
2. Cholelithiasis, rule out choledocholithiasis.

(Continued)

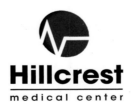

**Hillcrest**
medical center

DISCHARGE SUMMARY

Patient Name:  Victor Peterson
Patient ID:  973577
Date of Consult:  10/16/----
Page 2

Thank you very much for allowing us to participate in the care of your patient. We
will follow her along with you as necessary.

_____

Mary Wells, MD

MW:xx
D:10/16/----
T:10/17/----

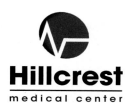

# Proofreading Exercise 8

**HISTORY AND PHYSICAL EXAMINATION**

**Patient Name**:  Maria Elena Ramirez

**Patient ID**:  158376

**Room No.**:  532

**Date of Admission**:  10/20/----

**Admitting Physician**:  Hal Seggerman, MD

**Admitting Diagnosis**:  Rule out adenomyosis of uterus.

CHIEF COMPLAIN:  Exceedingly heavy and painfully menses.

PRESENT ILLNESS:  Patient is a 35-year-old mildly obese Hispanic female, gravida 5, para 4-1-0-4, whose younger child is 13 years old. Patient states that over the past years or so she has had increasing difficulty with moodiness, depression, generalized fatigue, weight gain, and bloating premenstrually. The symptoms described preceed her menses by about a weak. She was seen by another physician and diagnosed as having menstrual endometrium.

PAST SURGICAL HISTORY:  She has had DNCs on two occasions five or six years ago for what sounds like menorrhagia/metrorrhagia. A sterilization procedure was done afterbirth of her last child.

ALLERGIES, PAST HISTORY, AND MEDICATIONS:  The patient is allergic to Ergotrate an iodine, especially in the forum of IVP die. Her only medication at present is Motrin used p.r.n. menstrual cramps. She has had the usual childhood diseases with no sequelae, no serious adult illnesses, no similar problems in her remote passed.

PHYSICAL EXAMINATION:  VITAL SIGN:  Completely within normal limits. HEENT:  Normocephalic. PERRLA. NECK:  No crepitus. Trachea is midline. No JVD. BREASTS are pendulous with a monilial-appearing rash between the breasts. No masses, tenderness, or discharge. Areola are darkly pigmented. ABDOMEN: Fatty abdominal apron with a well-heeled scar at the sight of her sterilization procedure. No hepatosplenomegaly. Positive bowel sounds. PELVIC/RECTAL: Introduction of speculum reveals the cervix to be multiparous and clean. No vaginal wall lesions are noted. On by manual exam, uterus is exquisitely tender to

(Continued)

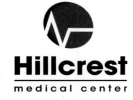
**Hillcrest**
medical center

# HISTORY AND PHYSICAL EXAMINATION

Patient Name:  Maria Elena Ramirez
Patient ID:  158376
Date of Admission:  10/20/----
Page 2

compression and is retroversion in position. Adnexa are negative for masses but are moderately tender. BUS negative. Rectal exam confirmatory with some internal and external hemorrhoid. SKIN:  Patient has had some itching between her breasts and on her inner thighs due to apparent Monilia. NEUROLOGIC:  No focale deficits.

## IMPRESSING
1. Cyclic edema inadequately compensated.
2. Probable adenomyosis of the uterus.
3. Monilia.
4. Internal and external hemorrhoids.

_____
Hal Seggerman, M.D.

HS:xx
D:10/20/----
T:10/21/----

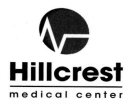

**Hillcrest**
medical center

# PROOFREADING EXERCISE 9

STUDENT _____ (20 ERRORS)

### HISTORY AND PHYSICAL EXAMINATION

**Patient Name**:  Christina Youngblood

**Patient ID**:  712102

**Room No.**:  418

**Date of Admission**:  06/24/----

**Admitting Physician**:  Cynthia Richards, MD

**Admitting Diagnosis**:  Cystocele, prolapsed uterus, B9 cyst of vulva.

CHIEF COMPLAINT:  Painful menstrual flew; urinary incontinence.

PRESENT ILLNESS:  This 38-year-old Native American female presented with increased menstrual flow and stress urinary incontinence over the last too years. No other complaints.

PAST MEDICAL HISTORY:  Essentially negative except for pyelonefritis as a child with no sequelae. Scarlet fever at age 19 with subsequent tonsilectomy. Has had "sinus trouble" in the past, which cleared after she stopped smoking. (Smoked approximate a pack a day between the ages of 16 and 26 years.)

MEDICATIONS:  None. No allergies save for a reaction to ASA.

FAMILY HISTORY:  Mother has COPD. Father has hearing lost and elevated cholesterol. One sibling with hearing loss. Maternal aunt with type 2 diabetes mellitos.

SOCIAL HISTORY:  Divorced. Formal smoker (see PMH). Drinks wine socially. Two daughter, ages 6 and 15, in good healthy.

PHYSICAL EXAMINATION:  In general, a Well-developed, well-nourished, obese American Indian woman with stable vitals. HEENT:  Normocephalic, atraumatic. No neck masses. CHEST:  Clear to PNA. HEART:  Not enlarge, regular rate and rhythm. No murmurs. BREASTS:  No masses. ABDOMEN:  Soft, nontender. No organomegalo. PELVIC:  Six centimeter superficial cyst, right upper labia minora.

(Continued)

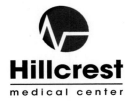

**Hillcrest**
medical center

HISTORY AND PHYSICAL EXAMINATION

Patient Name:  Christina Youngblood
Patient ID:  712102
Date of Admission:  06/24/----
Page 2


Cystocele. Uterus normal size with mile prolapse. Cervix oval, clean. Adnexa, cul de sac clean.
RECTAL:  Confirmatory. EXTREMITIES:  Pulses 2+, no edema. NEUROLOGIC
EXAM:  Cranial nerves II thru XII intact as tested.

DISPOSITION:  Admit for possible urinary bladder repair and hysterectomy.


_____

Cynthia Richards, MD

RC:xx
D:06/24/----
T:06/25/----

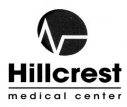

**Hillcrest**
medical center

# PROOFREADING EXERCISE 10

STUDENT _____ (18 ERRORS)

## DISCHARGE SUMMARY

**Patient Name**:  Kurt G. Kinsey

**Patient ID**:  314988

**Admitted**:  07/21/----

**Discharged**:  07/26/----

**Consultations**:    Jean W. Mooney, PA
Physical Medicine/Rehab

**Procedures**:  Bilateral correction of hallux valgus with osteotomy, right;  Mayo procedure, left.

**Complications**:  None.

**Admitting Diagnoses**:  Bilateral hallux valgus.

This 15-year-old young men was admitted for scheduled surgery as listed above.

DIAGNOSTIC DATA ON ADMISSION:  WBC 6.5, RBC 4.53, hemoglobin 14.1, hematocrit 41, MCV 92, MCH 31.1, MCHC 3.2, platelets 26100; differential, 42 polys, 40 limps, 3 bands, 10 monos, 5 eos. Urinalysis, clear yellow with specific gravity 1.025, PH 5, glucose negative, keytones negative, bilirubin negative. No red cells, no white cells, urobilinogen normal. RPR nonreactive. Preoperative chest film normally.

HOSPITAL COURSE:  Patient response to anesthesia uneventfully. Postoperatively patient was hemodynamically stable, afebrile. Physical therapy was instituted with Jean Mooney, PA, during hospital stayed. Therapist taught the patient to use crutches, including on stares and at curbs. Patient did well postoperatively and with the visual therapy.

DISCHARGE DX:  Bilateral hallux valgus, corrected.

(Continued)

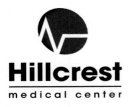

DISCHARGE SUMMARY

Patient Name: Kurt G. Kinsey
Patient ID: 314988
Discharge Date: 07/26/----
Page 2

DISCHARGE INSTRUCTIONS: He was discharged on postoperative day 5 in improved condition to be seen in the office or dressing check in 1 week. He was given Tylenol No. 3 p.r.n. pain. Diet regular. Activities: Crutches, no weightbearing, keep upper limbs iced and elevation as much as possible. Patient voiced understanding of the plan as described above. Both he and his parents agreed to the plan and scheduled follow up.

_____
Bill Perry, MD

BB:xx
D:07/26/----
T:08/02/----

C: Reed Phillips, MD, Pediatric Services
   Jean W. Mooney, PA, Physical Medicine/Rehab

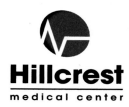

**Hillcrest**
medical center

# PROOFREADING EXERCISE 11

STUDENT _____ (25 ERRORS)

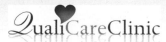

**QUALI-CARE CLINIC SOAP NOTE**

**Patient Name**:  Joan Barnett                    **PCP**:  David S. Duke, MD

**Date of Birth**:  02/08/----          **Age**:  27                **Sex**:  Female

**Date of Exam**:  12/03/----

SUBJECTIVE:  This is a pleasant 27-year-old white female who is new to the
practice.  She presents today for a couple of medications.  She was given a script for
Patanol by her eye doctor to help with some allergic conjunctivitis issues.  She also
has been prescribed Metrogel by her dermatologist for acne rosacea.  She denies any
acute concerns at this time.  Patient is due for her anual healthcare maintenance and
gynecologic care after the first of the year.  She is going to have records from her
other providers sent here.  She is on no other medications at this time.  Denies any
known medication allergies.  She is currently a nonsmoker, quit five years ago.  No
EtOH and no ellicit drug exposure.  Denies significant chronic medial problems.
Patient does have an aura on her left arm that she would like looked at by a
dermatologist, and she would like a referral to be evaluated by Dermatology here.
She describes a small mold that has been present for quite some time and may be
increasing slight in size.

0BJECTIVE:  Patient appears as a well-developed female in no specific distress.
Blood pressure134/86, pulse 85, weight 168 pounds.  Focused examination of the
right arm reveals a small, circular lesion on the anterior forearm, most consistent with
a seborrheic keratosis.  This is pigmented and is popular.

ASSESMENT:  Patient is a 27-year-old white female with a history of acne rosacea,
followed by Dermatology.  She has a script for Metrogel that she would like to have
filed.  She feels that controls things well.  She would like to continue care with
Dermatology here.  She has a pigmented legion on her left forearm, most consistent
with a seborrheic keratosis.  She would like to have this evaluated for possible
excision.  She will be establishing primary car within our clinic.

(Continued)

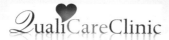

QUALI-CARE CLINIC SOAP NOTE

Patient Name:  Joan Barnett
PCP:  David S. Duke, MD
Date of Exam:  12/03/----
Page 2

PLAN:  At this time I have filled her Metrogel and Patanol prescriptions to be
continue as current.  I have referred her to Dermatology for continued care and further
evaluating and management.  She will call and arrange hat appointment.  She will
maintain routine followup with us and will have her record sent here.  She will
accomplish her maintenance care after the first of the years.  She will return to see me
as needed. Return precautions are reviewed.  I have reviewed these issues with the
patient to day.  She expresses comfort and understanding with the overall plan and
agrees to maintain followup.

_____
David S. Duke, MD
Family Practice

DD:xx
D:12/4/----
T:12/5/----

# PROOFREADING EXERCISE 12

STUDENT _____ (36 ERRORS)

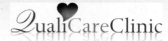

**QUALI-CARE OB/GYN CLINIC**

**Patient Name**: Amelia Sandmann                    **Surgeon**: Joshua Noll, MD

**Date of Birth**: 07/11/----          **Age**: 29                    **Sex**: Female

**Date of Procedure**: 02/24-----

**Preoperative Diagnosis**: Secondary infertility do to prior bilateral tubal ligations.

**Postoperative Diagnosis**: Secondary infertility due to prior bilateral tubal ligations.

**Procedures Performed**
1. Exam under anesthesia.
2. Diagnostic laparoscope.

**Anesthesia**: General endotrachea by Dr. Avalon.

**Time Operation Began**: 0743 hours.

**Time Completed**: 0812 hours.

**Fluids**: 900 cc lactated Ringer's solution.

**Urine Output**: 150 cc.

**Estimated  Blood Loss**: Minimal.

**Complications**: Nine.

INDICATIONS:  The patient is a 29-year-old G3, P2-0-1-2, who is status post interval bilateral tubal ligations with Falope rings, now remarried, desiring restoration of fertility.  The patient has been counseled on the risks of the laparoscopic procedure to include possibility of funding insufficient fallopian tube segments for reanastomosis and operative risks.  Questions were answered and written informed consent was sighed, as the patient desired to proceed with the procedure.

FINDINGS:  Exam under anesthesia revealed a 4- to 6-week sized uterus that was motile and antiverted with no adnexal masses.  Laparoscopy revealed a normal abdomen and pelvic with a 6-week sized uterus with minimal to no pelvic adhesive

(Continued)

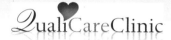

QUALI-CARE OB/GYN CLINIC

Patient Name: Amelia Sandmann
Surgeon: Joshua Noll, MD
Date of Procedure: 02/24-----
Page 2

disease. The appendix was normal and retrocecum. There was a normal liver edge and gallbladder with normal bilateral ovaries. The tubes had two Falope rings bilaterally with a left proximal segment of 3 cm, left distal segment of 2 cm, right distal segment of 3 cm, and right proximal segment of 1.5 cm. These findings were judged to be adequate for an attempt at bilateral tubal re-anastomosis.

DESCRIPTION OF OPERATION: Patient was taken to the OR where general endotracheal anesthesia was found to be adequate. She was placed in the dorsal lithotomy position, prepped and draped in the usual sterile manor, and exam under anesthesia was preformed with the findings noted above.

An operative speculum was placed in the patient's vagina, and a single-toothed tenaculum was used to graft the anterior lip of the cervix. A Cohen uterine manipulator was placed into the cervical os and attached to the single-toothed tenaculum. The operative speculum was removed. A Foley catheter, placed in the urethra without difficulty, drained clear, yellowed urine.

Attention was turned to the abdomen, where approximately 6.5 mL of 0.5% Marcaine was instilled in an area approximately 2 cm above the pubic symphysis and an area just inferior to the umbilicus. A 1-cm vertical incision was made in the inferior umbilicus.

This was extended down to the level of the fascia with blunt dissection. The fascia was grasped, tented up, and entered sharply with curved Mayo scissors. A 1-0 Vicryl tag was placed on either side of the cut edges of fascia. Additional blunt dissection was performed until the perineum was identified, grasped, and tented up. This was entered sharply with Metzenbaum scissors, and a 10 mm Hasson trocar was placed intraperitoneally. Carbon dioxide insufflated was performed per protocol, and laparoscope confirmed intraperitoneal placement. Diagnostic laparoscopy was performed with findings as noted above. A second 5 mm incision was made in the skin at the suprapubic cyte. A 5 mm trocar was placed under laparoscopic visualization.

(Continued)

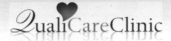

QUALI-CARE OB/GYN CLINIC

Patient Name:  Amelia Sandmann
Surgeon:  Joshua Noll, MD
Date of Procedure:  02/24-----
Page 3

Blunt probe was used to aide digital manipulation and diagnostic laparoscopy. Once the diagnostic procedure was completed, the 5 mm suprapubic port was removed under direct laparoscopic visualization with good hemostatis noted. The Hasson trocar was also removed under direct laparoscopic visualization, and the fascial tags were used to closed the fascial defect in the umbilicus.  The skin was closed with 4-0 Monocryl in a running subcuticular fashion.  Thin the suprapubic incision was closed with 4-0 Monocryl in a single interrupted subcuticular stitches.  Mastisol & Steri-Strips, sterile gauze & occlusive dressings were applied to the skin incisions.

Patient tolerated the procedures well.  Sponge, lap, and instrument counts were correct x3.  All instruments were removed from the patients' vaginal.  Good hemostasis was assured.  The patient was taken to PACU awake, extubated, and in stable condition.  The patient had received 2 g of cefotetan I.V. prior to the start of the procedure.

_____
Joshua Noll, MD
Obstetrics/Gynecology

JN:xx
D:02/25/----
T:02/24/----

# COMMON DICTATION ERRORS

... and how transcriptionists use medical language and editing skills to correct them, leaving their doctors' dictation medically intact yet grammatically correct and suitable for the legal and insurance fields, government agencies, research purposes, etc,

OR

why verbatim transcription is a myth.

## Key:

Grammar/usage error = G
Sentence structure error = SS
Inappropriate words = IW
Dictionary or reference needed = DN
Medical Transcription Style = STY

| | Type of error |
|---|---|
| **D:** The distal common iliac artery on the right and the external iliac artery was recanalized. | G |
| **T:** The distal common iliac artery on the right and the external iliac artery were recanalized. | |
| **D:** 7 cc was used. | STY |
| **T:** Some 7 mL was used. | |
| (**NOTE:** Do not start a sentence with a number. "Seven milliliters" would be okay here, too.) | |
| **D:** 30 cc of local anesthetic were ... | G, STY |
| **T:** Then 30 mL of local anesthetic was ... | |
| **D:** ...right common femoral and right profunda femoral artery ... | DN, G |
| **T:** ...right common femoral and profunda femoris arteries .. | |
| **D:** Purulent secretions from the trachea was removed. | G |
| **T:** Purulent secretions from the trachea were removed. | |
| **D:** ...with cap refill <2 sec. | STY |
| **T:** ...with capillary refill less than 2 seconds. | |
| **D:** ...although it only measured 2.4 mm by duplex examination. | G |
| **T:** ...although it measured only 2.4 mm by duplex examination. | |
| **D:** The peroneal muscles were dissected off of the lateral aspect. | G |
| **T:** The peroneal muscles were dissected off the lateral aspect | |
| **D:** Left nare was examined with ... | IW |
| **T:** Left naris was examined with ... | |

| | Type of error |
|---|---|
| **D:** The tubes were taken bilaterally from the cornea down the mesosalpinx. | DN |
| **T:** The tubes were taken bilaterally from the cornua down the mesosalpinx. | |
| (**NOTE:** GYN surgery, not ophthalmologic surgery) | |
| **D:** ...dissected superiorly towards the upper limit ... | G |
| **T:** ...dissected superiorly toward the upper limit ... | |
| **D:** ...vena comitantes ... | DN |
| **T:** ... venae comitantes ... | |
| **D:** The patient said she couldn't move her legs. | G |
| **T:** The patient said she could not move her legs. | |
| **D:** He was supposed to see his orthopod ... | IW |
| **T:** He was supposed to see his orthopedist ... | |
| **D:** ...sustained an injury in August 2006 at work to his lower back. | SS |
| **T:** ...sustained an injury to his lower back at work in August 2006. | |
| **D:** ...workup is inclusive for ... | G |
| **T:** ...workup is inclusive of ... | |
| **D:** ...potassium three five, hemoglobin twelve five ... | DN, STY |
| **T:** ...potassium 3.5, hemoglobin 12.5... | |
| **D:** ...forty to fifty percent stenosis... | STY |
| **T::** ...40% to 50% stenosis... | |
| **D:** ...The collateral ligaments were tested, and they were intact; medial and lateral collateral ligaments. | SS |
| **T:** The medial and lateral collateral ligaments were tested, and they were intact. | |

| | Type of error |
|---|---|
| **D:** It was probed with a forcep. | DN, IW |
| **T:** It was probed with a forceps. | |
| **D:** The bed, however, of the wound... | SS |
| **T:** The bed of the wound, however,... | |
| **D:** It is my gut feeling is that she will be admitted. | IW |
| **T:** It is my feeling that she will be admitted. | |
| **D:** Psychiatric: Negative except for hard-headedness. | IW |
| **T:** Psychiatric: Negative except for "hard-headedness." | |
| **D:** Since that time patient is without complaints. | G |
| **T:** Since that time patient has been without complaints. | |
| **D:** The patient moves all four upper extremities freely. | IW |
| **T:** The patient moves _____ freely. (There is no way to check this dictation other then by asking the dictator of the report. The report should be flagged using the medical transcriptionist's normal procedure for flagging reports.) | |

# APPENDIX

# PROOFREADER'S MARKS

*Transcription ⎫ open*
*Dictionary ⎬ Book*

| Defined | Examples |
|---|---|
| Paragraph ⁋ | ⁋Begin a new paragraph at this point. Insᵉrt a letter here. |
| Insert a character ∧ | |
| Delete ℓ | Delete these words. Disregard the previous correction. To |
| Do not change *stet or* ⋯⋯⋯ | |
| Transpose *tr* | transpose is to around turn. |
| Move to the left [ | ⸢Move this copy to the left. |
| Move to the right ] | ⸤Move this copy to the right. |
| No paragraph *no* ⁋ | *no* ⁋ Do not begin a new paragraph here. Delete the hyphen from |
| Delete and close up ⁀ | preᵉmpt and close up the space. |
| Set in caps *caps or* ≡ | a sentence begins with a capital letter. This Ⱳord should not be |
| Set in lower case *lc* | |
| Insert a period ⊙   *colon, semicolon* | capitalized. Insert a period⊙ |
| Quotation marks ⁝⁝  ⁝⁝ | ᵛQuotation marks and a comma should be placed here he said. |
| Comma ⁁ | |
| Insert space # | Space between these words. An |
| Apostrophe ⌄ | apostrophe is whats needed here. |
| Hyphen ＝ | Add a hyphen to African⹀American. Close |
| Close up ⌒ | up the extra spa⌒ce. |
| Use superior figure ⌄ | Footnote this sentence. Set |
| Set in italic *ital. or* ___ | the words, sine qua non, in italics. |
| Move up ⎴ | This word is too low. That word is |
| Move down ⎵ | too high. |

*Finals*

2 _ _ _ _ _  *subscript*

# CHALLENGING MEDICAL WORDS, PHRASES, PREFIXES

Each of the following words and abbreviations can be difficult or confusing. Some sound alike yet have different meanings, whereas others do not sound alike but are often used and spelled incorrectly. When listening to dictation, MTs should be aware of regional accent pronunciation as well as foreign accent pronunciation. Be prepared to spell, transcribe, and use *each* of the following terms and abbreviations correctly:

ACE—angiotensin-converting enzyme (most often dictated in the phrase "ACE inhibitor"), adrenocortical extract, plus several other medically related abbreviations

Ace—brand name for an elastic bandage

affect—noun; a state of mind or mood; countenance; pronounced with accent on the first syllable

affect—verb; to influence, to produce an effect upon; pronounced with accent on the second syllable

effect—noun; result, impression

effect—verb; to result in, bring about, to accomplish

ala nasi—singular noun meaning naris or opening of the nasal cavity

alae nasi—plural noun meaning nares or openings of the nasal cavity

angle—a corner, like a right angle (hard g)

angel—a heavenly body, like angels on our shoulders (soft g)

a lot—two words that refer to having many things; e.g., having a lot of symptoms or taking a lot of medicine

allot—verb meaning to distribute or to assign as a share or portion (remember that the verb is 1 word and the phrase above is 2 words)

ante—prefix meaning before, in front of, prior, earlier

anti—prefix meaning against, opposite, over

anterior—in front of, forward part of, toward the head

inferior—below, beneath, directed downward, lower surface

interior—inside, inward, inner part or cavity

appose—to place side by side or next to; before, beside, or on

oppose—to place opposite or against something, so as to provide resistance, counterbalance, or contrast

arteritis—inflammation of an artery

arthritis—inflammation of a joint

aura—subjective evidence of the beginning of either a seizurelike episode or a migraine headache

aural—relating to the ears or to an aura

oral—relating to the mouth

auxiliary—subordinate, secondary

axillary—referring to the underarm area (sometimes temperature is taken here)

bases—plural of basis

basis—the lower, basic, or fundamental part of an object

basil—an herb, a seasoning

basal—forming the base, arising from the base; the foundation; e.g., basal ganglia, basal cell, basal metabolic rate

bile—fluid secreted by the liver

bowel—intestine

Betagan—trade name for an ophthalmologic medication (eye drops)

Betagen—trade name for a surgical scrub, an antiseptic ointment, or a vitamin supplement

bisect—to cut in half

resect—to cut out a large portion

transect—to cut across

dissect—to cut up, as at autopsy (note the double "s")

BMP—basic metabolic profile (panel of 8 lab tests)

BNP—brain natriuretic peptide; sometimes dictated proBNP, which refers to the NT-proBNP or N-terminal fragment brain natriuretic peptide

caliber—the diameter of a hollow, tubular structure (like a bullet)

caliper—instrument used for measuring diameters, like pelvic diameters cancer—cellular tumor, usually malignant

carcinoma—malignant new growth (synonym for cancer)

CA—abbreviation for carcinoma or cancer but can also stand for cardiac arrest, coronary artery, and other phrases

Ca—chemical symbol for calcium

callous—adjective meaning hard or bony

callus—noun meaning bone

Carrisyn (generic is acemannan)—an antiviral AIDS drug

Carrasyn Hydrogel (brand name)—a wound dressing, over the counter

chord—there is a chord incision; there can be "multiple chords" (dissecting lines) in radiology

cord—an anatomic word, e.g., spinal cord

cor—an anatomic word, the heart

chorda—any cord or sinew, e.g., chorda tympani nerve (originating from the facial nerve)

chordae—plural of chorda, as in chordae tendineae (heart)

chordee—associated with hypospadias (downward bowing of the penis)

cirrhosal—adjective describing a diseased liver

serosal—adjective describing a membrane covering certain cavities of the body

clavicle—collarbone

pedicle—stalk

coarse—rough

course—route, plan

descent—noun meaning downward trajectory, as in descent of the fetal head during birth or descent of the pelvic organs into the vagina when ligaments and attachments in the pelvis become stretched (called pelvic prolapse)

decent—adjective meaning fairly good, acceptable, appropriate, as in a decent, hard-working person

defer—to put off or delay, as in "exam was deferred"

differ—to be unlike or distinct; different

diaphysis—the elongated cylindrical portion of a long bone; a tube of compact bone

diastasis—separation of two normally joined parts, as in diastasis recti, which is abnormally separated abdominal wall musculature; a period of slow filling of the ventricle of the heart

diathesis—a condition of the body that makes a person more susceptible to certain diseases

diffuse—adjective meaning scattered, not localized, e.g., diffuse infiltrates

defuse—verb meaning to make a situation less harmful, to calm a crisis

diploic—adjective meaning double

diploë—noun meaning loose bony tissue between the cranial bones

discreet—showing good judgment, prudent

discrete—made up of separate parts, not blended; e.g., a discrete mass

(NOTE: Discrete and separate both end in "te")

disease—morbid process with identifiable signs and symptoms

sign—evidence of disease that is seen (objective)

symptom—evidence of disease not seen (subjective)

syndrome—a set of symptoms

diverticulum, datum, labium, and medium are each singular nouns taking singular verbs

diverticula, data, labia, and media are each plural nouns—don't forget the plural verb

DNC—did not come

D&C—dilation and curettage

efflux—outward flow

reflux—backward or return flow

endogenous—growing, developing, or originating from within

exogenous—developing or originating from the outside, e.g., exogenous obesity

enterocleisis—closure of an intestinal wound

enteroclysis—injection of a nutrient or medicinal liquid into the bowel etiology—cause, origin; e.g., the cause of a disease or abnormal condition

ideology—the manner of thinking; characteristic of an individual, group, or culture

Eurax—a dermatologic cream, ointment

Urex—a urologic tablet, anti-infective

excise—to cut out or off

incise—to cut into

extirpation—to remove entirely, as in extirpation of varicose veins

extubation—to remove a tube, like a nasogastric tube, from a patient

expiration—synonym for death; breathing out or exhalation

en bloc—(French, "ahn bloc") in a lump, whole

en face—(French, "ahn fahs") in front or head on; e.g., an x-ray taken both in profile and en face

fecal—adjective meaning related to feces

thecal—pertaining to a case, covering, or sheath

fetal—of or relating to a fetus (developing human); also fetal position, fetal alcohol syndrome, fetal hemoglobin, etc.

fundus—bottom or base; the part of a hollow organ farthest from its mouth, e.g., the fundus of the stomach

fungus—any one of a class of mushrooms, yeasts, molds

gait—(noun) a manner of walking or moving on foot

gate—(noun) an opening in a wall or a fence

hemostasis—surgical procedure of the stoppage of bleeding

homeostasis—internal metabolic stability

healed—(verb) cured, restored to health

heeled—(verb) to furnish with a sole, to move along at someone's heels

in situ—in its normal place, confined to the site of origin

in toto—totally

in vivo—within the living body

in vitro—within a test tube (glass)

glans—(singular) a small, rounded mass of glandlike body, e.g., end of penis

glands—(plural) aggregation of cells specialized to secrete or excrete

graft—tissue for implantation (grafting)

graph—a written record, diagram

grasp—grab hold of or seize, as with a surgical instrument

gravida—a pregnant woman (gravida 1 = primigravida)

multiparous—having had 2 or more pregnancies, resulting in viable offspring (para 2 or para 3, etc.)

nulligravida—never having been pregnant

nulliparous—never having given birth to a viable infant

(NOTE: Gravida 5, para 3-1-1-3 refers to a woman who has been pregnant 5 times, resulting in 3 full-term deliveries, 1 premature birth, 1 abortion or miscarriage, and 3 living children. The 3-1-1 above equals 5, which is correct. The number of living children makes no difference in the equation.)

HNP—herniated nucleus pulposus

H&P—history and physical

hypo—prefix meaning beneath, under, or deficient

hyper—prefix meaning above, beyond, or excessive

illicit—adjective meaning illegal, as in illicit drugs

elicit—verb meaning to bring out, as to elicit a response or reaction

inflamed, inflammatory, inflammation—(the way the body responds to infection, irritation, or injury)—same root word; note the spelling difference

ilium—bone (iliac crest)

ileum—portion of the small intestine

ileus—disease (obstruction of small intestine)

(NOTE: There is both an iliac artery and an iliac vein.)

inter—prefix meaning situated or occurring between

intra—prefix meaning situated or occurring within

infra—prefix meaning situated or occurring beneath

intubated—having had a tube inserted (as into the larynx for providing oxygen)

incubated—placed in an optimal situation for development

it's—it is or it has (contraction); e.g., It's too late, it's already been done

its—possessive form relating to it or itself; e.g., newspaper proud of its objectivity

lavage—to wash out or irrigate

gavage—forced feeding, especially through a tube

lienal—pertaining to the spleen, as in gastro-lienal ligament

renal—pertaining to the kidneys

ligament—a band of tissue connecting bones, supporting viscera

ligature—a thread or wire (suture) for tying vessels

ligate—a verb meaning to sew, tie, or bind with ligature, as after a surgical procedure

liver—the largest gland in the body

livor—the discoloration of the skin on the dependent parts of a corpse

livid—discolored as from a contusion, congestion, or cyanosis

L&D—abbreviation for labor and delivery

LND—abbreviation for lymph node dissection, living nondirected donors

loose—adjective meaning not tight, as in loose clothes

lose—verb meaning to miss from a customary place, as in "Did you lose the book?"

malleus (pl. mallei)—pertaining to the outer-most and largest of the 3 bones in the ear

malleolus (pl. malleoli)—pertaining to the bony prominences on either side of the ankle joint

manner—(noun) a customary way of acting, conduct, or deportment

manor—(noun) large house on an estate

melena—blood in the stool, remember *melenic stools* is a proper phrase

melanin—dark brown to black pigment

melanotic—pertaining to the presence of melanin or dark pigment in the skin, hair, etc., and has nothing to do with stool

metacarpal—relating to the hand

metatarsal—relating to the foot between the instep and the toes

mucus—noun meaning the free slime of the mucous membrane

mucous—adjective meaning pertaining to or resembling mucus

occur/recur and occurrence/recurrence—something either occurs or recurs; we have an occurrence or a recurrence (Remember, "reoccur" and "reoccurrence" are *not* acceptable, even if dictated. Transcribe recur or recurrence instead.)

ophthalmologist—a physician specializing in the care of the eyes; note spelling, as "ophthal" is often mispronounced and misspelled

os (pl. ora)—the mouth; any opening into a hollow organ or canal; e.g., cervical os or medication taken per os

os (pl. ossa)—bone; e.g., os pubis (pubic bone) or ossa cranii (cranial bones)

ostium—(pl. ostia) a small opening

ostiomeatal—*not* osteo, it denotes an opening and has nothing to do with bone

pachymetry—a measure of central corneal thickness (ophthalmology)

pachymeter—instrument for measuring the thickness of the cornea

palpation—to touch or feel, examine with the hand(s)

palpitation—rapid and/or irregular pulsations of the heart

PAP—positive airway pressure (pulmonary)

Pap—Papanicolaou smear (gynecology)

para—prefix meaning beside, beyond

peri—prefix meaning around

pedal—(noun) a lever pressed by the foot, as a foot pedal used in transcription; (adjective) of or relating to the foot, as in pedal edema—pee'dul uhdee'ma

petal—the leaf of a flower, as in a rose petal

perineum—genital area, perineal area (between anus and scrotum or vulva)

peritoneum—covering of viscera, lining of abdominopelvic wall

peroneal—pertaining to the fibula, lateral side of the leg, or to the tissues present there

per<u>form</u>—verb meaning to achieve, carry out, discharge, execute, accomplish, etc.

<u>pre</u>form—verb meaning to form or shape beforehand, as in preformed back brace

plane—a flat surface

plain—unadorned

pleural—referring to the pleural cavity (lungs)

plural—meaning more than one

presence—noun meaning here, in this place at this time; the fact or condition of being present, e.g., "His presence was comforting."

presents—noun meaning gifts, e.g., "We like to receive birthday presents."

prostate—the male gland surrounding the urethra

prostrate—overcome (prostrate with grief) or lying in a horizontal position

proximal—nearest, closer to any point of reference, a location

approximate—verb meaning to bring close together, as to approximate the edges of a wound

approximately—adverb meaning estimation

pruritic—adjective describing itchy skin, as a pruritic incision site

pruritus—noun meaning an itchy skin condition

purulent—adjective meaning containing, consisting of, or forming pus, as in a purulent wound site

radicle—an anatomic word, the radicles are the smallest branches

radical—going to the root or source of disease, as in radical dissection at surgery

regimen—strictly regulated scheme of diet, exercise, medication, therapy, or training

regime—same as above but pronounced and spelled differently; also used to refer to a government

regiment—a military unit; to organize rigidly

retroperitoneal—adverb meaning behind the peritoneum (a direction)

reperitonealize—verb meaning to cover again with peritoneum

rigid—not flexible; hard; stiff; as in a rigid spine

ridged—having a ridge or ridges

shoddy—inferior goods, hastily or poorly done, as in shoddy work

shotty—like shot, lead pellets used in shotguns (usually used in reference to lymph nodes, e.g., shotty nodes)

sight—noun meaning something that is seen or visualized; e.g., injury was in sight

site—noun meaning a specific place or position; e.g., sutures at the surgical site

cite—verb meaning to quote, to call upon, to summon; e.g., to cite poetry

(NOTE: He cited that the site was in sight.)

-cyte—combining form meaning cell

sulfa—pertaining to the sulfonamides, the sulfa drugs

sulfur—brimstone, an element, the chemical symbol for which is S

tendon—noun meaning a band of connective tissue

tendinous—adjective meaning resembling a tendon

tendinitis—noun meaning inflammation of a tendon or tendons (note spelling)

tenia (pl. teniae)—any anatomic bandlike structure

tinea—ringworm, which is a fungus

tinnitus—abnormal noises in the ears, such as ringing or booming or whistling

TNA—abbreviation for total nutrient admixture

T&A—abbreviation for tonsils and adenoids and also for tonsillectomy and adenoidectomy

Tonsil, tonsillectomy—same root word; note spelling difference.

track—(noun) a path or groove, as in needle tracks, railroad tracks, losing track of time, staying on track

tract—(noun) system of body parts, as in the digestive tract, the respiratory tract; a bundle of nerve fibers having a common origin, termination, and function

umbo (pl. umbones)—a round projection, an orthopedic term

umbonate—knoblike

ureter—tube from kidney to bladder; there is a left and a right ureter

urethra—tube carrying urine out of the body; 1 urethra per person

vagus—noun meaning the 10th cranial nerve or vagus nerve

valgus—adjective meaning bent outward, twisted, deformed

vesicle—little blister or sac

vesical—urinary bladder *only*

verses—(noun) stanzas or verses of a poem, singular is verse; e.g., "chapter and verse"

versus—(adverb) against, in contrast to, as in good versus evil, north versus south

villus (pl. villi)—noun meaning little protrusion

villous—adjective meaning shaggy with soft hairs

(NOTE:  There could be a villous villus.)

weather—(noun) the climate, the atmosphere; e.g., under the weather, to weather the storm

whether—(conjunction) used as a function word usually with "or"; e.g., whether black or white, whether he is alive or dead, whether to eat or to fast, whether to come or to go

womb—the uterus

wound—trauma to the body

xerosis—dryness

cirrhosis—liver disease

Z-lengthen (orthopedic surgery)

Z-plasty (plastic surgery)

*Reference material used in developing this list includes* Dorland's Illustrated Medical Dictionary, *31st edition;* Stedman's Medical Dictionary, *28th edition;* AMA Manual of Style, *9th edition;* Gregg Reference Manual, *10th edition;* Vera Pyle's Current Medical Terminology, *10th edition*; Tessier's The Surgical Word Book, *3rd edition*; AHDI Book of Style for Medical Transcription, *3rd edition,* Medical Abbreviations, *14th edition, by Neil M. Davis, and* Merriam Webster's Collegiate Dictionary, *11th edition.*

# SAMPLE PATIENT HISTORY FORM

Patient Name:_____          Date:_____

| | DOCTOR OR THERAPIST USE ONLY |
|---|---|

1. PLEASE CHECK THE AREA OF YOUR MAJOR COMPLAINT.
   ☐ HEADACHE  ☐ NECK  ☐ BETWEEN SHOULDERS  ☐ LOW BACK
   ☐ SHOULDER  ☐ HIP  ☐ ARM  ☐ LEG

2. HOW DID THIS EPISODE BEGIN (CHECK APPROPRIATE ANSWER)?
   ☐ LIFTING       ☐ HIT IN BACK
   ☐ TWISTING      ☐ AUTO ACCIDENT  →DATE OF INJURY:_____
   ☐ PUSHING       ☐ ON THE JOB      →DATE OF INJURY:_____
   ☐ PULLING       ☐ UNKNOWN
   ☐ BENDING       ☐ OTHER:_____
   _____

3. WHEN DID THIS EPISODE OF PAIN BEGIN?_____

4. HAVE YOU HAD A SIMILAR EPISODE BEFORE?  ☐ YES    ☐ NO

5. WHAT TESTS HAVE YOU HAD AND WHAT ARE THE RESULTS?
   1.
   2.
   3.
   4.

6. LIST DOCTORS AND THERAPISTS YOU HAVE SEEN, AND THE RESULTS.
   1.
   2.
   3.
   4.

7. WHAT HAVE YOU BEEN TOLD IS WRONG?
   ☐ PINCHED NERVE   ☐ ARTHRITIS
   ☐ SLIPPED DISC    ☐ NOT TOLD
   ☐ PULLED MUSCLE
   ☐ OTHER:_____

8. FOR YOUR NECK OR BACK, HAVE YOU EVER HAD
   ☐ HOSPITALIZATION  ☐ BONE SCAN
   ☐ X-RAYS           ☐ MYELOGRAM
   ☐ CAT SCAN         ☐ EMG
   ☐ MRI SCAN         ☐ NONE
   ☐ OTHER:_____

9. HAVE YOU TAKEN ANY MEDICINE FOR THIS PROBLEM?
   ☐ NONE       ☐ FELDENE    ☐ IBUPROFEN
   ☐ MOTRIN     ☐ MECLOMEN   ☐ ALEVE
   ☐ NALFON     ☐ ORUDIS     ☐ ASPIRIN
   ☐ NAPROSYN   ☐ ORUVAIL    ☐ TYLENOL
   ☐ CLINORIL   ☐ RELAFEN    ☐ CORTISONE:  STEROIDS
   ☐ INDOCIN    ☐ LODINE                   PREDNISONE
   ☐ TOLECTIN   ☐ ADVIL                    DECADRON
   ☐ OTHER:_____       MEDROL

10. HAVE YOU HAD

| | YES | NO | BETTER | WORSE | SAME |
|---|---|---|---|---|---|
| PHYSICAL THERAPY | ☐ | ☐ | ☐ | ☐ | ☐ |
| CORSET OR BRACE | ☐ | ☐ | ☐ | ☐ | ☐ |
| CHIROPRACTIC | ☐ | ☐ | ☐ | ☐ | ☐ |
| MASSAGE | ☐ | ☐ | ☐ | ☐ | ☐ |
| BACK SURGERY | ☐ | ☐ | ☐ | ☐ | ☐ |
| ACUPUNCTURE | ☐ | ☐ | ☐ | ☐ | ☐ |
| CORTISONE SHOT | ☐ | ☐ | ☐ | ☐ | ☐ |

(Continued)

Patient Name:_____

11.   USE THESE SYMBOLS TO SHOW AREA ON THE DRAWINGS WHERE YOU HAVE SYMPTOMS.

>>>ACHE          ☐ ☐  NUMBNESS          ☐ ☐  PINS AND NEEDLES          X X BURNING          //// STABBING

LEFT     RIGHT     RIGHT     LEFT     R     L     RIGHT     LEFT     RIGHT     LEFT     R     L

12.  ARE YOUR SYMPTOMS GETTING   ☐ BETTER   ☐ SAME   ☐ WORSE

13.  PLEASE CHECK ONE ANSWER IF IT APPLIES TO YOU.
     ☐ BACK (NECK) PAIN IS WORSE THAN LEG (ARM) PAIN
     ☐ BACK (NECK) PAIN EQUALS LEG (ARM) PAIN
     ☐ LEG (ARM) PAIN IS WORSE THAN BACK (NECK) PAIN

14.  PLEASE CHECK ALL OF THE FOLLOWING THAT BEST DESCRIBE YOUR PAIN.
     ☐ CONSTANT            ☐ WAKES YOU UP AT NIGHT
     ☐ DAILY               ☐ WORSE WITH COUGH OR SNEEZE
     ☐ WORSE IN MORNING    ☐ WORSE WITH ACTIVITY

15.  CHECK THE APPROPRIATE BOXES REGARDING YOUR PAIN.

|                         | WORSE | BETTER | NO CHANGE |
|-------------------------|-------|--------|-----------|
| SITTING                 | ☐     | ☐      | ☐         |
| STANDING                | ☐     | ☐      | ☐         |
| GETTING UP FROM SITTING | ☐     | ☐      | ☐         |
| BENDING FORWARD         | ☐     | ☐      | ☐         |
| LEANING BACKWARD        | ☐     | ☐      | ☐         |
| LIFTING                 | ☐     | ☐      | ☐         |
| WALKING                 | ☐     | ☐      | ☐         |
| REST                    | ☐     | ☐      | ☐         |
| LYING ON BACK           | ☐     | ☐      | ☐         |
| LYING ON STOMACH        | ☐     | ☐      | ☐         |
| MENSTRUAL PERIODS       | ☐     | ☐      | ☐         |

16.  HAVE YOU LOST CONTROL OF YOUR BOWELS OR BLADDER?
     ☐ YES   ☐ NO

DOCTOR OR THERAPIST USE ONLY

(*Delmar/Cengage Learning*)

# THE LUND-BROWDER CHART

The Burn Extent Estimator is a convenient method of estimating the percentage of a patient's burn, the total surface area of the patient's body in square feet, and the approximate surface area of the burn, in square feet.

Shade the burn areas on the figures shown, and use the table to estimate the percentage of the burn. The rule of nines is a method of estimating the extent of body surface that has been burned in an adult. The body surface is divided into sections of 9 percent or multiples of 9 percent.

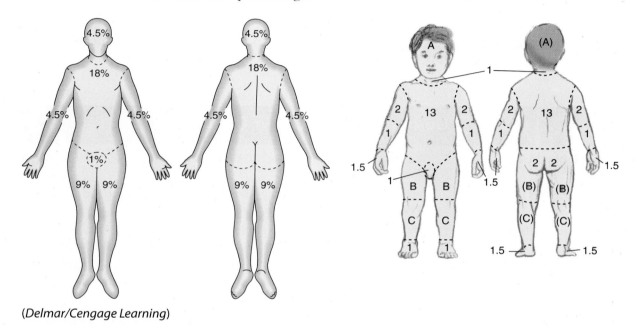

*(Delmar/Cengage Learning)*

| LUND AND BROWDER CHART | | | | | | |
|---|---|---|---|---|---|---|
| **Age** | **0** | **1** | **5** | **10** | **15** | **Adult** |
| A = Half of Head | 9.5 | 8.5 | 6.5 | 5.5 | 4.5 | 3.5 |
| B = Half of Thigh | 2.75 | 3.25 | 4.0 | 4.25 | 4.25 | 4.75 |
| C = Half of Leg | 2.5 | 2.5 | 2.75 | 3.0 | 3.25 | 3.5 |

| Region | Percentage of body surface |
|---|---|
| Head and neck | 9% |
| Anterior trunk | 18% |
| Posterior trunk | 18% |
| Left arm | 9% |
| Right arm | 9% |
| Left leg | 18% |
| Right leg | 18% |
| Genitalia and perineum | 1% |

# Laboratory Test Information

## Complete Blood Count (CBC)

This group of blood tests may be dictated as a hemogram, a blood count, a CBC, a CBC with diff, or a complete blood cell count with differential. In some labs, the differential is done automatically. A CBC includes several tests done on blood drawn from a vein. (For a standard laboratory request form on which the CBC is listed, see Hematology in this appendix.)

Segmented neutrophils (segs), basophils, (basos), eosinophils (eos), bands, lymphocytes (lymphs), and monocytes (monos) represent different types of white blood cells. Counting the types of WBCs is known as the white blood cell differential count (or "diff"). Analyzing the patterns of the differential can give information about many diseases. A "shift to the left" indicates an increase in the percentage of unsegmented (immature) neutrophils, also called band cells or bands. A "shift to the right" indicates an increase in the percentage of multisegmented (mature) neutrophils, also called segs.

| COMPLETE BLOOD COUNT (CBC) | |
|---|---|
| **hemoglobin (Hgb)** | The hemoglobin and hematocrit (H&H) results give different measures of red blood |
| **hematocrit (Hct)** | cell volume. Low levels indicate anemia. Hemoglobin is reported in grams or g/dL; hematocrit is reported as a percent. |
| **white blood cells (WBCs)** | White cells (leukocytes) fight infection, and high levels can indicate infection. Low levels can be due to medication or even bone marrow suppression. |
| **red blood cells (RBCs)** | Red cells are erythrocytes, and this is a measure of red blood cells in a certain volume of blood. |
| **platelets** | Platelets are components essential for coagulation (clotting). |
| **MCV, MCH, MCHC** | Known as the red blood cell indices, the MCH, MCV, and MCHC describe the size of the red blood cells and the amount of hemoglobin in the red cells. For example, iron-deficiency anemia and pernicious anemia would have different indices. The initials stand for mean corpuscular volume (MCV), mean corpuscular hemoglobin (MCH), and mean corpuscular hemoglobin concentration (MCHC). |

## Urinalysis (UA)

Testing some chemical reactions in the urine and looking at centrifuged debris (sediment) under the microscope gives information about different diseases, including those of the kidney and urinary bladder.

| URINALYSIS (UA) | |
|---|---|
| **glucose (sugar)** | The presence of glucose may indicate diabetes mellitus. |
| **protein** | The presence of protein may indicate kidney disease but is also seen with recent exercise, dehydration, heart failure, and multiple myeloma. |
| **specific gravity** | This is a measurement of the concentration of urine, being low after consuming abundant fluids and being high with dehydration. |
| **pH** | This measures the acidity of urine, always transcribed pH. |

## Microscopic Urinalysis

White blood cells (WBCs) in urine seen under a microscope can be due to infection in the kidney or in the urinary bladder.

Red blood cells (RBCs) in urine seen under a microscope may be due to infection, stones, or even a malignancy.

The presence of bacteria in urine seen under a microscope may indicate a urinary tract infection. If a specimen has been sitting out for a time before being tested, however, bacteria could be present from sitting too long, with no true urinary tract infection present.

## Prothrombin Time with INR and the Partial Thromboplastin Time

The PT/PTT blood tests are used to track anticoagulation, and the results are often dictated together. The prothrombin time or pro time (PT) can be used to keep track of Coumadin levels. The partial thromboplastin time (PTT) can be used to keep track of heparin levels. Coumadin and heparin are both blood thinners. PT/PTT results can be abnormal with blood abnormalities, liver disease, hemophilia, etc.

The PT and INR results (International Normalized Ratio) may be dictated without the PTT. (Example: PT is 16.5 seconds with an INR of 1.4%.) The INR is a method of improving prothrombin time tests despite variations in the properties of different batches of thromboplastin used in the test.

## Sedimentation Rate (Sed Rate)

A nonspecific test that indicates inflammation anywhere in the body, the sed rate may be elevated in the presence of infection, malignancy, trauma, and/or certain types of rheumatism. Like an elevated temperature, the sedimentation rate indicates a problem but defines neither the location nor the type of problem. This test is also known as the ESR (erythrocyte sedimentation rate).

## Thyroid Function Tests (TFTs)

$T_3$, $T_4$ (sometimes transcribed T3, T4), and TSH are the usual screening tests for thyroid disease.

$T_3$ (triiodothyronine) is an organic, iodine-containing hormone compound secreted in small amounts by the thyroid gland.

$T_4$ (thyroxine) is the principal hormone manufactured by the thyroid gland. If elevated, it may indicate an overactive thyroid (hyperthyroidism). If low, underactive thyroid disease (hypothyroidism) may be the cause.

TSH (thyroid-stimulating hormone) is manufactured by the pituitary gland and directs the thyroid gland to either increase or decrease production of thyroxine ($T_4$). In the usual form of hypothyroidism, the $T_4$ is low, and the TSH is high. Low $T_4$ *and* TSH levels may indicate hypothyroidism secondary to pituitary disease. $T_3$, $T_4$, and TSH may be decreased by either an acute or a chronic illness, by fasting, or by severe stress.

## Prostate-Specific Antigen (PSA)

Prostate-specific antigen is a substance produced in the prostate gland. Normal levels are between 0 and 4. The most common cause of an elevated PSA (>4) is prostate enlargement, known as benign prostatic hyperplasia (BPH). An elevated PSA, however, can also indicate prostatic cancer. Being a nonspecific test, a diagnosis may require additional studies, including ultrasound and/or needle biopsy of the prostate.

## Chemistry Profile (CHEM Profile)

A chemistry profile is a group of blood studies that provide information about internal bodily function and disease. It is an effective and economical study using a small blood sample and performed on a machine (sometimes called a SMAC or a Coulter) that runs the tests simultaneously. A chemistry profile is known as a "screening procedure" and is designed to uncover common diseases that might be missed on physical examination. It usually provides no definite answers, since most diagnoses require more specific tests and correlation with the physician's history and physical exam. The blood tests and their significance are discussed in the following table.

(See the standard laboratory request forms included in this appendix.)

| BLOOD TEST | SIGNIFICANCE |
|---|---|
| glucose | Sugar in the blood, high levels of which can indicate diabetes mellitus. |
| cholesterol<br>cholesterol/HDL<br>triglycerides<br>cholesterol/LDL | Known as the lipid (fat) profile, the pattern of results provides information about fat metabolism. Abnormal patterns can indicate a tendency for coronary artery disease. Generally, lower levels of cholesterol, triglycerides, and LDL are ideal. With HDL, the "good" cholesterol, however, higher levels are better than lower levels. |
| blood urea nitrogen and creatinine | The BUN and creatinine measure kidney function; their results are usually dictated together. |
| uric acid | Commonly high with gout, the uric acid level is abnormal in kidney disease, with tissue breakdown, dehydration, and in other disease conditions. |
| calcium and phosphorus | Abnormal levels can indicate disease of the bone, parathyroid gland, kidneys, and other diseases. |
| bilirubin, alkaline phosphatase, AST (SGOT), ALT (SGPT), LDH, and GGPT | This group of chemistry tests is commonly referred to as a liver function panel or the liver function tests (LFTs). The bilirubin is a yellow pigment and can be abnormal with liver and gallbladder disease, plus certain blood diseases. The alkaline phosphatase (often dictated alk phos) is an enzyme that indicates bone disease, cancer, or other disease. AST, ALT, and LDH are enzymes that can be abnormal with liver, muscle, or heart disease. (AST and ALT are preferred usage over SGOT and SGPT, but you may hear any one of them on dictation. You should transcribe what you hear.)<br><br>LDH: Cardiac enzyme isoform used in the diagnosis of myocardial infarction (MI). GGPT distinguishes liver disease from other disease. |
| protein and albumin-globulin ratio | These provide a picture of general nutrition, liver function, and acute or chronic inflammation. |
| sodium, potassium, chloride, and bicarbonate (electrolytes) | This group of 4 chemistry tests is known as the electrolytes (often dictated "lytes"). They can be abnormal with kidney disease, liver or respiratory failure, dehydration, and diuretic therapy (water pills). |

Chemistry terminology also heard on dictation includes:

BMP (basic metabolic profile)

CMP (complete metabolic profile)

SMAC-8 (8 chemistry tests)

SMAC-21 (21 chemistry tests)

Chem-12 (panel of 12 chemistry tests)

*Disclaimer: Each of the above descriptions is meant to provide some basic information about the many tests done in the clinical laboratory. Normal results do not always assure good health; abnormal results do not always indicate disease. The human body is very complex, and different results in different people can have different meanings. Therefore, interpretation and/or evaluation by your physician is essential.*

# Sample Forms for Ordering Laboratory Tests, Scheduling Radiology Tests, and Consults for Physical Therapy, Sleep Studies, etc.

☐ Fax
☐ Call
☐ Mail

Send additional copy of report to:

Client Number/Physician's Name

Phone/Fax Number ( )

Physician's Address    City, State, Zip

0800.01

| Patient's Legal Name (Last, First, MI) | Sex | Date of Birth MO DAY YR | Collection Time : AM PM | Fasting ☐ Yes ☐ No | Collection Date MO DAY YR | Urine hrs/vol hrs___ vol___ |

| NPI | UPIN | Physician's ID # | Patient's SS # | Patient's ID # |

Physician's Name (Last, First)    Physician's Signature   X

Hospital Patient Status: ☐ In-Patient ☐ Out-Patient ☐ Non-Patient

**Diagnosis/Signs/Symptom in ICD-9 Format (Highest Specificity)**
R E Q U I R E D

PATIENT

Patient's Address    Phone
City    State    ZIP

Name of Policy Holder (if different from patient)
Address of Policy Holder    APT #
City    State    ZIP

I hereby authorize the release of medical information related to the service described herein and authorize payment directly to. I agree to assume responsibility for payment of charges for laboratory services that are not covered by my healthcare insurer.

X _____
Patient's Signature    Date

**MEDICARE ADVANCE BENEFICIARY NOTICE (ABN)**
Refer to Determining Necessity of ABN Completion on reverse.

RESP. PARTY

| PRIMARY BILLING PARTY | SECONDARY BILLING PARTY |
| --- | --- |
| Insurance Carrier * | Insurance Carrier * |
| ID # | ID # |
| Group # | Group # |
| Insurance Address | Insurance Address |
| Name of Insured Person | Name of Insured Person |
| Relationship to Patient | Relationship to Patient |
| Employer Name | Employer Name |
| *If Medicaid State | Physician's Provider # | Workers Comp ☐ Yes ☐ No |

INDIVIDUAL COMPONENTS OF TEST COMBINATIONS / PROFILES LISTED IN THE SECTION ABOVE CAN BE ORDERED BELOW

**TRAVEL LOG ID**

| LAB USE ONLY | STAT ☐ 998074 | VENIPUNCTURE ☐ 998085 | NON LABCORP ☐ 998239 | VERBAL ORDER ☐ 998250 | CHART ORDER ☐ 998261 | HANDWRITTEN ☐ 998272 | 24 HR TUV ☐ 998283 | PST/PSC # | PST HR# | DATE | LOG# |

## ORGAN OR DISEASE PANELS
See reverse for components

| | | | |
| --- | --- | --- | --- |
| 322744 | Acute Hepatitis Panel | 80074 | RED |
| 322758 | Basic Metabolic Panel (8) | 80048 | GEL |
| 322000 | Comp Metabolic Panel (14) | 80053 | GEL |
| 303754 | Electrolyte Panel | 80051 | GEL |
| 322755 | Hepatic Function Panel (7) | 80076 | GEL |
| 303756 | Lipid Panel | 80061 | GEL |
| 235010 | Lipid Panel w/LDL/HDL Ratio | 80061 | GEL |
| 221010 | Lipid Panel w/TC:HDL Ratio | 80061 | RED |
| 343925 | Lipid Panel w/Non-HDL Cholesterol | 80061 | GEL |
| 322777 | Renal Function Panel | 80069 | GEL |

### HEMATOLOGY

| | | | |
| --- | --- | --- | --- |
| 005009 | CBC w Diff w Plt | 85025 | LAV |
| 115907 | CBC w Diff w/o Plt | see reverse | LAV |
| 028142 | CBC w/o Diff w Plt | 85027 | LAV |
| 005017 | CBC w/o Diff w/o Plt | reverse | LAV |
| 005058 | Hematocrit | 85014 | LAV |
| 005041 | Hemoglobin | 85018 | LAV |
| 005249 | Platelet Count | 85049 | LAV |
| 005033 | RBC Count | 85041 | LAV |
| 005025 | WBC Count | 85048 | LAV |
| 005090 | WBC Differential | 85004 | LAV |

### ALPHABETICAL/COMBINATION TESTS

| | | | |
| --- | --- | --- | --- |
| 006049 | ABO and Rh | see reverse 86900 86901 | LAV |
| 001081 | Albumin | 82040 | GEL |
| 001107 | Alkaline Phosphatase | 84075 | GEL |
| 001545 | ALT (SGPT) | 84460 | GEL |
| 001396 | Amylase | 82150 | GEL |
| 164855 | Antinuclear Antibodies | 86038 | GEL |
| 001123 | AST (SGOT) | 84450 | GEL |
| 000810 | B₁₂ and Folate | see reverse 82607 82746 | GEL |
| 001099 | Bilirubin, Total | 82247 | GEL |

### ALPHABETICAL/COMBINATION TESTS CON'T

| | | | |
| --- | --- | --- | --- |
| 001040 | BUN | 84520 | GEL |
| 006627 | C-Reactive Protein (CRP), Quant | 86140 | RED |
| 120766 | hsCardiac C-Reactive Protein (CRP) | 86141 | RED |
| 001016 | Calcium | 82310 | GEL |
| 007419 | Carbamazepine (Tegretol®) | 80156 | SER |
| 002139 | CEA | 82378 | GEL |
| 804500 | Cholesterol Profile | 83701 84478 | |
| 001065 | Cholesterol, Total | 82465 | GEL |
| 001370 | Creatinine | 82565 | GEL |
| 007385 | Digoxin (Lanoxin®) | 80162 | SER |
| 004515 | Estradiol | 82670 | GEL |
| 004598 | Ferritin | 82728 | GEL |
| 028480 | FSH and LH | see reverse 83001 83002 | |
| 001958 | GGT | 82977 | GEL |
| 001818 | Glucose, Plasma | 82947 | GRY |
| 001032 | Glucose, Serum | 82947 | GEL |
| 001693 | Glycohemoglobin, Total | 83036 | LAV |
| 004556 | hCG, Beta Subunit, Qual (Serum Pregnancy) | 84703 | GEL |
| 004416 | hCG, Beta Subunit, Quant | 84702 | GEL |
| 001925 | HDL Cholesterol | 83718 | GEL |
| 006734 | Hep A Antibody, IgM | 86709 | GEL |
| 006395 | Hep B Surface Antibody | 86706 | GEL |
| 006510 | Hep B Surface Antigen | 87340 | GEL |
| 143991 | Hep C Antibody* | 86803 | GEL |
| 001453 | Hemoglobin A₁c | 83036 | LAV |
| 083824 | HIV-1/0/2 Antibodies* | 86703 | GEL |
| 180836 | H pylori Urea Breath | 83013 | |
| 180764 | H pylori Stool Antigen | 87338 | Fecal Transp |
| 001321 | Iron and IBC | see reverse 83540 83550 | GEL |
| 001115 | LDH | 83615 | GEL |

### ALPHABETICAL/COMBINATION TESTS CON'T

| | | | |
| --- | --- | --- | --- |
| 007708 | Lithium (Eskalith®) | 80178 | SER |
| 001537 | Magnesium | 83735 | GEL |
| 006189 | Mononucleosis Test, Qual | 86308 | GEL |
| 884247 | NMR LipoProfile | 80061 83704 | RED |
| 007823 | Phenobarbital (Luminal®) | 80184 | SER |
| 007401 | Phenytoin (Dilantin®) | 80185 | SER |
| 001024 | Phosphorus | 84100 | GEL |
| 001180 | Potassium | 84132 | GEL |
| 004465 | Prolactin | 84146 | GEL |
| 010322 | PSA | 84153/G0103 | GEL |
| 480947 | Prostate-specific Antigen (PSA), Free: Total Ratio* | 84153 84154 | RED |
| 005199 | Prothrombin Time (PT)/INR | 85610 | BLU |
| 020321 | PT and PTT Activated | 85610 85730 | BLU |
| 005207 | PTT Activated | 85730 | BLU |
| 006502 | Rheumatoid Arthritis Factor | 86431 | GEL |
| 006072 | RPR | 86592 | GEL |
| 006197 | Rubella Antibodies, IgG | 86762 | GEL |
| 005215 | Sed Rate, Westergren | 85652 | LAV |
| 001198 | Sodium | 84295 | GEL |
| 004226 | Testosterone, Total | 84403 | RED |
| 007336 | Theophylline | 80198 | SER |
| 330015 | Thyroid Cascade Profile | see reverse | |
| 001149 | Thyroxine (T₄) | 84436 | GEL |
| 001172 | Triglycerides | 84478 | GEL |
| 002188 | Triiodothyronine (T₃) | 84480 | GEL |
| 001156 | T₃ Uptake | 84479 | GEL |
| 004259 | TSH, 3rd generation | 84443 | GEL |
| 001057 | Uric Acid | 84550 | GEL |
| 003038 | Urinalysis | Microscopic on Positives 81003 | URN |
| 081950 | Vitamin D, 25-Hydroxy | 82306 | RED |

## MICROBIOLOGY See Reverse Side

☐ ENDOCERVICAL ☐ THROAT ☐ URINE
☐ STOOL ☐ URETHRAL
OTHER    INDICATE SOURCE

| | | | |
| --- | --- | --- | --- |
| 008649 | Aerobic Bacterial Culture † | 87070 | |
| 183194 | Chlamydia/GC by Nucleic Acid Amplification Testing | 87491 87591 | OPTMA Transp |
| 008482 | Fungus Culture | 87101 | |
| 008334 | Genital Culture, Routine † | 87070 | |
| 008540 | Gram Stain | 87205 | SLS |
| 188128 | Group B Strep Colonization Detection Cult/DNA Probe | 87081 87149 | Red Transp |
| 180810 | Lower Respiratory Culture † | 87070 | Red Transp |
| 182949 | Occult Blood, Fecal, IA | 82274 | |
| 008623 | Ova and Parasites | 87177 87209 | O & P Vial |
| 008144 | Stool Culture † | 87045 87046, 87427 | Fecal Transp |
| 008169 | Throat, Beta-Hemolytic Strep Cult, Group A | 87081 | Red Transp |
| 008342 | Upper Respiratory Culture, Routine † | 87070 | Red Transp |
| 008847 | Urine Culture, Routine † | 87086 | Uri Cul Transp |

† = ID / Susceptibility at Additional Charge
* = Confirmation at Additional Charge

**Clinical Information/Comments**

**OTHER TESTS / INDIVIDUAL PROFILE COMPONENTS**
TEST #    TEST NAMES

NOTE: WHEN ORDERING TESTS FOR WHICH MEDICARE OR MEDICAID REIMBURSEMENT WILL BE SOUGHT, PHYSICIANS SHOULD ONLY ORDER TESTS THAT ARE MEDICALLY NECESSARY FOR THE DIAGNOSIS OR TREATMENT OF THE PATIENT. COMPONENTS OF THE ORGAN OR DISEASE PANELS/COMBINATIONS PRINTED ABOVE ARE SHOWN ON THE REVERSE SIDE AND MAY ALSO BE ORDERED INDIVIDUALLY ABOVE. COMPONENTS MAY BE BILLED SEPARATELY PER CARRIER POLICY.

*(Adapted from the Laboratory Corporation of America® http://www.labcorp.com)*

**BILL TO:**
- [ ] MY ACCOUNT
- [ ] PATIENT
- [ ] MEDICARE
- [ ] RAILROAD MEDICARE
- [ ] MEDICAID
- [ ] Lab Card/Select
- [ ] OTHER INSURANCE

PRINT PATIENT NAME (LAST, FIRST, MIDDLE)

REGISTRATION # (IF APPLICABLE) | DATE OF BIRTH | M M D D YEAR | SEX

PATIENT SOCIAL SECURITY # | OFFICE / PATIENT ID #

**DID YOU REMEMBER...**

**TO INCLUDE DIAGNOSIS CODE(S)?**

**TO REQUEST OR MARK TEST(S)?**

**TO PROVIDE ORDER CODE(S) FOR HANDWRITTEN TESTS?**

**TO CHECK "BILL TO" BOX ABOVE?**

ROOM # | LAB REFERENCE # | PATIENT PHONE # ( )

PRINT NAME OF INSURED/RESPONSIBLE PARTY (LAST, FIRST, MIDDLE) - IF OTHER THAN PATIENT

PATIENT STREET ADDRESS (OR INSURED/RESPONSIBLE PARTY) | APT. # | KEY #

CITY | STATE | ZIP

ACCOUNT #:
NAME:
ADDRESS:
CITY, STATE, ZIP
TELEPHONE #:

MEDICARE NUMBER | SUFFIX

DATE COLLECTED | TIME : [ ] AM [ ] PM | TOTAL VOL/HRS. _____ ML _____ HR | [ ] Fasting [ ] Non Fasting

**PRIMARY INSURANCE**

MEDICAID 1 NUMBER | STATE
RELATIONSHIP TO INSURED: [ ] SELF [ ] SPOUSE [ ] DEPENDENT
PRIMARY INSURANCE CO. NAME

MEMBER / INSURED ID # | GROUP #

INSURANCE ADDRESS

CITY | STATE | ZIP

EMPLOYER NAME/EMPLOYER # | INSURED SOCIAL SECURITY # (if not patient)

NPI/UPIN ORDERING/SUPERVISING PHYSICIAN AND/OR PAYORS (MUST BE INDICATED)

[ ] ADDIT'L PHYS.: Dr. _____ NPI/UPIN _____
NON-PHYSICIAN PROVIDER: NAME _____ I.D. # _____

[ ] Fax Results to: ( ) _____
Send Duplicate Report to: Client # OR NAME: _____
ADDRESS: _____
CITY: _____ STATE _____ ZIP _____

**Medicare Limited Coverage Tests**
@ = May not be covered for the reported diagnosis.
F = Has prescribed frequency rules for coverage.
& = A test or service performed with research/experimental kit.
B = Has both diagnosis and frequency-related coverage limitations.

**Provide signed ABN when necessary**

**ICD9 Codes (enter all that apply)**

## ORGAN / DISEASE PANELS

| Code | Test | |
|---|---|---|
| 34392 | [ ] **ELECTROLYTE PANEL** (Na, K, Cl, CO2) | S |
| 10256 | [ ] **HEPATIC FUNCTION PANEL** (Alb, TBili, DBili, AP, AST, ALT, TP) | S |
| 10165 | [ ] **BASIC METABOLIC PANEL w/eGFR** (Na, K, Ca, Cl, CO2, Glu, BUN, Cr) | S |
| 10231 | [ ] **COMP METABOLIC PANEL w/eGFR** (Na, K, Cl, CO2, Glu, BUN, Cr, Ca, TP, Alb, TBili, AP, AST, ALT) | S |
| B 7600 | [ ] **LIPID PANEL** (Fasting Specimen) (TChol, Trig, HDL, calc. LDL) | S |
| B 14852 | [ ] **LIPID PANEL W/REFLEX DLDL** (TChol,Trig, HDL, calc. LDL or DLDL when Trig >400) | S |
| 20210 | [ ] **OBSTETRIC PANEL W/REFLEX** (ABO/Rh, Antibody Scr RBC w/reflex, CBC, RPR (DX) w/reflex confirm, HbsAg w/reflex confirm, Rubella IgG Ab) | 2L,S |
| @ 10306 | [ ] **HEPATITIS PANEL, ACUTE W/REFLEX** (HBsAg w/reflex confirm, HC Ab, HA Ab IgM, HBcAb IgM) | S |

## HEMATOLOGY

| Code | Test | |
|---|---|---|
| @ 510 | [ ] HEMOGLOBIN | L |
| @ 509 | [ ] HEMATOCRIT | L |
| @ 1759 | [ ] CBC (Hgb, Hct, RBC, WBC, Plt) | L |
| @ 6399 | [ ] CBC w/DIFF (Hgb, Hct, RBC, WBC, Plt, Diff) | L |
| B 8847 | [ ] PT WITH INR | B |
| @ 763 | [ ] PTT, ACTIVATED | B |

## OTHER TESTS

| Code | Test | |
|---|---|---|
| 7788 | [ ] ABO GROUP & RH TYPE | L |
| 223 | [ ] ALBUMIN (Alb) | S |
| 234 | [ ] ALKALINE PHOSPHATASE (AP) | S |
| 823 | [ ] ALT (SGPT) | S |
| 243 | [ ] AMYLASE | S |

ADDITIONAL TESTS: (INCLUDE COMPLETE TEST NAME AND ORDER CODE)

## OTHER TESTS (continued)

| Code | Test | |
|---|---|---|
| 249 | [ ] ANA W/REFLEX TITER | S |
| 795 | [ ] ANTIBODY SCR, RBC W/REFLEX ID | L |
| 822 | [ ] AST (SGOT) | S |
| 285 | [ ] BILIRUBIN, DIRECT (DBili) | S |
| 287 | [ ] BILIRUBIN, TOTAL (TBili) | S |
| 4420 | [ ] C-REACTIVE PROTEIN | S |
| @ 29256 | [ ] CA 125 | S |
| 303 | [ ] CALCIUM (Ca) | S |
| 310 | [ ] CARBON DIOXIDE (CO2) | S |
| B 10124 | [ ] CARDIO CRP | S |
| B 978 | [ ] CEA | S |
| 330 | [ ] CHLORIDE (Cl) | S |
| B 334 | [ ] CHOLESTEROL, TOTAL (TChol) | S |
| 375 | [ ] CREATININE (Cr) w/eGFR | S |
| @ 418 | [ ] DIGOXIN | SR |
| B 8293 | [ ] DIRECT LDL | S |
| @ 457 | [ ] FERRITIN | S |
| B 466 | [ ] FOLIC ACID | S |
| 470 | [ ] FSH | S |
| B 482 | [ ] GGT | S |
| 8477 | [ ] GLUCOSE, GEST. SCR. | GY |
| B 484 | [ ] GLUCOSE, PLASMA | GY |
| B 483 | [ ] GLUCOSE, SERUM (Glu) | S |
| 8435 | [ ] HCG, SERUM, QUAL | S |
| B 8396 | [ ] HCG, SERUM, QUANT | S |
| B 608 | [ ] HDL | S |
| B 496 | [ ] HEMOGLOBIN A1C | L |
| 512 | [ ] HEP A AB, IGM | S |
| 4848 | [ ] HEP B CORE AB, IGM | S |
| 499 | [ ] HEP B SURFACE AB QUAL | S |
| 498 | [ ] HEP B SURFACE AG W/REFLEX CONFIRM | S |
| 8472 | [ ] HEP C VIRUS AB | S |
| B 19728 | [ ] HIV-1/HIV-2 SCR W/REFLEXES | S |
| @ 7573 | [ ] IRON (TOT), IBC% SAT | S |

**Reflex tests are performed at an additional charge.**

| Code | Test | |
|---|---|---|
| @ 571 | [ ] IRON, TOTAL | S |
| 593 | [ ] LDH | S |
| 599 | [ ] LEAD (B) | TN |
| 615 | [ ] LH | S |
| 613 | [ ] LITHIUM | S |
| 622 | [ ] MAGNESIUM | S |
| 6517 | [ ] MICROALBUMIN, RANDOM URINE W/CREAT | |
| 4555 | [ ] MICROALBUMIN, 24 HOUR URINE, W/O CREAT | |

**OCC BLD, FECES - GUAIAC**

| Code | Test | |
|---|---|---|
| B 35301 | [ ] DX | |
| F 35306 | [ ] MCR SCR | |

**OCC BLD, FECES - FIT, InSure®¹**

| Code | Test | |
|---|---|---|
| B 11290 | [ ] DX | |
| F 11293 | [ ] MCR SCR | |

| Code | Test | |
|---|---|---|
| 713 | [ ] PHENYTOIN | SR |
| 718 | [ ] PHOSPHORUS | S |
| 733 | [ ] POTASSIUM (K) | S |
| 745 | [ ] PROGESTERONE | S |
| 746 | [ ] PROLACTIN | S |
| 754 | [ ] PROTEIN, TOTAL (TP) | S |
| B 5363 | [ ] PSA, TOTAL | S |
| 4418 | [ ] RHEUMATOID FACTOR | S |
| 799 | [ ] RPR (MONITORING) W/REFLEX TITER | S |
| 36126 | [ ] RPR (DX) W/REFLEX CONFIRM FTA | S |
| 802 | [ ] RUBELLA IGG AB | S |
| 809 | [ ] SED RATE BY MOD WEST | L |
| 836 | [ ] SODIUM (Na) | S |
| 873 | [ ] TESTOSTERONE, TOTAL | S |
| B 896 | [ ] TRIGLYCERIDES (Trig) | S |
| B 899 | [ ] TSH | S |
| B 36127 | [ ] TSH W/REFLEX T-4, FREE | S |
| 859 | [ ] T-3, TOTAL | S |
| B 861 | [ ] T-3 UPTAKE | S |
| B 867 | [ ] T-4 (THYROXINE), TOTAL | S |

| Code | Test | |
|---|---|---|
| B 866 | [ ] T-4 (THYROXINE), FREE | S |
| 6448 | [ ] UA, DIPSTICK ONLY | U |
| 7909 | [ ] UA, DIPSTICK W/REFLEX TO MICROSCOPIC | U |
| 5463 | [ ] UA, COMPLETE (DIPSTICK & MICROSCOPIC) | U |
| @ 3020 | [ ] UA, COMPLETE, REFLEX TO CULTURE | |
| 294 | [ ] UREA NITROGEN (BUN) | S |
| 905 | [ ] URIC ACID | S |
| 916 | [ ] VALPROIC ACID | SR |
| B 7065 | [ ] VITAMIN B12/FOLIC ACID | S |
| B 927 | [ ] VITAMIN B12 | S |

## MICROBIOLOGY

SOURCE (REQUIRED) _____

| Code | Test | |
|---|---|---|
| 4485 | [ ] CULTURE, GP. A STREP* | |
| 5617 | [ ] CULTURE, GP. B STREP* | |
| 4558 | [ ] CULTURE, GENITAL* | |
| 394 | [ ] CULTURE, THROAT* | |
| @ 395 | [ ] CULTURE, URINE, ROUTINE* (INC. INDWELLING CATH.) | |
| @ 8502 | [ ] CHLAMYDIA DNA PROBE, ENDOCX OR M/URET | |
| @ 8501 | [ ] N. GONORRHOEAE (GC) DNA PROBE, ENDOCX OR M/URET | |
| @ 6919 | [ ] CHLAMYDIA & N. GONORRHOEAE W/REFLEX ID, DNA PROBE, ENDOCX OR M/URET | |

**Amplified Specimen Type (please check one)**
[ ] Endocervical  [ ] Urethral  [ ] Urine

| Code | Test | |
|---|---|---|
| @ 17303 | [ ] Chlamydia DNA, SDA | |
| @ 17304 | [ ] N. gonorrhoeae (GC) DNA, SDA | |
| @ 17305 | [ ] Chlamydia & N. gonorrhoeae DNA, SDA | |

**Stool Pathogens**

| Code | Test | |
|---|---|---|
| 10045 | [ ] CULTURE, STOOL (CAMPYLOBACTER SALMONELLA/SHIGELLA)* | |
| 4475 | [ ] CULTURE, CAMPYLOBACTER* | |
| 10019 | [ ] CULTURE, SALMONELLA/SHIGELLA* | |
| 30264 | [ ] E. COLI SHIGA TOXINS, EIA | |
| 681 | [ ] O & P W/PERMANENT STAIN | |

\* Additional charge for ID and Susceptibilities

All other marks - ®¹ and "™" are the property of their respective owner. QD20354K-TX. Revised 8/08.

COMMENTS, CLINICAL INFORMATION:

**TOTAL TESTS ORDERED** [  ]

1 Physician Signature (Required for PA, NY, NJ & MA)
_____

For any patient of any payor (including Medicare and Medicaid), only order those tests which are medically necessary for the diagnosis and treatment of the patient.

*(Adapted from Quest Diagnostics® www.questdiagnostic.com)*

Patient Name: _____

Appointment Date: _____ Time: _____ DOB: _____ Auth.#: _____ Phone #: _____ Today's Date: _____

Referring Physician: _____ Follow Up Appt. Date: _____ Previous Films & Locations: _____

Diagnostic / Clinical indicators: _____ ICD-9 Code: _____

☐ Please Schedule with Patient   ☐ Patient to Hand carry Film
☐ Fax Stat Prelim Report to: _____   ☐ Films with Report to Office
☐ Call Stat Report to: _____   ☐ Disc with Report to Office

(NPO) Nothing by mouth after midnight
♦ Drink 32oz. water 1 hr. prior to exam (DO NOT VOID)
♣ Prep. Kit Required
✤ Nothing by mouth 4 hours prior to exam
◆ Special Prep

## MRI SCANS

IV Contrast: ☐ If Needed ☐ With & Without Contrast ☐ Without Contrast

**BUN ___ Creatinine ___ Date: ___**
(Required for MRI IV contrast studies If: Diabetic, Renal Failure / Disorder, or Hypertension)

☐ Abdomen (NPO) specify organ _____
☐ Brain
☐ IAC's (Separate Indication Required)
☐ Pituitary/Sella (Separate Indication Required)
☐ Breast (Downtown and North Central Only)
☐ Implant ☐ Tumor
☐ Cervical Spine
☐ Chest
☐ Lumbar Spine

☐ MRCP (NPO) (High Field Only)
☐ Neck (Soft Tissue)
☐ Orbits
☐ Pelvis specify organ
☐ Spectroscopy (Medical Center Only)
☐ Thoracic Spine
☐ Other / specify

### MR ARTHROGRAPHY

☐ Left ☐ Right ☐ Bilateral

| | | |
|---|---|---|
| ☐ Ankle | ☐ Hand/Finger | ☐ Shoulder |
| ☐ Elbow | ☐ Hip | ☐ Wrist |
| ☐ Foot/Toe | ☐ Knee | ☐ Extremity |

## MRA / CTA SCANS

☐ MRA ✤ ☐ CTA

☐ Abdominal Aorta
☐ Brain (COW)
☐ Carotids
☐ Chest for PE
☐ Mesenteric Vessels
☐ Pelvis

☐ Renal
☐ Run Off
☐ Thoracic Aorta
☐ Other/specify

## CT SCANS

Contrast: ☐ With IV ☐ Without IV ☐ With Oral ☐ Without Oral

**BUN ___ Creatinine ___ Date: ___**
(Required with IV if: Diabetic, Renal Failure / Disorder, Hypertension or Over 50 yrs. old)

☐✤ Abdomen Only
☐✤ Abdomen / Pelvis
☐ Cervical Spine
☐✤ Chest
☐ Chest High Resolution
☐ Enterography (Small Bowel) w/ IV
☐ Extremities Rt. ___ Lt. ___ specify area
☐ Head

☐ Lumbar Spine
☐ Neck (Soft Tissue)
☐ Orbits
☐ Pelvis Only
☐ Pelvis Orthopedic (Bone)
☐ Sinuses
☐ Limited ☐ Complete
☐ Temporal Bone
☐ Thoracic Spine
☐ Other / specify
☐ Sagittal / Coronal Reconstruction
☐ With 3-D Reconstruction

## P.E.T. / CT

◆ ☐ PET/CT Brain
◆ ☐ PET/CT Body
*NOPR Registered Site*

See CT Section to order a Diagnostic CT Study.

## DEXA

☐ Bone Densitometry (DEXA)

## DIAGNOSTIC XRAYS (NO APPOINTMENT REQUIRED)

☐ Abdomen (KUB)
☐ Abdomen Flat & Upright
☐ Acute Abdominal Series
☐ Bone-Age
☐ Bone Survey
☐ Cervical Spine AP & LAT
☐ Cervical Spine with Flex. & Ext.
☐ Cervical Spine with OBL
☐ Chest ☐ 1 View ☐ PA & LAT

☐ Facial Bones
☐ Finger / specify
☐ Lumbar Spine PA & LAT
☐ Lumbar Spine with Flex. & Ext.
☐ Lumbar Spine with OBL
☐ Mandible
☐ Nasal Bones
☐ Neck (Soft Tissue)
☐ Paranasal Sinuses

☐ Pelvis
☐ Sacrum / Coccyx
☐ Skull
☐ Spine - Scoliosis Series
☐ Sternum
☐ Thoracic Spine
☐ Toe / specify
☐ Other / specify

☐ Left ☐ Right ☐ Bilateral

| | | |
|---|---|---|
| ☐ AC Joints | ☐ Elbow | ☐ Hand |
| ☐ Ankle | ☐ Femur | ☐ Hip |
| ☐ Calcaneous (Heel) | ☐ Foot | ☐ Humerus |
| ☐ Clavicle | ☐ Forearm | ☐ Knee - 2 Views |

☐ Knee - 3 Views or more
☐ Knee (Standing)
☐ Orbits
☐ Ribs
☐ Scapula
☐ Shoulder
☐ Tibia / Fibula
☐ Wrist
☐ SI Joints

## FLUOROSCOPY

☐ Arthrography
  * See MRI for MR Arthrogram
☐ Barium Enema w/ Air (NPO)
☐ Barium Enema Single Contrast
☐ Barium Swallow / Esophagram
☐ Cystogram
☐ Hysterosalpingogram (HSG)
☐ IV Pyelogram (NPO)
✤ Creatinine (required if > 50 yrs.)
Serum Creat ___ Date ___

☐ Small Bowel Series (NPO)
☐ T-tube Cholangiogram (NPO)
☐ UGI Series (NPO)
☐ Voiding Cystourethrogram
☐ Other / specify

## SPECIAL PROCEDURES

☐ *Joint Aspiration
☐ *Joint Injection

## NUCLEAR MEDICINE

☐ Bone Scan Limited ☐ w/ SPECT
☐ Bone Scan, Whole Body ☐ w/ SPECT
☐ Bone Scan, 3 Phase specify area
☐ Breast Scan (Miraluma)
☐ Gastric Emptying (NPO) ☐ Solid ☐ Liquid
☐ Gallium
☐ HIDA Scan (NPO)
  ◆ ☐ w/ CCK ☐ w/o CCK

☐ Indium Scan ☐ w/ SPECT
☐ Liver / Spleen
☐ Meckel's Scan (NPO)
☐ MUGA Scan
☐ Myocardial (MI) Scan
☐ RBC Hemangioma w/ SPECT
☐ RBC GI Bleed Scan
◆ ☐ Renal Scan Including ☐ Lasix ☐ GFR

☐ SPECT
☐ Testicular Scan
◆ ☐ Thyroid
    ☐ Scan Only
    ☐ Uptake & Scan
    ☐ I-131 Whole Body for Mets
☐ Other / specify

## MAMMOGRAPHY

☐ Diagnostic Rt. ___ Lt. ___
  (Ultrasound if indicated)
☐ Screening (w/ return work-up and/or Ultrasound if indicated)
☐ Implant
☐ Previous Mammogram ☐ Yes ☐ No
  where ___
  when ___

## ULTRASOUND (Sonograms)

☐ Abdominal Aorta w/ Doppler (NPO)
☐ Abdominal Complete (NPO)
☐ Abdominal Doppler (NPO)
  ☐ Hepatic ☐ Mesenteric
  ☐ Portal ☐ Renal
☐ Axillary Rt. ___ Lt. ___
☐ Breast Rt. ___ Lt. ___ Both ___
☐ Carotid
☐ Vertebral Doppler
☐ *Cyst Aspiration

☐ Extremity ☐ Upper ☐ Lower
  ☐ Arterial Rt. ___ Lt. ___
  ☐ Ankle Brachial Index (ABI)
  ☐ Venous Doppler Rt. ___ Lt. ___
☐ Fetal Biophysical Profile
☐ Gallbladder (NPO)
☐ Liver (NPO)
☐ OB Ultrasound (Transvaginal, if indicated)
☐ Pancreas (NPO)

☐ Pelvic Evaluation Transabdominal
☐ Pelvic Evaluation Transvaginal
☐ Renal Artery Doppler
☐ Renal Bil. (Retroperitoneum) (NPO)
☐ Right Upper Quadrant (NPO)
☐ Right Lower Quadrant (NPO)
☐ Testicular with Doppler
☐ Thyroid
☐ Other / specify

(Adapted from Baptist M&S Imaging, San Antonio, Texas www.baptisthealthsystem.com)

## □ STAT

□ Call Report: #:

□ Fax Prelim.: #:

□ Films with Patient
□ Deliver Films with Report
□ Deliver Report
□ Fax Report: #:

Referring Physician: _____ Contact: _____

**Physician Follow-Up Appointment: Date:** _____ Time: _____

Pt. Name: _____ D.O.B. _____

Pt. Home Phone #: _____ Alternate #: _____

Diagnosis: _____

Previous Study/Surgery: _____

Special Instructions: _____

Date of Study: _____

Time: _____ □ am □ pm

□ Call Patient to Schedule

Insurance Co.: _____

**Pre-Cert/Authorization Obtained?**
□ Yes □ No

Pre-Cert/Authorization #: _____

Diabetic/Kidney Problems: □ Yes □ No

Sedation: □ IV □ PO

## ■ HI FIELD MRI  ■ OPEN MRI

(w/ = With Contrast  w/o = Without Contrast
prn = Contrast Per Radiologist Discretion)

**prn w/w/o**
□□□ Brain
□□□ Brain Stem
□□□ Brain w/ Perfusion
□□□ Brain w/ Diffusion
□□□ Brain Spectroscopy (Hi-Field Only)
□□□ Alzheimers □ Tumors
□□□ Shunt Flow Study
□□□ CSF Flow Study
□□□ IAC's
□□□ Pituitary
□□□ Posterior Fossa
□□□ Sella
□□□ Orbits
□□□ Soft Tissue Neck
□□□ TMJ (Hi-Field Only)
□□□ Cervical Complete
□□□ Cervical Limited
□□□ Thoracic Complete

□□□ Thoracic Limited
□□□ Lumbar Complete
□□□ Lumbar Limited
□□□ Sacrum
□□□ SI Joints
□□□ Chest
□□□ Bilateral Breast/s
       (Hi-Field Only)
       □ LT □ RT
□□□ Abdomen*
□□□ Abdomen Only*
□□□ Pelvis
□□□ (MRCP) Abdominal
       (Hi-Field Only)*
□□□ Other: _____

**EXTREMITIES:**
**L  R**
□□ Shoulder
□□ Arm (specify): _____
□□ Elbow
□□ Wrist
□□ Hip
□□ Leg (specify): _____
□□ Knee
□□ Ankle
□□ Foot
□□ Other: _____

### MRA

**w/o**
□□ Intracranial
       (Head / Circle of Willis)
□□ Extracranial (Neck/Carotids)
□□ Femoral Arteries & Run Off
       (Hi-Field Only)
□□ Renals (Hi-Field Only)*
□□ Other: _____

### NUCLEAR MEDICINE

□ Bone Scan
□ Total Body
□ Multi Area (specify): _____
□ Limited (one area; specify): _____
□ 3 Phase (specify): _____
□ SPECT (specify): _____
□ Liver Scan w/ SPECT
□ Liver/Spleen Scan
□ RBC Liver Hemangioma
□ Hepatobiliary (HIDA) w/ CCK*
□ Hepatobiliary (HIDA) fatty meal*
□ Cardiac MUGA Scan
□ Urea Breath Test*
□ Other: _____

□ Gastric Emptying*
□ I-131 Whole Body Scan
□ Gallium Scan
□ Indium Scan
□ Thyroid Uptake & Scan *
□ Thyroid Uptake Only*
□ Thyroid Scan Only*
□ Renal Scan*
□ With Flow & Function
□ With Lasix Washout
□ For Residual Urine
□ Parathyroid Scan

## CT

(w/ = With Contrast  w/o = Without Contrast
prn = Contrast Per Radiologist Discretion)

**prn w/w/o**
□□□ Brain
□□□ Sinuses
□□□ Sinuses Limited - Coronal
□□□ Orbits
□□□ Temporal Bones
□□□ IAC's
□□□ Soft Tissue Neck
□□□ Chest
□□□ Abdomen/Pelvis*
□□□ Abdomen Only*
□□□ Pelvis Only*
□□□ Bony Pelvis
□□□ Renal/Adrenals

□□□ Facial Bones
□□□ Liver
□□□ C-Spine (levels): _____
□□□ T-Spine (levels): _____
□□□ L-Spine (levels): _____
□□□ 3-D Reconstruction
□□□ Sagittal/Coronal Recon.
□□□ Other: _____
**L  R**
□□ Upper Extremity
       (specify): _____
□□ Lower Extremity
       (specify): _____

### CTA

□ Renals
□ Peripheral Run Offs
□ Carotids
□ Intracranial
□ Other: _____

### SCREENING EXAMS

♡ Heart (Cardiac Scoring)
□ Lung
□ Full Body CT
□ BMD (QCT)

### ULTRASOUND

□ Abdomen*
□ Gallbladder*
□ RUQ*
□ Liver*
□ Aorta*
□ Testicular w/ Doppler
□ Renal □ BILAT □ UNILAT
□ Other: _____

□ Renal Transplant Evaluation
□ Extremity Non-Vascular
□ Thyroid
□ Pelvic* (w/ Transvaginal if indicated)
□ Transvaginal / Pelvic *
□ Breast □ LT □ RT
□ OB Limited (w/ Transvaginal if indicated)*
□ OB Complete (w/ Transvaginal if indicated)*

### VASCULAR ULTRASOUND

**□ ARTERIAL**
□ Upper Extremity □ LT □ RT
□ Lower Extremity □ LT □ RT
□ Carotid
□ Abdominal Aorta*
□ Dialysis Fistula/Graft Loc.
□ Claudication ABI - Screen
□ Renal Vascular*

**□ VENOUS**
□ Hepatic
□ Renal
□ Portal
□ Mesenteric
□ Other: _____

*EXAMS REQUIRING SPECIAL PREPARATION

## RADIOGRAPHY

**HEAD:**
□ Skull
□ Facial Bones
□ Nasal Bones
□ Mandible
□ Sinuses
□ Waters View Only
□ TMJ's

**CHEST:**
□ PA & Lateral
□ Ribs □ LT □ RT □ BIL.
□ Sternum

**ABDOMEN:**
□ AP (KUB)
□ AP & Upright

**PELVIS:**
□ AP

**TOMOGRAPHY:**
□ Specify: _____

**SPINE:**
□ Cervical □ Thoracic □ Lumbar
□ 5 Views □ 3 Views
□ AP & Lateral Only
□ Flex & Extension Only
□ C-Spine Davis (7 Views)
□ L-Spine Davis (7 Views)
□ Sacroiliac Joints
□ Sacrum/Coccyx
□ Bone Survey
□ Scoliosis Series
□ Weight Bearing
□ Other: _____

**UPPER EXTREMITIES:**
**L  R**
□□ Clavicle
□□ Shoulder
□□ A-C Joints
□□ Humerus
□□ Elbow
□□ Forearm
□□ Wrist
□□ Bone Age
□□ Hand
□□ Finger (specify): _____

**LOWER EXTREMITIES:**
**L  R**
□□ Hip
□□ Femur
□□ Knee
□□ Tibia/Fibula
□□ Foot
□□ Ankle
□□ Toe (specify): _____

## FLUOROSCOPY

□ Barium Enema w/ Air*
□ Upper GI w/ Air*
□ Small Bowel Series*
□ Barium Swallow (Esophagus)*
□ IVP*
□ Lumbar Puncture*

## ARTHROGRAPHY

**L  R**
□□ Knee*
□□ Shoulder*
□□ Wrist*
□□ Hip*
□□ Other: _____

## MYELOGRAPHY

□ Cervical*
□ Thoracic*
□ Lumbar*
□ Entire Spine*
□ Special Instructions: _____

## DEXA (BONE DENSITY STUDY)

□ Hip/Spine*  □ Wrist/Forearm*

(Adapted from Sendero Imaging & Treatment Center, San Antonio, Texas www.senderoimaging.com)

Patient Name: _____

D.O.B.: _____   Referring Physician: _____

Diagnosis/Clinical History: _____

**Follow Up Doctor Appointment Date:** _____  **Time:** _____  Previous Films & Location: _____

○ Films with Report to Office   ○ Fax Preliminary Report:
○ Patient to Hand Carry Films   Call Report: ○ to MD   ○ to Office

**Appt. Date :** _____
**Appt. Time:** _____

## BREAST IMAGING/SPECIAL PROCEDURES

○ **Screening Mammogram - w/ return work-up and/or Ultrasound if indicated**
○ Diagnostic Mammogram (with Ultrasound if indicated)
○ Implant Mammogram (with Ultrasound if indicated)
○ Unilateral Mammogram (with Ultrasound if indicated)   ○ LT  ○ RT
○ Breast Ultrasound
○ Fine Needle Aspiration

○ Cyst Aspiration
○ Needle Localization
○ Stereotactic Core Biopsy *
○ Galactography
○ Sentinel Node Localization
○ Hysterosalpingogram *
○ Fallopian Tube Recan.   ○ LT  ○ RT

## PAIN MANAGEMENT/SPECIAL PROCEDURES

○ Epidural Steroid (ESI)
○ Facet Injection *
○ Nerve Root Block *
○ Lumbar Puncture *
○ Joint Injection *

○ Discogram *
○ Cervical   ○ Thoracic   ○ Lumbar
○ Myelogram *
○ Cervical   ○ Thoracic   ○ Lumbar
○ Venogram

Other/Special Instructions _____

## RADIOGRAPHY

**HEAD**
○ Skull
○ Facial Bones
○ Mandible
○ Sinuses
○ Waters View

**CHEST**
○ PA & Lateral
○ Ribs   ○ LT  ○ RT
○ Sternum

**SPINE**
○ Cervical   ○ Thoracic   ○ Lumbar
○ 5 Views   ○ 3 Views
○ AP & Lateral Only
○ Flex & Extension
○ Davis (7 Views)
○ Scoliosis Study
○ Sacrum/Coccyx
○ Metastatic/Skeletal Survey

Other/Special Instructions _____

**ABDOMEN**
○ Flat/Upright
○ KUB

**PELVIS**
○ AP

**FLUOROSCOPY**
○ Barium Swallow
○ Upper GI *
○ Small Bowel *
○ Barium Enema
   ○ W/ Air Contrast *
○ IVP *   ○ VCUG
○ Cystogram
○ IVP   ○ LT  ○ RT

**JOINT**
○ Arthrogram
   ○ LT  ○ RT

**LEFT**        **RIGHT**        **BILATERAL**
○ Shoulder   ○ Femur     ○ TMJ
○ Humerus    ○ Knee      ○ Clavicle
○ Forearm    ○ Tibia/Fibula  ○ Ribs
○ Elbow      ○ Ankle     ○ Hip
○ Wrist      ○ Foot
○ Hand       ○ Toe
○ Finger  ○ Bone Age  Other/Special Instructions

## PET CT

○ Whole Body with CT Fusion
○ Brain with CT Fusion
○ Alzheimer's/Dementia

**See CT section to order a complete CT study**

## NUCLEAR MEDICINE

○ Bone Scan
   ○ Total Body
   ○ Multi Area
   ○ Limited
○ Liver SPECT
○ Liver/Spleen Scan
○ RBC Liver Hemangioma
○ Hepatobiliary (HIDA) *
   ○ w/CCK *
○ Cardiac MUGA Scan
○ Meckels Scan *
○ Gastric Emptying *
○ Urea Breath Test (H-Pylori)
○ Gallium Scan

○ Indium Scan (Ceretec)
○ Lung Scan - Vent/Perfusion
○ I-131 Whole Body Scan
○ Thyroid Uptake
   ○ 6 hr.   ○ 24 hr.
○ 3 Phase
○ SPECT
○ Thyroid Scan
   ○ I-123  ○ 99mc Tc
○ Parathyroid Scan
○ Renal Scan
   ○ W/ Lasix Washout

**THERAPY**
○ I-131 _____ mCi

Other/Special Instructions _____

## ULTRASOUND

○ Abdomen *
○ Abdominal Aorta *
○ Extremity   ○ LT  ○ RT
○ Gallbladder
○ Liver - Follow Up *

○ Thyroid
○ Kidney - Bilat.
○ Kidney   ○ LT  ○ RT
○ Renal Transplant Eval.
○ Pelvic *
   (w/ Trans-vaginal if Indicated)

○ Complete OB *
○ Follow-up OB *
○ Fetal Viability
   (w/ Trans-vaginal Ultrasound)
○ Hysterosonography *
○ Testicular *
○ Prostate *

○ Biopsy
○ Fine Needle Aspiration
○ Cyst Aspiration

Other/Special Instructions _____

## VASCULAR ULTRASOUND

○ **Arterial**        ○ **Venous**
○ Carotid
○ Vertebral
○ Doppler Aorta *
○ Upper Extremity   ○ LT  ○ RT
○ Lower Extremity   ○ LT  ○ RT
○ Dialysis Graft Evaluation

○ Abdominal Doppler *
○ Hepatic *
○ Renal *
○ Mesenteric *
○ Portal *
○ Pseudo Aneurysm

Other/Special Instructions _____

## BONE DENSITY STUDY (DEXA)

○ Osteoporosis Scan with One View Lumbar

**\* EXAMS THAT REQUIRE SPECIAL PREPARATION**

## MRI

○ Intra-articular Gadolinium (Joint)   ○ IV Gadolinium Enhancement

**Per Radiologist**
○ Brain
○ Brain with IAC's
○ Brain Spectroscopy
○ Alzheimers
○ Tumor
○ Post Fossa
○ Pituitary
○ IAC's

○ Orbits
○ TMJ
○ Neck (Soft Tissue)
○ C-Spine
○ T-Spine
○ L-Spine
○ Chest
○ Abdomen *

○ Pelvis *
○ Pelvis (soft tissue) *
○ Liver
○ Prostate
○ MRCP
○ Cardiac MRI
○ Morphology
○ Function

**LEFT**   **RIGHT**   **BILATERAL**
○ Breast-Tumor   ○ Wrist       ○ Knee
○ Breast-Implant ○ Hand/Finger ○ Ankle
○ Shoulder       ○ Hip w/ Limited Pelvis  ○ Mid Foot
○ Elbow          ○ Extremity ____  ○ Toes

Other/Special Instructions _____

## MR/CT ANGIOGRAPHY

○ **MR Angiography**   ○ **CT Angiography**
○ **Coronary CTA \* (64 Detector)**
(CT Chest w/. / CTA Coronary Arteries w/Calcium Scoring, Ejection Fraction)

○ Intracranial Arteries (Head)
○ Extracranial Arteries (Neck)
○ Dural Sinuses & Veins (Head)
○ Portal Vein - Inf. Vena Cava
○ CSF Flow Study

○ Aorta - Thoracic
○ Aorta - Abdominal
○ Renal Arteries
○ Femoral Arteries & Runoff
○ Mesenteric Arteries
○ Extremity _____

Other/Special Instructions _____

## CT

**CONTRAST:**  ○ Per Radiologist   ○ Oral & IV   ○ IV   ○ No Oral   ○ W/O & W/IV

○ Brain
○ Sinuses (Coronal)
○ Sinuses (Axial & Coronal)
○ Sinuses (Landmarx™)
○ Facial Bones
○ Temporal Bones
○ Orbits

○ Neck Soft Tissue
○ Abdomen/Pelvis
○ Pelvis Only
○ Chest
○ Chest w/Upper Abd. *
○ Chest/Abd./Pelvis *
○ Hematuria Evaluation *
○ Urography

○ Renal (WO/W IV) *
○ Liver *
○ Virtual Colonoscopy *
○ C-Spine w/Recon
○ T-Spine w/Recon
○ L-Spine w/Recon
○ Extremity w/ Reconstruction ____

Other/Special Instructions _____

○ Calcium Scoring        ○ Lung Cancer Screening
○ Whole Body Screening

(Adapted from stric [South Texas Radiology Imaging Centers], San Antonio, Texas www.stric.com)

# Mockingbird Physical Therapy
# & Sports Rehab

☐ **Miami (Metro)**  ☐ **Dorall (At airport)**  ☐ **Kendall (At 5-points)**

1 Plaza Dr Ste 422    22398 NW 36th St    1200 SW 67th Ave

Call 305.555.7790    Call 305.555.1990    Call 305.555.1200

Fax 305.555.7791    Fax 305.555.1995    Fax 305.555.1202

Patient Name: _____    Date: _____

Phone #: _____    Cell #: _____

Diagnosis: _____    Diagnosis Code(s): _____

Surgery: _____

Physical Therapy for:    1    2    3    4    5    visits per week for    1    2    3    4    5    6    weeks

---

☐    Evaluate   and   Treat   as   indicated: _____

### Therapeutic Exercise/ Activities
☐ PROM/AAROM/AROM
☐ Strengthening
☐ Flexibility
☐ Neuromuscular Re-ed
☐ Proprioceptive Training
☐ Gait Training
☐ Pre-op exercise
☐ Other:_____

### Manual Therapy
☐ Joint Mobilization
☐ Soft Tissue Mobilization
☐ Myofascial Release
☐ Other:_____

### Industrial Rehabillitation
☐ Functional Capacity Evaluation (FCE)
☐ Back School/Body Mechanics

### Modalities
☐ Hot/Cold Pack
☐ Ultrasound
☐ Electrical Stimulation
☐ NMES
☐ Traction
☐ Other:_____

Iontophoresis: Dexamethasone 4 mg / ml, 1-2 cc per treatment for _____ total treatments
MD Signature: _____

Phonophoresis: Hydrocortisone 10% / aquasonic gel 20 gms with _____ refills
MD Signature: _____

---

_____/_____/_____/_____

**Physician Name (please print)**          **Signature**          **Date**          **Phone**

I certify that the prescribed treatment is an appropriate course of treatment and the services prescribed are medically necessary.

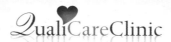

# FAX TO 305.555.2244

## Quali-Care Clinic
## SLEEP CENTER

> *Patient Referral
> Form for
> Consultation and
> Sleep Evaluation*

Patient Name: _____ DOB: _____

Patient Telephone Number: (_____)_____

Referring Physician: _____ UPIN: _____

Referring Physician Phone: (_____)_____

*Authorization for sleep consultation and evaluation. Your patient will be called
and scheduled promptly. Thank you!*

Please fax top portion to Quali-Care Clinic Sleep Center at 305.555.2244.
Please give bottom portion to patient.

You have been referred to Quali-Care Clinic Sleep Center for sleep evaluation. We
will call you to set up an appointment, or you may call us at 305.555.2242. We are
located on Medical Blvd next to Hillcrest Medical Center.

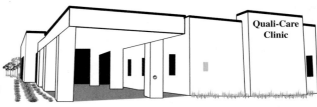

## Quali-Care Clinic
## SLEEP CENTER
Ten Medical Blvd Suite 100
Miami FL 33130

### Hillcrest Sleep Disorders Center
1500 Wood Trail • Miami FL 33130
Call 305.555.7498 • Fax 305.555.7499

# Physician's Order for Sleep Study

Patient Name: _____ DOB: _____

Home Phone: _____ Work Phone: _____ Cell Phone: _____

Service Requested (Please Check):

☐ **Standard evaluation (1-2 nights of polysomnography) for possible obstructive sleep apnea (OSA).** If the Apnea + Hypopnea Index (AHI) is greater that 15/hour in the first 2 hours of recording, a titration trial of CPAP will be initiated. If the baseline sleep study demonstrated significant sleep apnea (AHI >5/hour) but the patient does not qualify for CPAP after 2 hours, the patient will be scheduled for a second sleep study for a full night of CPAP titration.

☐ **Baseline study with CPAP titration after 2 hours regardless of AHI**

☐ **Baseline without any CPAP intervention**

☐ **CPAP titration study** (for patients with documented obstructive sleep apnea by previous sleep study)

☐ **Multiple Sleep Latency Test (MSLT)** with a baseline study the night before

☐ **Other** (please specify): _____

Brief History: _____

_____

**Check if Present:**

**1) Respiratory Dysfunction**
    ☐ Witnessed apneas
    ☐ Audible snoring
    ☐ Morning headaches

**2) Daytime Somnolence**
    ☐ Mild (sleepy during the day but does not sleep inappropriately)
    ☐ Moderate (naps if possible; falls asleep sitting up if permitted)
    ☐ Severe (requires naps; falls asleep while driving)

**3) Sleep Disturbance**
    ☐ Abnormal movements during sleep      ☐ Three or more awakenings per night

**4) Relevant History**

| | | | |
|---|---|---|---|
| ☐ OSA | ☐ Home Oxygen | ☐ UPPP | ☐ CVA |
| ☐ COPD | ☐ CPAP | ☐ Tonsillectomy | ☐ Obesity (BMI >30) |
| ☐ CHF | ☐ BiPAP | ☐ Tracheostomy | ☐ Overweight (BMI >27 <30) |
| ☐ Depression | ☐ Hypertension | ☐ CAD | ☐ Nocturia |
| ☐ Other:_____ | | | |

**Ordering Physician:**

Name: _____ UPIN: _____

Signature: _____ Date: _____

Address: _____ Phone: _____

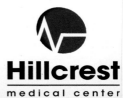

**Hillcrest**
medical center

# BUILDING A REFERENCE LIBRARY

Medical transcriptionists recognize the importance of maintaining a personal library of reference material. Keeping current is an ongoing and expensive effort; however, having current editions and up-to-date reference material is critical to the accuracy of medical transcription. These purchases are valid business tax deductions. Many of the current medical reference books are offered online, both in a CD version and in hard copy. Some considerations for building and maintaining a personal library of reference materials are as follows:

1. Build a basic library before branching out to the specialty areas, unless you happen to work in one of the specialty or subspecialty areas.

2. Have available both unabridged and collegiate editions of dictionaries, preferably with copyright dates within the past 5 years.

3. The word book(s) you choose should illustrate proper word division, i.e., hyphenation at the end of a line for both English and medical words.

4. Medical transcription is a mixture of technical writing and business writing—obtain reference books that will familiarize you with both areas.

5. Contact medical publishing companies and pharmaceutical companies and ask that your name be added to their mailing lists. You might be able to sign up for news, coupons, and product updates. Locate these companies online through Google. Also, your local library will have contact information on companies that publish allied health reference material.

6. Read reviews of newly published editions and ask your peers, coworkers, and professional associates about them before you purchase additional reference books for your personal library. Some publishing companies offer a trial period on newly purchased volumes.

7. Before you purchase any dictionary or reference work, check for the most recent copyright date. Publishing company personnel can tell you if they plan to have a revision on the market soon; if possible, wait and purchase the new edition.

8. If you enroll in an anatomy and physiology, medical terminology, medical transcription, grammar review, proofreading or editing class, keep your textbooks; these are excellent reference books to add to your personal library.

9. Medical transcriptionists constantly edit and proofread; therefore, become familiar with the basics in these areas by enrolling in classes and obtaining and reading reference material. (See the basic proofreading marks in this appendix.)

10. Association for Healthcare Documentation Integrity AHDI (http://www.ahdionline.org) has developed the BenchMark KB*, a completely online reference for a yearly subscription that includes electronic membership to AHDI. The KB offers a wide variety of tools, including the AHDI *Book of Style for Medical Transcription*, 3rd ed., and the Stedman's Rainbow reference book collection in online versions. See the link below to read about everything offered in this valuable new aid.

11. *Postal Addressing Standards,* the United States Postal Service publication 28, is available at no charge from your post office. Business addressing standards are discussed in detail along with other important post office regulations. (Available online at http://pe.usps.gov/text/pub28/welcome.htm.)

*KB stands for Knowledge Base. http://www.ahdionline.org/BenchmarkKBOnline/tabid/283/Default.aspx

# A Healthcare Controlled Vocabulary

*From* Medical Abbreviations: 30,000 Conveniences at the Expense of Communication and Safety, *14th edition, (ISBN: 978-0-931431-14-2) by Neil M. Davis, MS, PharmD, FASHP (www.medabbrev. com), printed with permission.*

Presently there are no standards for abbreviations used in prescribers' orders, consultations, written prescriptions, standing orders, computer order sets, nurse's medication administration records, pharmacy profiles, hospital formularies, etc. Because in the healthcare field everyone does their own thing, there are many variations. These variations in the way abbreviations are expressed are not always understood and at times are misinterpreted. They cause delays in initiating therapy, cause accidents, waste time for everyone in clarifying these documents, lengthen the time it takes to train those working in the healthcare field, lengthen hospital stays, and waste money.

A controlled vocabulary similar to what is used in the aviation industry is needed. Everyone in the aviation industry "follows the book," and uses a controlled vocabulary. All pilots and air traffic controllers say, "alfa", "bravo", "charlie." They do not go off on their own and say "adam", "beef", "candy!" They say "one three," not thirteen, because thirteen sounds like thirty. Radio transmission in the aviation industry is not easy to decipher, yet because precision is critical, everything possible is done to eliminate error. To prevent errors all radio transmissions are given only in English, every transmission is given in the same order and must be immediately repeated by the receiver to make sure it was heard correctly. Written and oral communication in the medical professions are just as critical and are also not easy to decipher, so establishing a controlled vocabulary is also necessary in this industry.

Listed below are some of the organizations that have ongoing projects related to standardizing medical terminology:

The United States Pharmacopeial
Convention, Inc.
12601 Twinbrook Parkway
Rockville, MD 20852

National Library of Medicine
Unified Medical Language Systems
8600 Rockville Pike
Bethesda, MD 20894

Council of Biological Editors, through their Scientific Style and Format: The *CBE Manual for Authors, Editors, and Publishers*, 6th Ed. Council of Biological Editors; Cambridge University Press, Cambridge UK, New York, Victoria Australia: 1995

American Medical Association, through their *AMA Manual of Style*, 10th Edition. AMA, Chicago, 2008

Computer-Based Patient Record Institute, Inc.
1000 East Woodfield Rd. Suite 102
Schuamburg, IL 60173-5921
http://www.CPRI.org

Association for Healthcare Documentation Integrity through their *The Book of Style for Medical Transcription*, 3rd ed., 2008, Association for Healthcare Documentation Integrity, Modesto CA

The following is the start of a Healthcare Controlled Vocabulary. The basis for this controlled vocabulary is established standard terminology and the result of 41 years of studying medical errors by this author.

It is anticipated that a Healthcare Controlled Vocabulary, with professional organizations' input and backing, will grow and someday evolve into an "official standard." Your suggestions and comments are vital to this growth and eventual recognition. It is always safest to avoid the use of abbreviations unless they are well known in your work environment.

## EXAMPLES OF A CONTROLLED VOCABULARY

| Standard | What not to use or do | Comments |
|---|---|---|
| 100 mg (100 space mg) | 100mg (100 no space mg) | The USP* standard way of expressing a strength is to leave a space between the number and its units. Leaving this space makes it easier to read the number as can be seen below.<br><br>1mg    1 mg<br>10mg   10 mg<br>100mg  100 mg |
| 1 mg | 1.0 mg | This is a USP standard. When a trailing zero is used, the decimal point is sometimes not seen when working from handwritten copies or when the decimal point falls on a line thus causing a tenfold overdose. These overdoses have caused injury and death. A "trailing zero" may be used only where required to demonstrate the level of precision of the value being reported, such as for laboratory results, imaging studies that report size of lesions, or catheter/tube sizes. It may **NOT** be used in medication orders or other medication-related documentation. |
| 0.1 mL | .1 mL | When the decimal point is not seen, this is read as 1 mL, causing a ten fold overdose. |
| once daily (Do not abbreviate.) | The abbreviation OD | The classic meaning for OD is right eye. Liquids intended to be given once daily are mistakenly given in the right eye. |
| | The abbreviation QD | When the Q in QD is dotted too aggressively it looks like Q.I.D. and the medication is given four times daily. When a lower case q is used, the tail of the q has come up between the q and the d to make it look like qid.<br><br>In the United Kingdom, Q.D. means four times daily |
| unit (Do not abbreviate. Write "unit" using a lower-case u.) | The abbreviation U | The handwritten U is mistaken for a zero when poorly written causing a 10 fold overdose (i.e. 6 U regular insulin is read as 60). The poorly written U has also been read as 4, 6, and cc. Write "unit," leaving a space between the number and the word unit. |
| mg (lower case mg with no period) | mg., Mg., Mg, MG, mgm, mgs | The USP standard expression is the mg |
| mL (lower case m with a capital L, no period) | mL., ml, ml., mls, mLs, cc | The USP standard expression is the mL for the measurement of liquids |
| Use generic names or brand names | Do not abbreviate drug names or combinations of drugs, such as CPZ, PBZ, NTG, MS, MSO₄, 5FC, MTX, 6MP, MOPP, ASA, HCTZ, etc. | Abbreviated drug names and acronyms are not always known to the reader; at times they have more than one possible meaning, or are thought to be another drug.<br><br>When the chemical name "6 mercaptopurine" has been used, six doses of mercaptopurine have been mistakenly administered. The generic name, mercaptopurine, should be used. MgSO₄ (magnesium sulfate) has been read as morphine sulfate. |
| Do not use shortened names or chemical names in patient-related documents | | When an unofficial shortened version of the name norfloxacin, norflox was used, Noflex was mistakenly given.<br><br>An order for Aredia was read as Adriamycin, as some professionals abbreviated the name Adriamycin as "Adria" which looks like Aredia. |

(Continued)

# Examples of a Controlled Vocabulary

| Standard | What not to use or do | Comments |
|---|---|---|
| The metric system | The apothecary system (grains, drams, minims, ounces, etc.) | The Apothecary system is so rarely used it is not recognized or understood. The symbol for minim (m) is read as mL; the symbol for one dram (3 T) is read as 3 tablespoons, and gr (grain) is read as gram. |
| Use properly placed commas for numbers above 9999, as in 10,000, or 5,000,000 | 5000000 | Some healthcare workers have difficulty in reading large numbers such as 5000000. The use of commas helps the reader to read these numbers correctly. |
| 600 mg  When possible, do not use decimal expressions.  25 mcg | 0.6 g  0.025 mg | A USP standard. The elimination of decimals lessens the chance for error.  Mistakes are made when reading numbers less than 1 with decimals. |
| Use specific concentrations and the time in which intravenous potassium chloride should be administered. | Do not use the term "bolus" in conjunction with the administration of potassium chloride injection. | Some physicians will erroneously indicate that potassium chloride injection should be "bolused" or be given "IV push," vaguely meaning that it should not be dripped in slowly. Many deaths have been reported when prescribers have been taken literally and the potassium chloride was given by bolus or IV push for fluid-restricted patients. Orders should be specific such as, "20 mEq of potassium chloride in 50 mL of 5% dextrose to run over 30 minutes." |
| use "and" | Do not use a slash (/) mark or the symbol "&" | A slash mark looks like a one. An order written "6 units regular insulin/20 units NPH insulin," was read as 120 units of NPH insulin.  The symbol "&" has been read as a 4. |
| Orally transmitted medical orders should be read back as heard for verification. | Do not assume that one has spoken or heard correctly. | During oral communications, speakers misspeak and/or transcribers mishear. To minimize these errors, the transmitter must speak clearly and slowly, the transcriber must repeat what was transcribed, and the transmitter must listen attentively when this is being done. Errors are less likely to occur when the prescription is complete. When spelling out words, use the phonetic alphabet used in the aviation industry. Oral orders should be avoided whenever possible. |
| When prescriptions are written or orally transmitted they must be complete.<br>• dosage form must be specified<br>• strength must be specified<br>• directions must be specified<br>• included in the directions must be the purpose or indication. | Incomplete orders | Prescribers on occasion think of one drug and mistakenly order another. Nurses and pharmacists on occasion misread prescriptions because of error, poor handwriting or poor oral communications, or look-alike or sound-alike drugs.[1]<br><br>When the prescription is complete and the purpose or indication is included, these errors are less likely to occur. Listing the purpose or indication on the prescription label will assist in increasing patient adherence. |
| Written communications must be legible. | Illegible handwriting | Those who cannot or will not write legibly must print (if this would be legible), type, use a computer, or have an employee write for them and then immediately verify and sign the document. |

## EXAMPLES OF A CONTROLLED VOCABULARY

| Standard | What not to use or do | Comments |
|---|---|---|
| Prescribe specific doses. | Do not prescribe 2 ampuls or 2 vials | There is often more than one size or concentration of drug available. Failing to be specific will lead to unintended doses being administered. |
| As required by The Joint Commission establish a list of dangerous abbreviations which should not be used | Use dangerous abbreviations. | See Chapter 2 of this book "Dangerous, Contradictory, and/or Ambiguous Abbreviations." |
| Use h or hr for hour | ° | An order written as q 4° has been read as q 40 or the symbol° has not been understood. |
| Specify amount of drug to be given in a single dose.[2] | Specify total amount of drug to be administered over a period of time. | Orders such as . . . 1600 mg over 4 days have caused death when mistakenly given as a single dose. Order should state . . . 400 mg once daily for four days (2-1-08 to 2-4-08) |

*USP = United States Pharmacopeia

1. Davis NM. Look-alike and sound-alike drug names. Hosp Pharm 2006, Supplement Wall-chart (Call 1-800-223-0554)
2. Kohler D. Standardizing the expression & nomenclature of cancer treatment regimens. Am J Health-System Pharm. 1998;55;137–44

Source: From Medical Abbreviations: 30,000 Conveniences at the Expense of Communication and Safety, 14th ed. (ISBN: 978-0-931431-14-2) by Neil M. Davis , MS, PharmD, FASHP (www.medabbrev.com), printed with permission.

# OFFICIAL "DO NOT USE" LIST FROM THE JOINT COMMISSION

| Do Not Use | Potential Problem | Use Instead |
|---|---|---|
| U (unit) | Mistaken for "0" (zero), the number "4" (four) or "cc" | Write "unit" |
| IU (International Unit) | Mistaken for IV (intravenous) or the number 10 (ten) | Write "International Unit" |
| Q.D., QD, q.d., qd (daily) | Mistaken for each other | Write "daily" |
| Q.O.D., QOD, q.o.d, qod (every other day) | Period after the Q mistaken for "I" and the "O" mistaken for "I" | Write "every other day" |
| Trailing zero (X.0 mg)* Lack of leading zero (.X mg) | Decimal point is missed | Write X mg Write 0.X mg |
| MS | Can mean morphine sulfate or magnesium sulfate | Write "morphine sulfate" Write "magnesium sulfate" |
| MSO$_4$ and MgSO$_4$ | Confused for one another | |

[1] Applies to all orders and all medication-related documentation that is handwritten (including free-text computer entry) or on pre-printed forms.

**\*Exception:** A "trailing zero" may be used only where required to demonstrate the level of precision of the value being reported, such as for laboratory results, imaging studies that report size of lesions, or catheter/tube sizes. It may not be used in medication orders or other medication-related documentation.

## Additional Abbreviations, Acronyms and Symbols
(For <u>possible</u> future inclusion in the Official "Do Not Use" List)

| Do Not Use | Potential Problem | Use Instead |
|---|---|---|
| > (greater than) < (less than) | Misinterpreted as the number "7" (seven) or the letter "L" Confused for one another | Write "greater than" Write "less than" |
| Abbreviations for drug names | Misinterpreted due to similar abbreviations for multiple drugs | Write drug names in full |
| Apothecary units | Unfamiliar to many practitioners Confused with metric units | Use metric units |
| @ | Mistaken for the number "2" (two) | Write "at" |
| cc | Mistaken for U (units) when poorly written | Write "mL" or "ml" or "milliliters" ("mL" is preferred) |
| µg | Mistaken for mg (milligrams) resulting in one thousand-fold overdose | Write "mcg" or "micrograms" |

*Source: © The Joint Commission, 2008. Reprinted with permission.*

# BIBLIOGRAPHY

## Books

American Medical Association. (2007). *American Medical Association manual of style* (10th ed.). New York: Oxford University Press.

Association for Healthcare Documentation Integrity. (2008). *The book of style for medical transcription* (3rd ed.). Modesto, CA: Author.

Chinyama, C.N. (2004). *Benign breast diseases: Radiology – pathology – risk assessment*. New York: Springer.

Davis, N.M. (2009). *Medical abbreviations: 30,000 conveniences at the expense of communication and safety* (14th ed.). Warminster, PA: Neil M. Davis Associates.

*Dorland's illustrated medical dictionary* (31st ed.). (2007). Philadelphia: Elsevier Saunders.

The Joint Commission. (2009). *Official "Do Not Use" list*. Terrace, IL: Author.

*Merriam-Webster's collegiate dictionary* (11th ed.). (2003). Springfield, MA: Merriam-Webster.

Pyle, V. (2005). *Vera Pyle's current medical terminology* (10th ed.). Modesto, CA: Health Professions Institute.

*Quick look drug book*. Philadelphia: Lippincott Williams & Wilkins.

Sabin, W.E. (2009). *The Gregg reference manual* (10th ed.). New York: McGraw-Hill.

Stedman, T.L. (2006). *Stedman's medical dictionary* (28th ed.). Philadelphia: Lippincott Williams & Wilkins.

Stedman, T.L. (2008). *Stedman's medical dictionary for the health professions and nursing* (6th ed.). Philadelphia: Wolters Kluwer Health/Lippincott Williams & Wilkins.

Tessier, C. (2004). *The surgical word book* (3rd ed.). Philadelphia: Elsevier Saunders.

United States Postal Service. (2006). *Postal addressing standards* (Publication 28). Washington, DC: Author.

Weinstein, S.L., & Buckwalter, J.A. (2005). *Turek's orthopedics: Principles and their application* (6th ed.). Philadelphia: Lippincott Williams & Wilkins.

## Websites

3M
http://solutions.3m.com

American Academy of Orthopaedic Surgeons
http://orthoinfo.aaos.org

American Heart Association
http://www.americanheart.org

American Red Cross
http://www.redcross.org

Animated-Teeth.com
http://www.animated-teeth.com

Biology Online
http://www.biology-online.org

Dressings.org
http://www.dressings.org

Drugs.com
http://www.drugs.com

The Eyes Have It
http://www.kellogg.umich.edu

The Free Dictionary's Medical Dictionary
http://medical-dictionary.thefreedictionary.com

HealthLinkBC
http://www.bchealthguide.org

HealthSquare.com
http://www.healthsquare.com

The Institute for Foot and Ankle Reconstruction
at Mercy
  http://footandankle.mdmercy.com

Johnson & Johnson Gateway
  http://www.jnjgateway.com

MedicineNet.com
  http://www.medterms.com

MediLexicon
  http://www.medilexicon.com

MedlinePlus
  http://www.nlm.nih.gov/medlineplus

The Merck Manuals Online Medical Library
  http://www.merck.com

MVS Cardiac Auscultation
  http://sprojects.mmi.mcgill.ca

The National Digestive Diseases Information
Clearinghouse
  http://digestive.niddk.nih.gov

National Institute of Mental Health
  http://www.nimh.nih.gov

Neuroexam.com
  http://www.neuroexam.com

The New York School of Regional Anesthesia
  http://www.nysora.com

Northeast Center for Special Care
  http://www.northeastcenter.com

Revolutionhealth
  http://www.revolutionhealth.com

Shoulder Pain Info
  http://www.shoulderpaininfo.com

University of Medicine & Dentistry of New Jersey
  http://vinst.umdnj.edu

WebMD
  http://www.webmd.com

WrongDiagnosis.com
  http://www.wrongdiagnosis.com

Yale University School of Medicine
  http://www.med.yale.edu

# INDEX

# E

# N

# T

## StudyWARE™ to Accompany
## Hillcrest Medical Center: Beginning Medical Transcription, 7th edition

### Minimum System Requirements

- Operating systems: Microsoft Windows XP w/SP 2, Windows Vista w/ SP 1, Windows 7

- Processor: Minimum required by Operating System

- Memory: Minimum required by Operating System

- Hard Drive Space: 90MB

- Screen resolution: 1024 × 768 pixels

- CD-ROM drive

- Sound card and listening device required for audio features

- Flash Player 10. The Adobe Flash Player is free, and can be downloaded from http://www.adobe.com/products/flashplayer/

- Microsoft Word 2003 or higher

### Setup Instructions

1. Insert disc into CD-ROM drive. The StudyWARE™ installation program should start automatically. If it does not, go to step 2.

2. From My Computer, double-click the icon for the CD drive.

3. Double-click the *setup.exe* file to start the program.

### Technical Support

Telephone: 1-800-648-7450
8:30 A.M. to 6:30 P.M. Eastern Time
E-mail: delmar.help@cengage.com

StudyWARE™ is a trademark used herein under license.

Microsoft® and Windows® are registered trademarks of the Microsoft Corporation.

Pentium® is a registered trademark of the Intel Corporation.